C0-AKA-988

Twin–Twin Tranfusion Syndrome

Twin–Twin Tranfusion Syndrome

Written and edited by

RUBÉN A QUINTERO MD
Professor and Director, Maternal Fetal Medicine
Department of Obstetrics and Gynecology
University of South Florida
Tampa, FL
USA

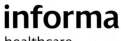

© 2007 Informa UK Ltd

First published in the United Kingdom in 2007 by Informa Healthcare,
4 Park Square, Milton Park, Abingdon, Oxon OX14 4RN.
Informa Healthcare is a trading division of Informa UK Ltd.
Registered Office: 37/41 Mortimer Street, London W1T 3JH.
Registered in England and Wales number 1072954.

Tel: +44 (0)20 7017 6000
Fax: +44 (0)20 7017 6699
Email: info.medicine@tandf.co.uk
Website: www.informahealthcare.com

All rights reserved. No part of this publication may be reproduced, stored in a retrieval system, or transmitted, in any form or by any means, electronic, mechanical, photocopying, recording, or otherwise, without the prior permission of the publisher or in accordance with the provisions of the Copyright, Designs and Patents Act 1988 or under the terms of any licence permitting limited copying issued by the Copyright Licensing Agency, 90 Tottenham Court Road, London W1P 0LP.

Although every effort has been made to ensure that all owners of copyright material have been acknowledged in this publication, we would be glad to acknowledge in subsequent reprints or editions any omissions brought to our attention.

Although every effort has been made to ensure that drug doses and other information are presented accurately in this publication, the ultimate responsibility rests with the prescribing physician. Neither the publishers nor the authors can be held responsible for errors or for any consequences arising from the use of information contained herein. For detailed prescribing information or instructions on the use of any product or procedure discussed herein, please consult the prescribing information or instructional material issued by the manufacturer.

A CIP record for this book is available from the British Library.
Library of Congress Cataloging-in-Publication Data

Data available on application

ISBN-10: 1 84214 298 4
ISBN-13: 978 1 84214 298 1

Distributed in North and South America by
Taylor & Francis
6000 Broken Sound Parkway, NW, (Suite 300)
Boca Raton, FL 33487, USA

Within Continental USA
Tel: 1 (800) 272 7737; Fax: 1 (800) 374 3401
Outside Continental USA
Tel: (561) 994 0555; Fax: (561) 361 6018
Email: orders@crcpress.com

Distributed in the rest of the world by
Thomson Publishing Services
Cheriton House
North Way
Andover, Hampshire SP10 5BE, UK
Tel: +44 (0)1264 332424
Email: tps.tandfsalesorder@thomson.com

Composition by Cepha Imaging Pvt Ltd, Bangalore, India.
Printed and bound in India by Replika Press Pvt. Ltd

Contents

Contributors

Mary H Allen RN CNOR
Tampa General Hospital
University of South Florida
Tampa, FL
USA

Victoria M Allen MD MSC FRCS(C)
Division of Maternal Fetal Medicine
Department of Obstetrics and Gynaecology,
Dalhousie University
Halifax, Nova Scotia
Canada

Kurt Benirschke MD
Department of Pathology
University of California San Diego
San Diego, CA
USA

Carlos Bermúdez MD
Unidad de Perinatología
Hospital Universitario de Caracas
Caracas
Venezuela

Patricia W Bornick RNC MSN
Tampa General Hospital,
University of South Florida
Tampa, FL
USA

Frank A Chervenak MD
Given Foundation Professor and Chairman,
Department of Obstetrics and Gynecology
The New York – Presbyterian Hospital
Weill Medical College of Cornell University
New York, NY
USA

Ramen H Chmait MD
Division of Maternal Fetal Medicine
Department of Obstetrics and Gynecology
University of Southern California
Los Angeles, CA
USA

Jan E Dickinson MD
School of Women's and Infants' Health
The University of Western Australia
Perth, Western Australia
Australia

James C Huhta MD
Professor of Pediatrics and Ob-Gyn
Daicoff-Andrews Chair of Perinatal Cardiology
University of South Florida College of Medicine
St Petersburg, FL
USA

Marc A Kaufman MD
Department of Anesthesia
St Joseph's Women's Hospital
Tampa, FL
USA

Eftichia V Kontopoulos MD
Department of Obstetrics and Gynecology
Division of Maternal–Fetal Medicine
University of South Florida
Tampa, FL
USA

Enrico Lopriore MD PhD
Division of Neonatology
Department of Pediatrics
Leiden University Medical Center
Leiden
The Netherlands

Samawal Lutfi MD CABP SSSP
Division of Neonatal–Perinatal Medicine and
Department of Pediatrics
Weil-Cornell University and
Hamad Medical Corporation
Doha
Qatar

Josep M Martínez MD PhD
Institut Clínic de Ginecologia
Obstetrícia i Neonatologia (ICGON)
Hospital Clínic, Universitat de Barcelona
Barcelona
Spain

Laurence B McCullough PhD
Professor of Medicine and Medical Ethics in the
Center for Medical Ethics and Health Policy
Baylor College of Medicine
Houston, TX
and
Adjunct Professor of Ethics in Obstetrics and
Gynecology and of Public Health
Weill Medical College of Cornell University
New York, NY
USA

Walter J Morales MD PhD
Florida Perinatal Associates
Tampa, FL
USA

Edwin Quarello MD
Department of Obstetrics and Gynecology
Universite Paris-Ouest
Poissy
France

Rubén A Quintero MD
Professor and Director, Maternal Fetal Medicine
Department of Obstetrics and Gynecology
University of South Florida
Tampa, FL
USA

Michael G Ross MD MPH
Department of Obstetrics and Gynecology
Harbor/UCLA Medical Center
Torrance, CA
USA

A Cristina Rossi MD
Department of Obstetrics and Gynecology
University of Foggia
Foggia
Italy

Daniel W Skupski MD
Weill Medical College of Cornell University
New York Hospital Queens
Flushing, NY
USA

Asli Umur PhD
Department of Micro-Array
Swammerdam Institute of Life Sciences
University of Amsterdam, Amsterdam
The Netherlands

Yves H Ville MD
Universite Paris-Ouest
Poissy
France

Masami Yamamoto MD
Unidad de Medicina Materno Fetal
Clinica Alemana de Santiago,
Hospital Padre Hurtado
Universidad del Desarrollo
Santiago
Chile

Martin JC van Gemert PhD
Laser Center and Department of Obstetrics
and Gynecology
Academic Medical Center
University of Amsterdam, Amsterdam
The Netherlands

Jeroen PHM van den Wijngaard PhD
Laser Center and Department of Obstetrics
and Gynecology
Academic Medical Center
University of Amsterdam, Amsterdam
The Netherlands

Foreword

Twin–Twin Transfusion Syndrome: A Success Story of Modern Obstetrics

The Twin–Twin Transfusion Syndrome was first described by Schatz in Germany in 1882, when he reported three cases of twin gestations with vascular anastomoses in the placenta. Schatz attributed the phenotype of the twins to the hemodynamic consequences of the vascular anastomoses which he termed 'the third circulation'.

Since that time, the Twin–Twin Transfusion Syndrome has remained a challenge in obstetrics, a condition requiring fundamental definition, diagnosis, classification, and treatment. Major developments in imaging and operative endoscopy have now allowed important breakthroughs in all these areas, and the diagnosis and treatment of Twin–Twin Transfusion Syndrome has become one of the success stories of modern obstetrics.

Imaging with ultrasound allowed the development of diagnostic criteria in the prenatal period, and several investigators contributed to the recognition of the importance of amniotic fluid volume (polyhydramnios and oligohydramnios) in the diagnosis. The next major contribution was the generation of a staging system that took into account the state of the bladder, Doppler velocimetry of the umbilical artery, vein and ductus venosus. Implicit in this staging system was that the disease was both heterogenous and dynamic. The lethality rate of fetuses with Stage IV (with hydrops) without treatment was approximately 95%, while those in Stage I (amniotic fluid volume abnormalities with a visible bladder and normal Doppler) was only 5%. This seminal observation had profound implications in the assessment of risk, and allowed examination of interventions on a rational basis. After the introduction of the staging system, not all Twin–Twin Transfusion Syndromes were the same.

A critical question of this fascinating and unique disease of pregnancy is its pathophysiology. The view that the syndrome is due to an imbalance of blood exchange between fetuses through vascular anastomoses in the placenta was a central hypothesis for more than a century. Moreover, even among those who accepted this mechanism of disease, the precise role of superficial and deep anastomoses remained unclear.

Laser photocoagulation was first introduced in the late 1980s for the treatment of this condition in the United States. However, the question of what vessels should be obliterated to cure the disease was unanswered. Some surgeons used the dividing membranes as a landmark to identify the vessels to be photocoagulated. This method identified many vessels suspected to participate in the process. This nonselective approach, however, could also result in the obliteration of vessels not participating in the disease process. A major step forward was the development of criteria to identify, during the course of an endoscopic procedure, the anastomotic from the non-anastomotic vessels. This was central to the major breakthrough: the development of selective photocoagulation for the treatment of the syndrome.

A multicenter European randomized clinical trial led by Professor Yves Ville of the Université Paris, France, demonstrated the superiority of selective laser photocoagulation over amnioreduction for the treatment of the syndrome. Photocoagulation was associated with improved neonatal survival and reduced neurologic injury. The results of this historical and pioneering trial have implications not only for patient care, but also provide evidence that "the third circulation" is responsible for the disease, as originally proposed by Schatz in 1882.

The challenges presented by the disease now include early diagnosis, refinement of the surgical technique, improving the pathophysiologic understanding and long-term prognosis of affected fetuses, as well as the training of a generation of fetal endoscopic surgeons capable of offering this treatment to patients worldwide.

Dr Ruben Quintero, now Director of Maternal-Fetal Medicine at the University of South Florida in Tampa, played a pioneering role in this success story. Therefore, it is fitting that he has undertaken editing a monograph designed to share with the biomedical community the information that talented investigators around the world have developed for the diagnosis, evaluation, and treatment of this syndrome.

This landmark contribution approaches the subject in a comprehensive manner and will be a reference point in the history of this disease.

Roberto Romero MD
Chief
Perinatology Research Branch
Program Director for Obstetrics and Perinatology
Intramural Division, NICHD, NIH, DHHS
Professor of Molecular Obstetrics and Genetics
Center for Molecular Medicine and Genetics
Wayne State University School of Medicine
Bethesda, Maryland and Detroit, Michigan
USA

Preface

One afternoon, in 1985, a patient arrived to the Labor and Delivery Suite at Yale New-Haven Hospital. Ultrasound showed a twin gestation with discordant amniotic fluid volume, one baby with polyhydramnios and the other with anhydramnios, 'stuck.' The diagnosis prompted a search into all possible management options, including cardiac tamponade of one of the fetuses. I will never forget the sense of hopelessness that the situation generated, despite being at an institution where nothing in obstetrics seemed impossible to accomplish.

Over the years, the controversies and challenges raised by twin–twin transfusion syndrome (TTTS) only contributed to my determination to tackle it. Testing the presumed pathophysiology, assessing the merits of a surgical approach to the disease combined with development of a specific surgical technique, overcoming technical obstacles such as bloody amniotic fluid discoloration and anterior placentas, and development of surgical instrumentation have all been part of a long-standing commitment to finding better ways to counsel and treat patients affected by TTTS.

A number of key developments in TTTS have taken place over the years. The definition of TTTS has gradually become standardized. Although previously used neonatal criteria of size discordance and hemoglobin differences still linger in the perinatal world, the sonographic definition of the disease in terms of specific amniotic fluid discordance has slowly gained wider acceptance. Indeed, acknowledgment of the ultrasound nature of the definition of the disease in-and-of itself constitutes a major achievement. The sonographic definition allowed distinction of TTTS from other conditions such as selective growth retardation. The sonographic nature of the definition, however, poses a serious epidemiological limitation, as the true incidence of the disease can only be known in countries with universal ultrasound screening.

Comparison of outcomes between series (particularly with older series) is similarly limited, as not all investigators may have used the same diagnostic criteria.

No issue has been more controversial than the treatment of TTTS. Perhaps the only undisputed aspect in this regard was the early knowledge that expectant or medical management played no role. The debate then centered on which form of invasive therapy was more appropriate. Interpretation of outcomes undoubtedly were marred by lack of standard diagnostic criteria, poor understanding of the natural history of the disease, and a laser surgical technique in evolution. Though to this date, there continues to be resistance to the overwhelming evidence supporting laser therapy over symptomatic treatment, the tides are finally changing. Unfortunately, many patients still do not receive optimal care due to logistic, political, or other non-scientific reasons. Moreover, the therapeutic short cut represented by the development of the bipolar coagulator, has had the potential of creating more harm than good. Nonetheless, the increasing number of physicians becoming adept in the performance of the selective laser technique in centers worldwide attests to the success of laser over any other form of therapy.

While a number of myths and truly unresolved scientific questions about TTTS still remain, most queries have been adequately and successfully addressed. This book brings together such knowledge for the benefit of patients and physicians alike.

I wish to take this opportunity to thank my research team in Tampa, Ms Mary Allen RN, Ms Patricia Bornick RN, our sonographers Ms Karen Pomeroy, Ms Lynette Cole, our operating room staff Mr Francisco Espejo, Ms Linda Roper, Ms Jennifer Townsend, and Ms Jennifer Weatherilt, our nurse anesthetist Ms 'Cookie' Neuman, Ms Laura Kersey from the administrative staff, and the support of Richard Wolf.

My most sincere gratitude to all of the contributors, who kindly accepted the invitation to share their knowledge on twin–twin transfusion with us all. Special thanks to Diane Spicer, Mary Torretta, and Rhonda Mabry for their assistance with the figures and illustrations. Lastly, I would like to thank Ms Patricia Bornick and the editorial staff of Informa Healthcare for their assistance in the preparation of this material, and without whom this book would not have been possible.

Rubén A Quintero

Color Plates

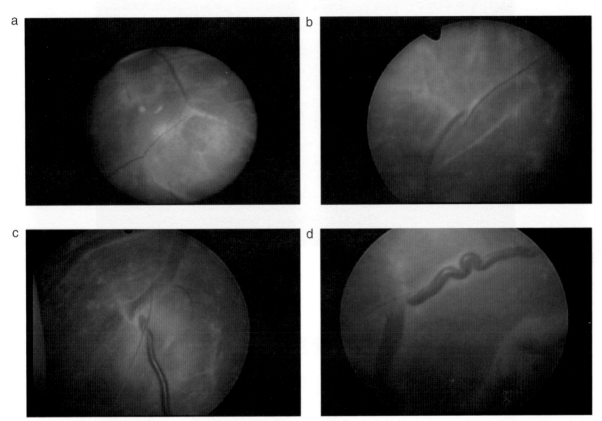

Figure 3.1 (a) Hair anastomosis. (b) Small anastomosis. (c) Medium anastomosis. (d) Large anastomosis.

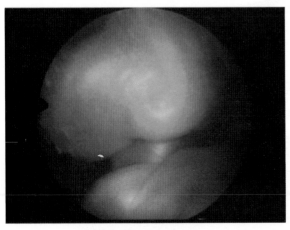

Figure 3.4 Double tight knot.

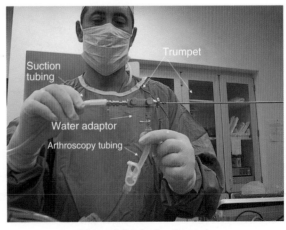

Figure 9.2 Irrigation trumpet.

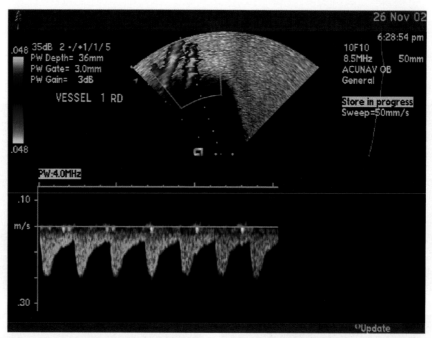

Figure 3.7 Color flow images and pulsed Doppler waveforms of the arterial component of the AV anastomoses. (Reproduced with permission from[7].)

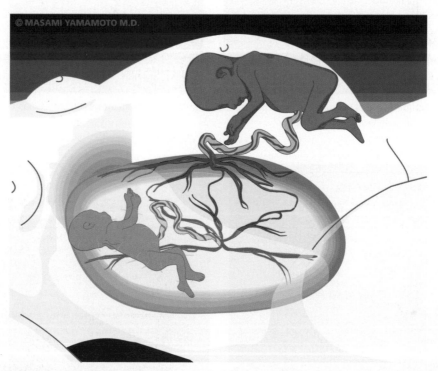

Figure 4.1 Characteristic features of polyhydramnios and oligohydramnios are due to hypervolemia and hypovolemia in recipient and donor twins, respectively.

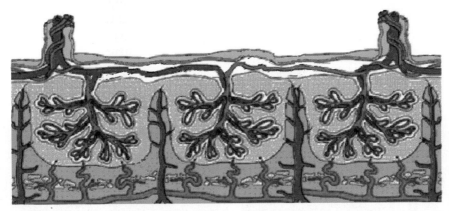

Figure 4.2 A monochorionic placenta is represented. The red vessels correspond to arteries and blue vessels to veins. One artery from the right cord irrigates a cotyledon that is drained by a vein from the left cord. This is a deep arteriovenous anastomosis.

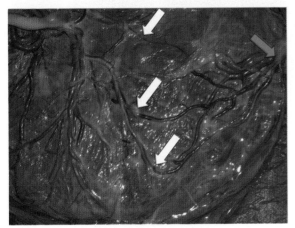

Figure 4.3 A monochorionic–diamniotic placenta with TTTS diagnosed at 25 weeks and delivered at 28 weeks treated only with amniodrainage. The intertwin membrane and amnios has been removed. Direct visualization of the chorionic plate after delivery shows the cord insertions of the donor (right) and the recipient (left). Three deep arteriovenous anastomoses were identified in this part of the chorionic plate, all directed from the donor to the recipient (white arrows). It is demonstrated that it comes from the donor's artery because it is directly connected to one of the thinner vessels in the cord (red arrow).

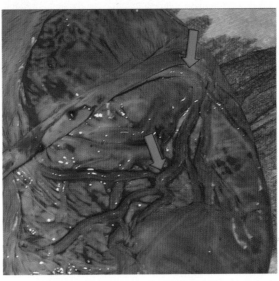

Figure 4.4 The same monochorionic–diamniotic placenta in the side of the donor with greater augmentation. The direct continuation of the anastomotic vessels with the artery in the cord is showed with the red arrows. The intertwin membrane is still in the placenta.

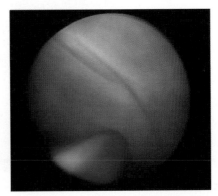

Figure 3.6 Placement of catheter. (Reproduced with permission from[7].)

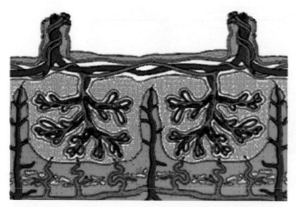

Figure 4.5 A monochorionic placenta with arterioarterial (red) and venovenous (blue) anastomoses. These correspond to direct communications between both cords, in which blood flow may be bidirectional. They may be present together or independently in monochorionic placentas.

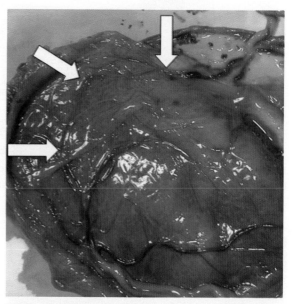

Figure 4.6 A monochorionic placenta from a TTTS with a superficial arterioarterial anastomosis. The white arrows show the passage of the vessel from one cord to the other. The donor (higher in the image) had a velamental insertion of the cord.

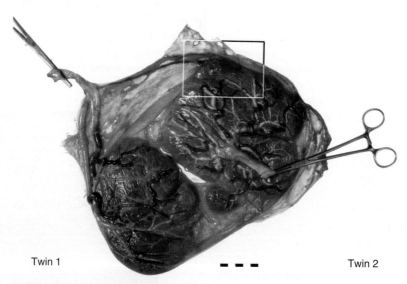

Twin 1   Twin 2

Figure 5.1 Bipartite monochorionic placenta after injection with colored dye. Arteries are injected with dark blue colored dye and veins with orange or yellow colored dye. (Reproduced with permission from[13].)

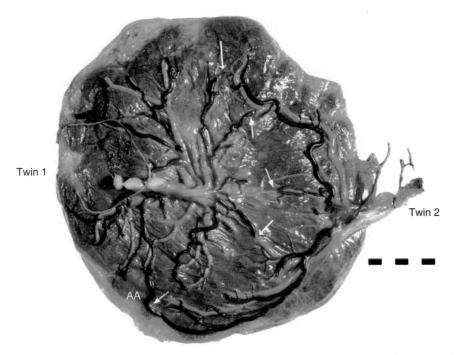

Figure 5.2 Placenta injection study with colored dye confirmed the presence of vascular communications confirming monochorionicity in this diamniotic twin placenta. This monochorionic twin gestation without twin-to-twin transfusion syndrome delivered after 38 weeks of gestation. Arteries are injected with dark-blue dye and veins with orange dye. The arrow at the bottom of the picture indicates an arterio-arterial anastomosis. Arterio-venous anastomoses from twin 2 to twin 1 are pointed out in the center of the picture, whereas an arterio-venous anastomosis from twin 1 to twin 2 is indicated at the top of the picture. (Not all anastomoses are labeled.) (Reproduced with permission from[15].)

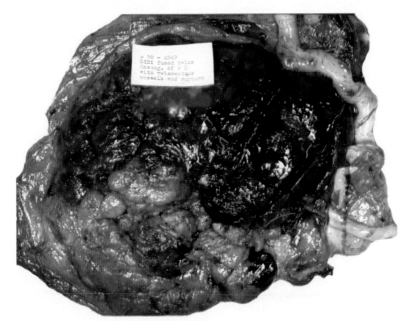

Figure 5.3 The chorionic side of a fused dichorionic-diamniotic placenta shows after exsanguination at the time of birth, which resulted in the pallor of Twin B's placenta. This allowed for a clear demarcation of the border between the fused placentas.

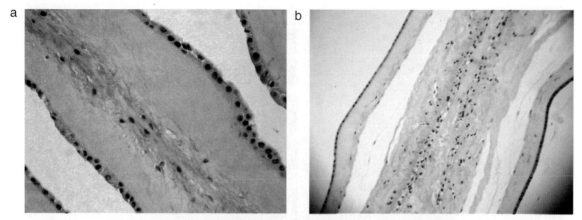

Figure 5.4 Histologic sections of the dividing membranes from a monochorionic diamniotic (a) and dichorionic diamniotic (b) twin gestations are shown. The monochorionic dividing membranes are composed of a layer of amnion and connective tissue only, in contrast to the dichorionic membranes which contain intervening chorions.

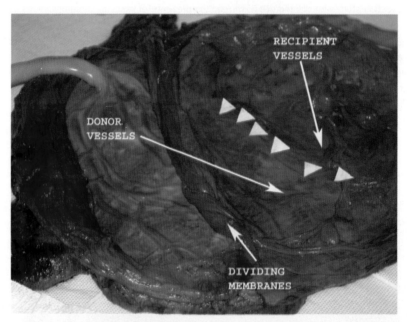

Figure 5.6 Dividing membranes pushed toward donor territory in this monochorionic placenta with TTTS, status post laser therapy. Small arrows point to laser photocoagulated areas and the vascular equator.

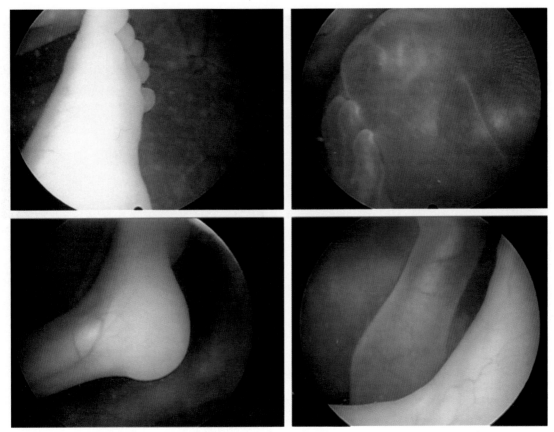

Figure 7.13 Stage V, defined as Intrauterine fetal demise of one or both twins. Feto–fetal results in a plethoric twin that has died and been transfused by the pale twin. (Reproduced with permission from[22].)

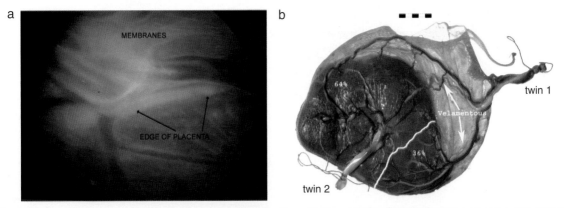

Figure 5.10 (a) Endoscopic view of a velamentous cord insertion with the vessels of the cord off the placenta, and instead embedded in the membranes. (b) Monochorionic placenta without TTTS. Twin 1 has a velamentous cord insertion and a placental share of 36%, whereas twin 2 has a paracentral cord insertion and a placental share of 64%. (Figure 5.10b reproduced with permission from Chapter 5, reference 40.

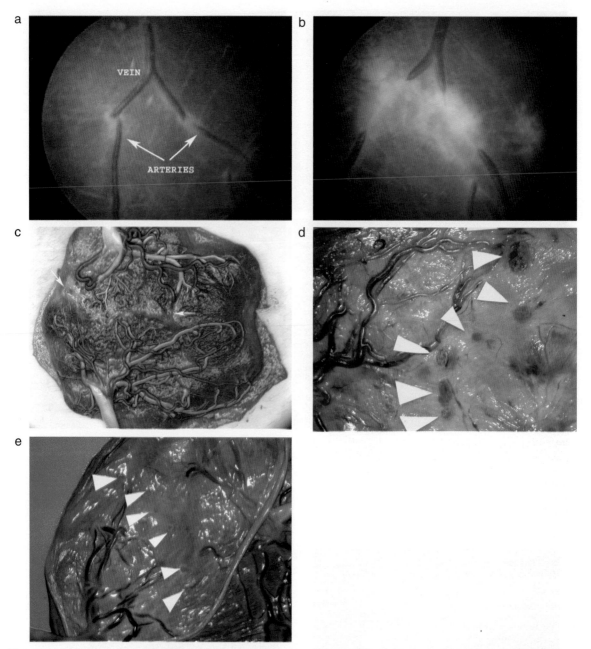

Figure 5.7 (a) Two artery-to-vein anastomoses, in a 'Y' shape, identified endoscopically in a pregnancy complicated by twin-twin transfusion syndrome. (b) The same vascular communication after laser ablation. (c) Functional dichorionization of a monochorionic-diamniotic placenta after laser therapy for TTTS. Arrows point to the lasered anastomoses. (d) and (e) Close up of monochorionic diamniotic placenta, status post laser therapy for TTTS. Arrows point to laser photocoagulated areas.

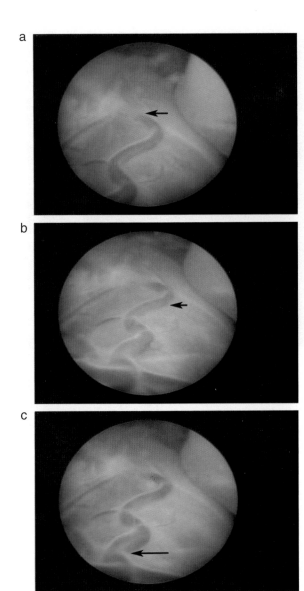

a

b

c

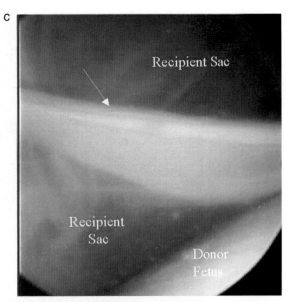

c

Recipient Sac

Recipient
Sac

Donor
Fetus

Figure 7.5 Cont'd (c) Endoscopic view of the cocoon sign. (Reproduced with permission from[20].)

Figure 5.9 This time sequence endoscopic view of an artery to artery anastomosis shows the collision front (arrows) between presumably oxygenated and less well oxygenated fetal blood: (a) collision front at the top of the vessel, (b) collision front half-way down the vessel, and (c) collision front at bottom of vessel.

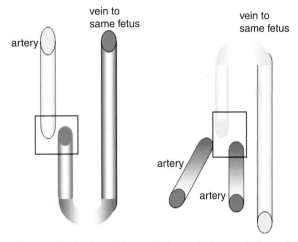

artery

vein to
same fetus

vein to
same fetus

artery

artery

Figure 7.18 Possible pitfalls using morphological criteria to assess deep AV anastomoses. The boxes show an artery and vein running in opposite directions.

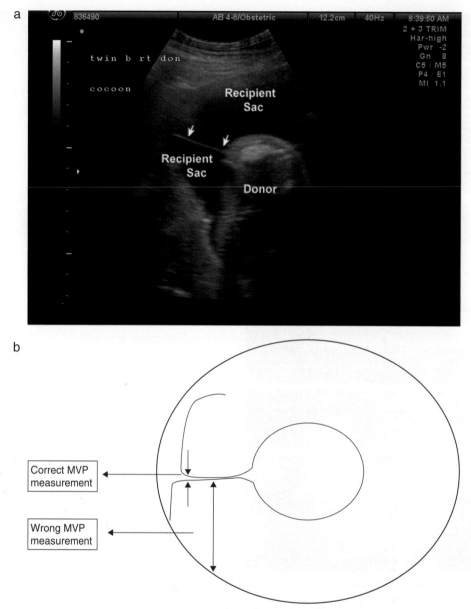

Figure 7.5 (a) Ultrasound view of the cocoon sign. (b) Correct and incorrect measurement of maximum vertical pocket (MVP) in the presence of the cocoon sign.

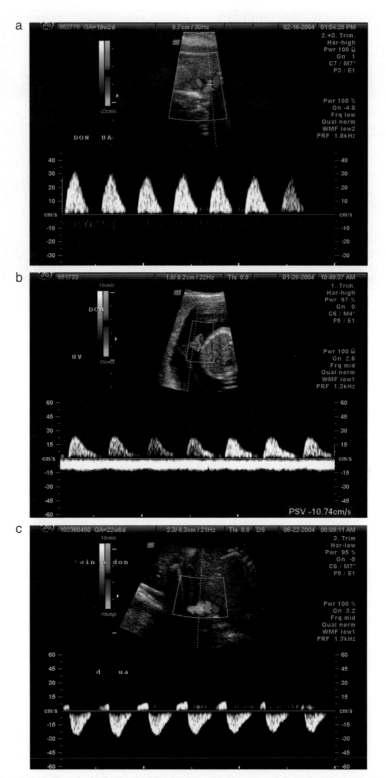

Figure 7.8 (a) Absent end-diastolic velocity in the umbilical artery. (b) Absent end-diastolic velocity in the umbilical artery and linear flow in the umbilical vein in the same view. (c) Reverse end-diastolic velocity in the umbilical artery.

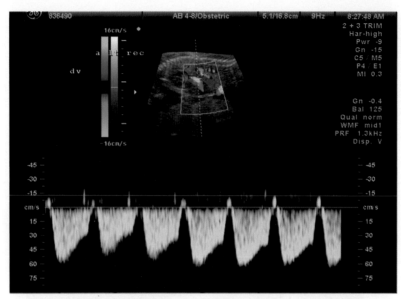

Figure 7.9 Reverse flow in the atrial contraction waveform of the ductus venosus.

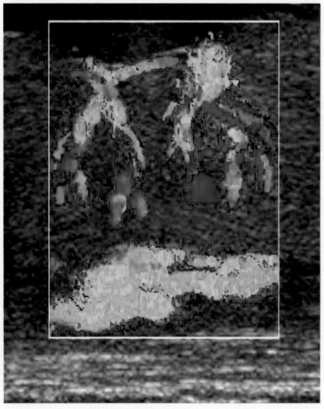

Figure 7.17 Color Doppler identification of an arterial vessel coming in one direction, and a venous drainage of the same cotyledon going in the opposite direction.

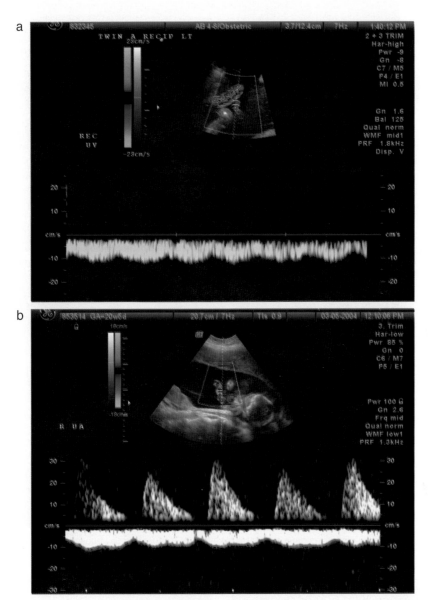

Figure 7.10 (a) Pulsatile umbilical venous flow. (b) Pulsatile umbilical venous flow in the umbilical vein and absent end-diastolic velocity in the umbilical artery in the same view.

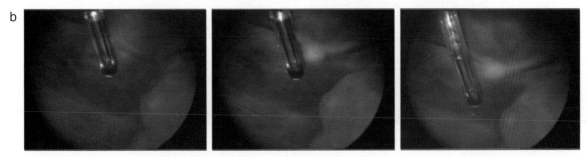

Figure 9.8 (b) Endoscopic view of side-firing laser fiber.

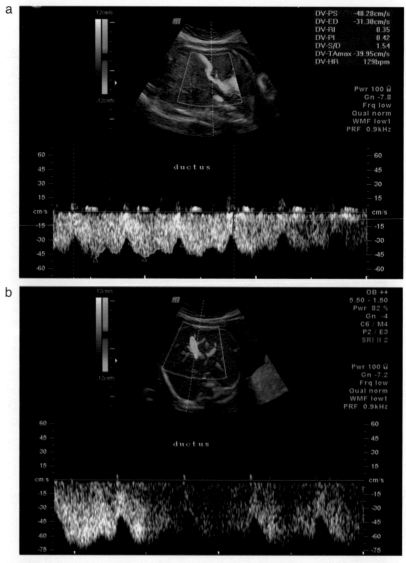

Figure 7.11 (a) Normal ductus venosus waveform, sagittal. (b) Normal ductus venosus waveform, transverse.

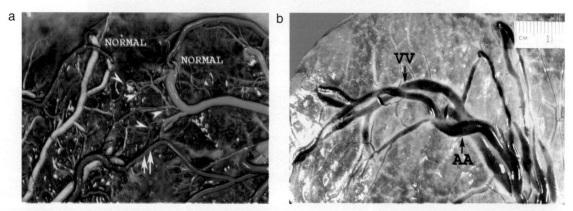

Figure 5.8 (a) This segment of placenta shows from bottom to top: 1) an artery to artery anastomosis (double arrows); 2) four artery to vein anastomoses designated by arrows; 3) two normally perfused cotyledons. (b) An artery to artery anastomosis (AA) courses toward the periphery with the AA crossing over its sister vein to vein anastomosis (VV) twice.

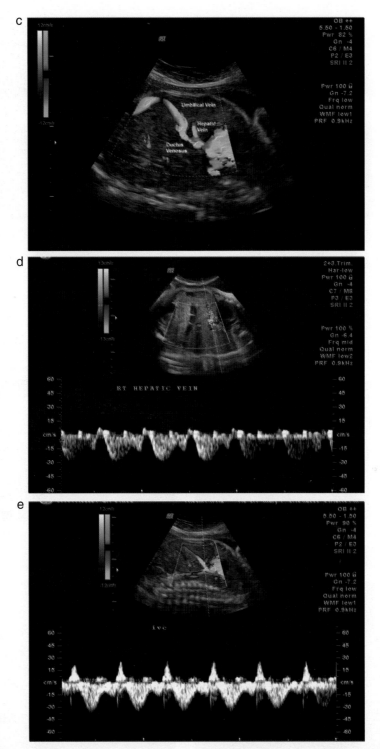

Figure 7.11 Cont'd (c) Normal ductus venosus, high resolution. (d) View of hepatic vein waveform. (e) View of inferior vena cava waveform.

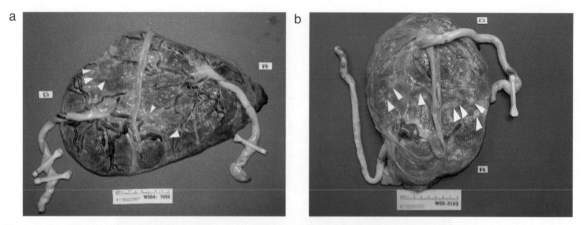

Figure 5.5 (a) Monochorionic-diamniotic placenta, status post laser therapy for TTTS, with the dividing membrane intersecting the vascular equator at a 45 degree angle to. Arrows point to lasered anastomoses. (b) Monochorionic diamniotic placenta, status post laser therapy for TTTS, with dividing membranes running perpendicular to the vascular equator. Arrows point to laser anastomoses.

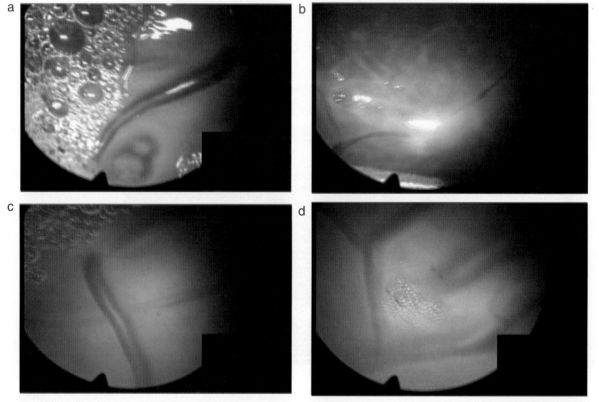

Figure 9.1 Vessels (a) and a lasered anastomosis (b) are clearly visualized within an air bubble. Anastomoses are difficult if not impossible to visualize through discolored amniotic fluid with debris from previous procedures (c and d).

1

The feto–fetal transfusion syndrome story, an historical perspective

Edwin Quarello and Yves H Ville

Introduction • The monochorionic placenta • The diagnosis • The pathophysiology • Vascular damage in feto–fetal transfusion syndrome • Prognostic factors • Management

INTRODUCTION

Despite significant improvements made in its management over the last decade, feto–fetal transfusion syndrome (FFTS) has remained an intriguing condition. Two periods should be individualized: before and after the 1980s. Before 1980, reports were mainly descriptive. The oldest medical description was reported in the Bible[1] with Esau and Jacob. Other examples can be found through the centuries, as in the 1617 painting 'The Swaddled Children' that depicted two babies, a red one and a white one.[2] Although the second period is shorter, it has coincided with dramatic improvements in the antenatal description, pathophysiology, and management of the syndrome.

THE MONOCHORIONIC PLACENTA

FFTS always develops from a monochorionic placenta which bears several intertwin vascular connections of different types on the chorionic plate. These transplacental communications were first described in 1687,[3] but their role was not suspected until 1882, when Schatz described the 'third circulation' and individualized all possible patterns of anastomoses.[3] Robertson[4] and Benirschke[5] using large ex-vivo placental dye injection studies refined the close relation between placental anastomoses and monochorionic placentation and described the

proportions of different types of sharing vessels. Vascular anastomoses are of three histological types: namely, artery-to-artery (AA), artery-to-vein (AV or VA), and vein-to-vein (VV) anastomoses. AA and VV are bidirectional and superficial anastomoses that indirectly connect the two fetal umbilical cords. These vessels run entirely, without interruption, on the surface of the chorionic plate. In contrast, AV and VA are deep anastomoses that always mediate a unidirectional blood flow.[6] AA and AV are the most frequent anastomoses (80% and 75%, respectively), unlike VV which are only present in 15% of monochorionic placentas. The specific role of each type of anastomosis in the development or non-development of FFTS is controversial. Some studies correlate the development of FFTS with a paucity of superficial anastomoses.[6] Recently, Wee et al,[7] using placental vascular casting, described another type of AV. These atypical deep AV anastomoses could be found in up to 90% of monochorionic placentas and could not be individualized either by endoscopy or dye injection. The possibility of cast artifacts makes it controversial. The paucity of and imbalance between the unidirectional (AV) and the bidirectional (AA or VV) are likely to influence the underlying pathophysiology.[6] The most commonly shared hypothesis is that FFTS develops when there is no effective means for AV blood to return from recipients to donors.

THE DIAGNOSIS

FFTS was initially diagnosed at birth using neonatal data and careful examination of the placenta. The diagnosis was supported by macroscopic and biological features. The red and plethoric neonate was called the recipient, whereas the donor was pale and often growth restricted. Herlitz in 1941[3] highlighted the volemia imbalances of the twins with the finding of anemia in one twin and polycythemia in its co-twin. In 1965, Rausen et al.[8] made a new attempt at defining the FFTS. They concluded that a neonatal hemoglobin difference greater than 5 g/dl was a good criterion. Tan et al, in 1979,[9] used an additional criterion with a difference in birth weight of at least 20% to differentiate between acute and chronic forms of the condition. Ex-vivo placental dye injection studies developed further to demonstrate the presence of vascular anastomoses between the two umbilical cords. However, all these criteria lacked both sensitivity and specificity. Indeed, at birth, a dead monochorionic twin can appear red, owing to the exsanguination of the survivor into the dead co-twin, irrespective of the initial status of donor or recipient. More recently, Denbow et al,[10] challenged the use of hemoglobin difference to establish the diagnosis of FFTS. In their series of 36 pregnancies complicated by FFTS, they found a mean hemoglobin difference of 3.6 g/dl and confirmed that large intertwin hemoglobin/hematocrit differences are infrequent in FFTS in utero. In addition, monochorionic twins complicated by weight discordance without FFTS often show significant hemoglobin differences. Danskin and Neilson[11] also reevaluted the diagnostic criteria of the syndrome. Intertwin differences in hemoglobin and in birth weight of more than 5 g/dl and of more than 20% respectively were equally found in monochorionic and in dichorionic twins. In placental injection studies, the presence of vascular anastomoses is found almost universally in monochorionic placentas[4] and cannot therefore establish the occurrence of FFTS.

Progress in imaging technology then allowed the diagnosis of the syndrome to shift from the postnatal to the antenatal period. Brennan et al[12] provided the first sonographic criteria to diagnose FFTS antenatally: fetal identical sexual phenotypes, disparity in size, single placenta, and evidence of hydrops in either twin or congestive cardiac failure in the recipient. The oligohydramnios–polyhydramnios sequence was described later in association with other sonographic findings, and was described as the 'stuck twin' phenomenon.[13] However this latter description created a long-lasting misunderstanding and a confusion between the finding of oligohydramnios in one twin and the diagnosis of FFTS. A stuck twin is not specific of FFTS, as it can equally occur in both monochorionic and dichorionic twins as part of numerous different conditions such as premature rupture of the membranes of one sac or bilateral renal agenesis in one twin. Amniotic fluid disparity reflects the imbalance in urine production. The bladder is most of the time empty in the donor, whereas it is distended in the recipient and the presence of polyuric polyhydramnios in the co-twin was confirmed to be critical to the diagnosis.[14]

THE PATHOPHYSIOLOGY

The pathophysiology of FFTS is still poorly understood. The shunting of blood from donor to recipient is a simplistic summary of the consequences of this syndrome. The donor and the recipient compensate this imbalance with oliguria and polyuria, respectively, that initiate the amniotic fluid disparity sequence. This theory is supported by higher ferritin concentrations in recipient fetuses,[15] but the same authors have challenged this latter hypothesis. They demonstrated the absence of iron overload in the recipient and depletion in the donor twins, and also that the total stainable liver iron was identical between twins pairs with and without FFTS. In utero and at birth, hematological analyses of 36 fetuses complicated by FFTS revealed that 75% of them do not show hemoglobin discordance ≥5 g/dl, with a mean hemoglobin difference of 3.6 g/dl.[10]

Bromley and co-workers[16] have usefully described the natural history of 12 monochorionic pregnancies complicated with the oligohydramnios/polyhydramnios sequence. Despite confusions in the definition, they have shown fluctuations in amniotic fluid and suggested that this phenomenon is a dynamic one.

This hemodynamic imbalance results in a net transfer of blood flow across placental vascular anastomoses from the donor to the recipient. It was described as mainly chronical and unidirectional, which could become acute and inverted.[17]

Sebire and co-workers[18] correlated this dynamic process to a random asymmetric reduction in the number of placental anastomoses. FFTS will occur when the random loss of these anastomoses ends up in an asymmetric flow resistance to interplacental transfusion. According to probabilistic calculations, they suggested that the chance for placental vascular circulation to become asymmetric will be greater in cases starting with several asymmetric connections. An initially asymmetric pattern may become symmetric, and an initially symmetric pattern may become asymmetric. This theory may explain why not all fetuses with discordant increased nuchal translucency will develop FFTS, and why some fetuses with initially normal nuchal translucency measurements will develop FFTS. Another hypothesis supported the fact that FFTS may develop as a consequence of a primary uteroplacental insufficiency affecting the donor side.[14] In this situation, the subsequent increase in peripheral resistance could trigger shunting of blood to the recipient. In 1993, Fries and co-workers[19] highlighted the role of a velamentous cord insertion in the genesis of FFTS. Velamentous cord insertions are more common in twins than in singletons, particularly in twins complicated by FFTS (63.6%), owing to the competition for uterine space by vascular placental territory. Velamentous cord insertion can easily be compressed, reducing the blood flow to its twin. It may contribute to the development of vascular imbalance and amniotic fluid discrepancy. Whether there is a pressure gradient between donors' and recipients' cavities or not has been debated. In 2000, Hartung and co-workers[20] and Quintero et al[21] demonstrated that intra-amniotic pressure was high in FFTS but equal in both cavities.

Because fetal urine is hypo-osmotic, a vicious cycle of hypervolemia–polyuria–hyperosmolality is established, leading to polyhydramnios and high-output cardiac failure in the recipient. Cardiac overload and ventricular dilatation in the recipient promote high atriopeptin (ANP) secretion by dilated atria. In addition, Mahieu-Caputo

and co-workers[22] speculated, supported by morphological studies, that fetal hypertension in the recipient might be partly mediated by the transfer of circulating renin originating from the donor through the placental vascular connections. The secretion of renin caused by hypovolemia in the donor may negatively affect both fetuses by worsening hypoperfusion in the donor and increasing blood pressure and cardiac afterload in the recipient.

Other metabolic pathways were suggested using fetal erythropoietin (Epo) and leptin concentration measurements.[23,24] First, fetal Epo concentrations were higher in the FFTS group than in the non-FFTS group but comparable between donors and recipients. Secondly, the leptin levels in the recipients were higher than in their siblings. Despite these provocative findings, no convincing explanation was given for these underlying mechanisms. These findings may therefore only reflect the consequences of FFTS rather than a trigger mechanism.

VASCULAR DAMAGE IN FETO–FETAL TRANSFUSION SYNDROME

The interdependency of the two fetal circulations is highly specific of monochorionicity. This is also the main anatomical and functional support for the development of vascular disruptive cerebral lesions. Two theories were suggested in the early 1960s and in the 1990s by Benirschke[5] and Larroche,[25] respectively, to explain the pathogenesis of these lesions. There are two main circumstances associated with cerebral lesions and FFTS syndrome when both twins are alive as opposed to when one fetus has died in utero.

In 1961, Benirschke proposed that pathological findings were compatible with an embolization phenomenon which could explain several visceral infarcts and lesions of necrosis. These could only be found in one surviving twin next to its dead co-twin.[5] This pathological mechanism suggested that necrotic debris and thrombocytoplastic substances elaborated in the dead twin or in its infarcted placenta could reach the surviving twin through placental vascular shunts, resulting in the occlusion of vessels or disseminated intravascular coagulation (DIC) and subsequent damage. Although this explanation was attractive, it was always based on postmortem or postnatal findings and it was never demonstrated in vivo. Necrotic emboli are therefore an unlikely phenomenon, owing to the dead twin's inability to disseminate emboli in the survivor and particularly against its active pressure and because blood flow stops shortly after the death of one twin. Thrombosis was only demonstrated by Yoshioka et al[26] in two infants, which were 5 and 12 months old at the time of diagnosis. These two infants were born next to their macerated co-twin. Occlusion of the cerebral vessels was identified using angiography and suggested an embolic origin of the thrombosis. However, they would have also been compatible with a vasospasm or thrombosis due to an acute drop in blood pressure and blood volume in the immature cerebral vessels. In-utero DIC has never been confirmed in vivo in any surviving twin. However, this simplistic image of one twin being poisoned by its dead co-twin has imprinted perinatologists' brains beyond generations and beyond reason owing to paragraphs copied from one textbook to the next and lacking critical analysis. In 1991, Fusi et al[27] even described one case of single intrauterine death in which no coagulation abnormality could be established in the survivor in utero using fetal blood sampling within days of the death of his sibling.

In 1990 Larroche et al[25] highlighted the state of hemodynamic imbalance related to the monochorionic condition. She supported the idea that this was the main and probably the only phenomenon involved in the development of brain lesions in monochorionic twins since it could occur just as well when both twins were alive. Although a chronic and overall unidirectional transfusion from one twin, the donor, to his sibling, the recipient, is likely to occur through placental vascular anastomoses, this can also evolve as an acute and massive[28] phenomenon, leading to feto–fetal exsanguination. Amnioreduction alters feto–fetal hemodynamics with acute changes in blood pressure both in donors and recipients.[27] This can also occur following incomplete laser coagulation. This hemodynamic theory was confirmed by the consistent diagnosis of severe anemia in single survivors irrespective of their initial status of donor or recipient and by the constant finding of polycythemia in the dead

twin both postnatally and in utero within hours following the death of one monochorionic twin.[25,29–33] Jou[34] and Gembruch[35] have visualized reversal of the transfusion initiated towards the agonizing twin, near the time of its death, using color and pulsed Doppler examination. The development of anemia in the surviving twin can accurately be monitored using V_{max} in the middle cerebral artery (V_{max}–MCA) by considering a cut-off value of greater than 1.5 MoM (multiple of the median) of the expected value. This avoids the need for fetal blood sampling in order to refine the risk to the survivor and it allows correction of severe anemia by intrauterine transfusion[36] to be more selectively targeted at cases of fetal exsanguination. Although this may appear a lifesaving procedure, its influence on the development of cerebral lesions in the survivor should be further investigated.[32,36]

PROGNOSTIC FACTORS

Several attempts have been made to identify objective prognostic markers to characterize the severity of FFTS: several factors such as amniotic fluid pressure, percentage of discordance in fetal growth, and visualization of the bladder in the donor have been initially proposed. In 1999, Quintero[37] established a classification for FFTS that consists of five stages reflecting different forms of the disease at presentation. This classification helps to homogenize the description of FFTS. However, it does not inform on the evolution or reflect the dynamic process in this condition. Taylor and co-workers[38] tentatively identified three independent factors to predict a poor survival in FFTS managed by amnioreduction: absent or reversed end-diastolic flow in the umbilical artery of the donor; abnormal pulsatility in the venous system of the recipient; and the absence of arterioarterial anastomosis on the chorionic plate.

MANAGEMENT

Despite many unanswered questions on the pathophysiology of FFTS, different therapeutic approaches have been developed to treat 'the visible part of the iceberg'.

First, indomethacin has been successfully used in the treatment of polyuric polyhydramnios in singleton and in twin pregancies. However, the presumed beneficial effects to the recipient may be opposed to its potential adverse effects on the donor's renal function and blood flow through the ductus arteriosus. Digoxin was also used in 1985 to treat FFTS complicated by heart failure.[39]

Secondly, together with the early description of the ultrasonographic features of FFTS by Elliott et al,[40] serial amnioreduction was proposed as a solution to treat amniotic fluid disparity by reducing the polyhydramnios in the recipient cavity. In 1980, Mills advocated that 'as much fluid as possible must be removed as quickly as possible and the procedure being repeated as often as necessary'.[41] This approach aimed initially at preventing preterm labor or preterm premature rupture of the membranes mediated by polyhydramnios, and therefore to prolong the pregnancy. However, it also reduces intra-amniotic pressure and may therefore improve uterine and cord blood flows. This is the simplest and most inexpensive method but it needs to be serially performed in up to 80% of cases[42] because of the lack of control of the underlying mechanism. Some cases of FFTS respond well to therapeutic amnioreduction, most do not. Bajoria[43] postulated that the presence of bidirectional (AA or VV) anastomoses may prevent reaccumulation of amniotic fluid in the recipient's sac following amnioreduction by compensating for hemodynamic imbalance set up by unidirectional vessels (AV).

Thirdly, the aim of deliberate septostomy was to allow amniotic fluid balance between the recipient's and donor's sacs. This approach was supported by a speculative 'low incidence of FFTS in monoamniotic twins'. Disruption of the inter-twin membrane was believed to allow correction of the polyhydramnios by filling the empty sac of the stuck twin. This technique was discovered unintentionally in 1995 by Hubinont and co-workers.[44] They noted normalization of the amniotic fluid volume in both sacs a few days following septostomy together with an improvement in fetal umbilical artery blood flow. All these changes seem to be mediated through changes in amniotic fluid pressure. Despite anecdotal good

results, both groups treated with amniodrainage or septostomy achieved similar survival rates when looking at outcomes reported in a multi-center randomized controlled trial comparing septostomy against amnioreduction.[45] Septostomy has since become obsolete. The initial postulate was then challenged by Quintero et al in 1998 and Hartung and co-workers,[46] in 2000, who documented that amniotic fluid pressures prior to amniodrainage were equally high in both sacs. Umur and co-workers,[47] using a mathematical model of twin–twin transfusion syndrome, demonstrated that septostomy allows amniotic fluid to be swallowed by the donor with minimal effects on donor growth and volemia. In addition, specific complications, such as cord entanglement or amniotic bands through the defect in the inter-twin membrane, have also been reported.[48]

Fourthly, based on the observation of the resolution of FFTS following spontaneous intrauterine death of one twin, selective feticide was suggested as a potential additional 'therapy'.[49] This, however, should be restricted to severe cases of FFTS in which one fetus demonstrates ominous signs of fetal demise. All techniques used must completely and permanently occlude all vessels in the umbilical cord in order to prevent acute exsanguination in the dead twin. Several methods have already been described in this situation: umbilical cord embolization using Histoacryl, thrombogenic coils, bipolar cord coagulation, interstitial laser coagulation, cord ligation, and ultrasonic cord transection. However, the technique which has been most consistently reported to be efficient in most indications is ultrasound-guided cord coagulation using a bipolar forceps.[50,51]

Finally, the revival of fetoscopy for laser coagulation of intertwin anastomoses on the chorionic plate allowed a significant step towards a more causative treatment of FFTS with the aim of changing the placenta from mono- to dichorionic. The original technique was described by De Lia et al in 1990,[52] and was only aimed at cases with a posterior placenta. It was performed under general anesthesia and required a maternal laparotomy to expose the uterus. A hysterotomy was then performed to insert the fetoscope. The approach was to coagulate only anastomotic vessels seen on the vascular equator of the placenta.

In 1992, Ville et al.[53] modified the technique radically into a minimally invasive approach. The fetoscope and laser fiber were introduced percutaneously under local analgesia and ultrasound guidance. Both anterior and posterior placentas can be operated upon with this technique. The intertwin membrane was used as an anatomical landmark for the identification of the communicating vessels. All crossing vessels were then non-selectively photocoagulated. This approach conferred the advantage of improving the reproducibility of the technique and the comparison of outcomes. However, the 'non-selective' photocoagulation of all crossing vessels could at least theoretically worsen placental vascular insufficiency of some donor twins, since the location of the dividing membrane on the surface of the placenta bears little relationship to the actual distribution of the vascular territories of the two fetuses and the cavity of the donor twin is often smaller. In order to preserve more of the non-shared cotyledons, in 1997 Quintero et al[54] proposed a 'selective' approach. All vessels that cross the membrane are assessed systematically and followed into the territory of the recipient twin.

This technique has become the standard in all centers performing laser for TTTS. Machin et al.[55] reported that AA anastomoses should be preserved, owing to their potential ability to prevent the development of FFTS. We believe that this could become an 'historitical' mistake. Indeed, any vessel left patent could favor the exsanguination of the survivor into its dead co-twin if surgery is followed by single fetal demise as happens in up to 33% of cases.[56]

The justification for using intrauterine surgery for TTTS had been questioned by the heterogeneous results reported with serial amnioreduction over the past 20 years. Indeed, with survival ranging from 20 to 80%, the advantage of using fetoscopy, which requires specific skills and equipment, had to be established.

This was achieved in 2004[57] with the coordination of the first randomized controlled trial showing a clear benefit of laser over amniocentesis benefit with fetal therapy. The advantages both in terms of improved survival as well as morbidity, is a milestone in the management of the disease.

The future will hopefully be the development of reliable methods to achieve preoperative mapping of the placental angioarchitecture. This is unlikely to come from ultrasound technology, which finds its limitation with the presence of polyhydramnios but possible rather from further developments of the magnetic resonance or other imaging (MRI) technologies.

An improvement in the management of FFTS is also likely to result from better follow-up of treated cases with the recognition of preoperative risk factors.[58,59] In addition, an understanding of postoperative complications such as feto–fetal chronic hemorrhage and its management is also likely to improve results.[60]

REFERENCES

1. Blickstein I, Gurewitsch‐ED. Biblical twins. Obstet Gynecol 1998; 91:632–4.
2. Berger HM, de Waard F, Molenaar Y. A case of twin–twin transfusion syndrome in 1617. Lancet 2000; 356:847–8.
3. Blickstein I. The twin–twin transfusion syndrome. Obstet Gynecol 1990; 76:714–22.
4. Robertson EG, Neer KJN. Placental injection studies in twin gestation. Am J Obstet Gynecol 1983; 170: 170–4.
5. Benirschke K. Twin placenta in perinatal mortality. NY State J Med 1961; 61:1499–507.
6. Bajoria R, Wigglesworth J, Fisk NM. Angioarchitecture of monochorionic placentas in relation to the twin–twin transfusion syndrome. Am J Obstet Gynecol 1995; 172: 856–63.
7. Wee LY, Taylor M, Watkins N et al. Characterisation of deep arterio-venous anastomoses within monochorionic placentae by vascular casting. Placenta 2005; 26:19–24.
8. Rausen AR, Seki M, Strauss L. Twin transfusion syndrome. A review of 19 cases studied at one institute. J Pediatr 1965; 66:613–28.
9. Tan KL, Tan R, Tan SH, Tan AM. The twin transfusion syndrome. Clin Pediatr 1979;18:111–14.
10. Denbow M, Fogliani R, Kyle P et al. Haematological indices at fetal blood sampling in monochorionic pregnancies complicated by feto–fetal transfusion syndrome. Prenatal Diagnosis 1998; 18:941–6.
11. Danskin FH, Neilson JP. Twin–twin transfusion syndrome: what are appropriate diagnostic criteria? Am J Obstet Gynecol 1989; 161:365–9.
12. Brennan JN, Diwan RV, Rosen MG, Bellon EM. Fetofetal transfusion syndrome: prenatal ultrasonographic diagnosis. Radiology 1982; 143:535–6.

13. Mahony BS, Petty CN, Nyberg DA et al. The 'stuck twin' phenomenon: ultrasonographic findings, pregnancy outcome, and management with amniocenteses. Am J Obstet Gynecol 1990; 163:1513–22.

14. Saunders NJ, Snijders RJM, Nicolaides KH. Twin–twin transfusion syndrome during the second trimester is associated with small intertwin differences. Fetal Diagn Ther 1991; 6:34–6.

15. Bajoria R, Lazda EJ, Ward S, Sooranna SR. Iron metabolism in monochorionic twin pregnancies in relation to twin–twin transfusion syndrome. Hum Reprod 2001; 16:567–73.

16. Bromley B, Frigoletto FD, Estroff JA, Benacerraf BR. The natural history of oligohydramnios/polyhydramnios sequence in monochorionic diamniotic twins. Ultrasound Obstet Gynecol 1992; 2:317–20.

17. Wee LY, Taylor MJO, Vanderheyden T et al. Reversal of twin–twin transfusion syndrome: frequency, vascular anatomy, associated anomalies and outcome. Prenat Diagn 2004; 24:104–10.

18. Sebire NJ, Talbert D, Fisk NM. Twin-to-twin transfusion syndrome results from dynamic asymmetrical reduction in placental anastomoses: a hypothesis. Placenta 2001; 22:383–91.

19. Fries MH, Goldstein RB, Kilpatrick SJ et al. The role of velamentous cord insertion in the etiology of twin–twin transfusion syndrome. Obstet Gynecol 1993; 81:569–74.

20. Hartung J, Chaoui R, Bollman R. Amniotic fluid pressure in both cavities of twin-to-twin transfusion syndrome: a vote against septostomy. Fetal Diagn Ther 2000; 15:79–82.

21. Quintero R, Quintero L, Morales W, Allen M, Bornick P. Amniotic fluid pressures in severe twin–twin transfusion syndrome. Prenat Neonat Med 1998; 3:607–10.

22. Mahieu-Caputo D, Dommergues M, Delezoide AL et al. Twin-to-twin transfusion syndrome. Role of the fetal renin angiotensin system. Am J Pathol 2000; 156:629–36.

23. Bajoria R, Ward S, Sooranna SR. Erythropoietin in monochorionic twin pregnancies in relation to twin–twin transfusion syndrome. Hum Reprod 2001; 16:574–80.

24. Bajoria R, Ward S, Sooranna SR. Discordant fetal leptin levels in monochorionic twins with chronic midtrimester twin–twin transfusion syndrome. Placenta 2001; 22:392–8.

25. Larroche JC, Droulle P, Delezoide AL, Narcy F, Nessmann C. Brain damage in monozygous twins. Biol Neonat 1990; 57:261–8.

26. Yoshioka H, Kadomoto Y, Mino M et al. Multicystic encephalomalacia in liveborn twin with a stillborn co-twin. Paediatr 1979; 95(5 pt 1):798–800.

27. Fusi L, McParland P, Fisk N, Nicolini U, Wigglesworth J. Acute twin–twin transfusion: possible mechanism for brain damaged survivors after intrauterine death of a monochorionic twin. Obstet Gynecol 1991; 78:517–20.

28. Gratacos E, Van Schoubroeck D, Carreras E et al. Impact of laser coagulation in severe twin–twin transfusion syndrome on fetal Doppler indices and venous blood flow volume. Ultrasound Obstet Gynecol 2002; 20:125–30.

29. Fusi L, Gordon H. Twin pregnancy complicated by single intrauterine death. Problems and outcome with conservative management. Br J Obstet Gynaecol 1990; 97:511–16.

30. Okamura K, Murotsuki J, Tanigawara S, Uehara S, Yajima A. Funipuncture for evaluation of hematologic and coagulation indices in the surviving twin following co-twin's death. Obstet Gynecol 1994; 83: 975–8.

31. Nicolini U, Pisoni MP, Cela E, Roberts A. Fetal blood sampling immediately before and within 24 hours of death in monochorionic pregnancies complicated by single intrauterine death. Am J Obstet Gynecol 1998; 179:800–3.

32. Tanawattanacharoen S, Taylor MJO, Letsky E et al. Intrauterine rescue transfusion in monochorionic multiple pregnancies with recent single intrauterine death. Prenat Diagn 2001; 21:274–8.

33. Senat MV, Bernard JP, Loizeau S, Ville Y. Management of single death in twin-to-twin transfusion syndrome: a role for fetal blood sampling. Ultrasound Obstet Gynecol 2002; 20(4):360–3.

34. Jou HJ, Ng KY, Teng RJ, Hsieh FJ. Doppler sonographic detection of reverse twin–twin transfusion after death of the donor. J Ultrasound Med 1993; 5:307–9.

35. Gembruch U, Viski S, Baganery K, Berg C, Germer U. Twin reversal arterial perfusion sequence in twin-to-twin transfusion syndrome after the death of the donor co-twin in the second trimester. Ultrasound Obstet Gynecol 2001; 17(2):153–6.

36. Senat MV, Loizeau S, Couderc S, Bernard JP, Ville Y. The value of middle cerebral artery peak systolic velocity in the diagnosis of fetal anemia after intrauterine death of one monochorionic twin. Am J Obstet Gynecol 2003; 189(5):1320–4.

37. Quintero RA, Morales WJ, Allen MH et al. Staging of twin–twin transfusion syndrome. Am J Perinat 1999; 19:550–5.

38. Taylor MJO, Denbow ML, Duncan KR, Overton TG, Fisk NM. Antenatal factors at diagnosis that predict outcome in twin–twin transfusion syndrome. Am J Obstet Gynecol 2000; 183:1023–8.

39. De Lia JE, Emery MG, Sheafor SA, Jennison TA. Twin transfusion syndrome: successful in utero treatment with digoxin. Int J Gynaecol Obstet 1985; 23: 197–201.

40. Elliott JP, Urig MA, Clewell WH. Aggressive therapeutic amniocentesis for treatment of twin–twin transfusion syndrome. Obstet Gynecol 1991; 77:537–40.

41. Mills WG. Letter to editor. Br J Obstet Gynaecol 1980; 87:255.

42. Huber A, Hecher K. How can we diagnose and manage twin–twin transfusion syndrome? Best Pract Res Clin Obstet Gynecol 2004; 18:543–56.

43. Bajoria R. Chorionic plate vascular anatomy determines the efficacy of amnioreduction therapy for twin–twin transfusion syndrome. Hum Reprod 1998; 13:1709–13.

44. Hubinont C, Bernard P, Mwebesa W, Magritte JP, Donnez J. Nd:YAG laser and needle disruption of the interfetal septum: a possible therapy in severe twin–twin transfusion syndrome. J Gynecol Surg 1996; 12:183–9.

45. Saade G, Moise K, Droman K et al. A randomized trial of septostomy versus amnioreduction in the treatment of twin oligohydramnios polyhydramnios sequence. Am J Obstet Gynecol 2002; 187:S54.

46. Hartung J, Chaoui R, Bollmann R. Amniotic fluid pressure in both cavities of twin-to-twin transfusion syndrome: a vote against septostomy. Fetal Diagn Ther 2000; 15:79–82.

47. Umur A, van Gemert MJC, Ross MG. Fetal urine and amniotic fluid in monochorionic twins with twin–twin transfusion syndrome: simulations of therapy. Am J Obstet Gynecol 2001; 185:996–1003.

48. Cook TL, Shaugnessy R. Iatrogenic creation of a monoamniotic twin gestation in severe twin-to-twin transfusion syndrome. J Ultrasound Med 1997; 16:853–5.

49. Wittmann BK, Farquharson DF, Thomas WDS, Baldwin VJ, Wadsworth LD. The role of feticide in the management of severe twin–twin transfusion syndrome. Am J Obstet Gynecol 1986; 155:1023–6.

50. Challis D, Gratacos E, Deprest J. Cord occlusion techniques for selective termination in monochorionic twins. J Perinat Med 1999; 27:327–38.

51. Robyr R, Yamamoto M, Ville Y. Selective feticide in complicated monochorionic twin pregnancies using ultrasound-guided bipolar cord coagulation. BJOG 2005; 112:1344–8.

52. De Lia JE, Cruikshank DP, Keye WR. Fetoscopic neodymium:YAG laser occlusion of placental vessels in severe twin–twin transfusion syndrome. Obstet Gynecol 1990; 75:1046–53.

53. Ville Y, Hecher K, Ogg D, Warren R, Nicolaides K. Successful outcome after Nd:YAG laser separation of chorioangiopagus twins under sonoendoscopic control. Ultrasound Obstet Gynecol 1992; 2:429–31.

54. Quintero RA, Morales WJ, Mendoza G et al. Selective photocoagulation of placental vessels in twin–twin transfusion syndrome: evolution of a surgical technique. Obstet Gynecol Surv 1998; 53:97S–103S.

55. Machin GA. The monochorionic twin placenta in vivo is not a black box. Ultrasound Obstet Gynecol 2001; 17:4–6.

56. Hecher K, Diehl W, Zikulnig L, Vetter M, Hackelöer BJ. Endoscopic laser coagulation of placental anastomoses in 200 pregnancies with severe mid-trimester twin-to-twin transfusion syndrome. Eur J Obstet Gynecol Reprod Biol 2000; 92:135–9.

57. Senat MV, Deprest J, Boulvain M et al. Endoscopic laser surgery versus serial amnioreduction for severe twin-to-twin transfusion syndrome. N Engl J Med 2004; 351:136–44.

58. Robyr R, Boulvain M, Lewi L et al. Cervical length as a prognostic factor for preterm delivery in twin-to-twin transfusion syndrome treated by fetoscopic laser coagulation of chorionic plate anastomoses. Ultrasound Obstet Gynecol 2005; 25:37–41.

59. Cavicchioni O, Yamamoto M, Robyr R, Takahashi Y, Ville Y. Intrauterine fetal demise following laser treatment in twin-to-twin transfusion syndrome. BJOG 2005; 113:590–4.

60. Robyr R, Lewi L, Yamamoto M, Deprest J, Ville Y. Permanent feto–fetal transfusion from the recipient to the donor twin. A complication of laser surgery in twin-to-twin transfusion syndrome. Am J Obstet Gynecol 2004; 191:S163.

2

The epidemiology of twin–twin transfusion syndrome

Samawal Lutfi and Victoria M Allen

Introduction • Incidence of twin–twin transfusion syndrome • Diagnosis • Twin–twin transfusion syndrome in monochorionic-monoamniotic twins • Twin–twin transfusion syndrome in higher multiple births • Predictors of twin–twin transfusion syndrome • Prognostic factors for adverse outcome • Summary

INTRODUCTION

Multiple births carry a high risk of antenatal and delivery complications to both mother and child.[1,2] These complications reflect directly and indirectly on additional social and economic costs borne by both the families and the respective healthcare system.[3,4] With the rising rates of twins and higher-order births worldwide, it is becoming more necessary to direct healthcare attention to challenges we have and will continue to face. Twins are the largest proportion of multiple births, constituting 94–98.5% of all multiple births.[5,6] The average twin rate in North America is estimated to be 9.6–26.8/1000 births (Figure 2.1a, b). Rates as high as 57.2/1000 births have been reported in Africa,[7] whereas Japan has quoted one of the lowest rates in the world at 4/1000 births.[8]

The rates of twin pregnancies in the United States have shown a 42% increase between 1980 and 1997[5] and a Canadian survey demonstrated a 35% increase between 1974 and 1990.[6] These increasing rates are believed to reflect the advancement in reproductive technology as well as advancing maternal age. The rise in twin rates may partly be explained by the relatively lower rate of singleton births despite the expanding population.[5] Recently, a significant proportion of deliveries following assisted reproductive technology have been multiple pregnancies (Table 2.1). In the majority of surveys, the rate of twins expressed per thousand births will obviously exclude the large numbers of multiple conceptions that are inadvertently lost prior to 20 weeks. In one survey early-stage pregnancy loss has accounted for 15–20% of conceptions.[6]

Monozygotic twinning occurs in 0.42% of all births.[9] Two-thirds of all monozygotic twin gestations are of monochorionic placentation. Placentation rather than zygosity is clinically relevant because of the increased risk of mortality and morbidity associated with monochorionicity.[10,11] Recently, monochorionicity in dizygous twin pregnancies has been reported.[12–15]

Monozygotic twinning appears to be increased after assisted reproductive technologies, including ovulation induction and in vitro fertilization,[16] and may be associated with blastocyst transfer compared with day 3 embryo transfer.[9]

INCIDENCE OF TWIN–TWIN TRANSFUSION SYNDROME

Twin-to-twin transfusion is a complication unique to monochorionic twin pregnancies. Although previously known by such terms as feto–fetal transfusion syndrome, autotransfusion syndrome, intrauterine parabiotic syndrome,[17] twin–twin transfusion syndrome (TTTS) is now commonly used. The incidence of TTTS ranges between 1.7% and 6.9% of twin pregnancies and between 5% and 15% of monochorionic twins,[18–21] although the incidence may be higher and may be

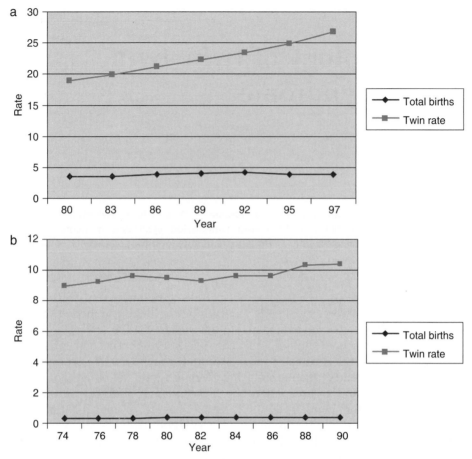

Figure 2.1 Total number of births expressed in millions and twin rate per thousand births in the United States (a) and Canada (b), extrapolated from work done by Martin and Park[5] and Millar et al,[6] respectively.

influenced by criteria used to establish the diagnosis of TTTS.[18,22,23] The purpose of this chapter is to evaluate the reported incidence rates as well as assessing predictors for the development of TTTS and prognostic factors for adverse outcomes.

DIAGNOSIS

The diagnosis of TTTS was originally based on the identification of anemia of one twin and polycythemia of the other with a growth-restricted donor twin,[24] birthweight discordance of greater

Table 2.1 Proportion of deliveries in the United States, Europe, and Canada following assisted reproductive technology (ART) by plurality

	Number of deliveries following ART	Singleton (%)	Twin (%)	Triplet (%)	Higher order (%)
United States[48]	25641	65	31	4	0.2
Europe[49]	34392	74	24	2	0.04
Canada[50]	2201*	68	29	3[†]	

* Number of ongoing pregnancies (pregnancy rate minus miscarriage rate).
[†] Higher-order pregnancies.

Table 2.2 Incidence of TTTS/twin births in cohort studies utilizing neonatal diagnostic criteria

Author	Total cohort	Gestational age range	Twins with TTTS	Incidence of TTTS	>5 g/dl Hb discordance*	Weight discordance*
Tan[25]	482	≥31–term	35	7%	100	26[§]
Shah[26]	49	24–28	10	20%	40[†]	60[†]
Rausen[27]	616	≥20–term	19	3%	100	0
Seng[20]	292	27–38	18	6.2%	56	56[†]

* Discordance calculated only in pregnancies with two liveborn and expressed as % occurrence in the TTTS group.
[†] Authors used 15% discordance.
[§] Authors used 20% discordance.
[†] Authors used >15% hematocrit difference.

than 20%, or a hemoglobin difference of >5 g/dl.[25] A number of hospital-based cohort studies adopted the neonatal criteria to evaluate the incidence and outcome of pregnancies diagnosed with TTTS (Table 2.2). In a retrospective review of 49 twin pregnancies, ≤28 weeks' gestation, Shah and Chaffin[26] used a hematocrit difference of 15% or a birthweight discordance of >15% in a histologically confirmed monochorial placenta. The incidence of TTTS was estimated to be 20% of all twins in this preterm population. Tan et al[25] used plethora and pallor color differences between liveborn twins in addition to a difference in hemoglobin of 5 g/dl and found an incidence of TTTS of 7% of all twin pregnancies. Rausen et al[27] used the clinical appearance of pallor and plethora, hemoglobin difference of >5 g/dl, weight and size discordance, and postmortem findings, and found an incidence of 3% of twin pregnancies (15% of monochorionic twins). This study may have been limited by inadequate clinical and placental data. Seng and Rajadurai[20] used pallor, plethora, birthweight discordance, and hemoglobin difference and found an incidence of 6.2% of twin birth.

However, neonatal findings may exist in the absence of TTTS, and antenatal ultrasound criteria have been adopted for the diagnosis of TTTS.[28] In addition, a staging system has been developed to describe the spectrum of severity of the disease.[29] In instances where antenatal ultrasound is not readily available, the cautious use of the neonatal criteria may still offer some guide in the management of these newborns. The incidence of TTTS using obstetrical diagnostic criteria[28,29] is summarized in Table 2.3. Cincotta et al[21] (hospital-based cohort) quoted an incidence of TTTS of 15% of monochorionic twins. Dickinson and Evans[19] (population-based study) found an incidence of 1.7% of all twins born in a single Western Australia tertiary center. In Qatar, an annual birth of >12 000 constituting >98% of birth of the Gulf state, are seen in one tertiary center. Over a

Table 2.3 Incidence of TTTS/twin births in studies utilizing obstetrical diagnostic criteria

Author	Year of study	Total number of twins	Gestational age range	Twins with TTTS	Incidence of TTTS
Lutfi[18]	Jan 1988 to Dec 2000	1,623	20–44	26	1.6%
Dickinson and Evans[19]	Jan 1992 to Jan 1999	2,433	>20	42	1.7%
HMC*	June 2002 to Dec 2004	522	24–39	6	1.1%

* Data extrapolated from Hamad Medical Corporation (Qatar).

30-month retrospective review of delivery records, only six twins of 522 twin sets born, were diagnosed as TTTS utilizing obstetrical criteria. This resulted in a TTTS incidence of 1.1% of all twin births (unpublished data). Lutfi et al[18] (population-based study), described an incidence of TTTS of 2.9% of all twins born >20 weeks' gestation, using both obstetrical ultrasound and neonatal criteria. The obstetrical ultrasonographic criteria used included confirming monochorionic placental mass using absence of the twin-peak sign, oligo- or anhydramnios in the donor using amniotic fluid pocket measurements (defined as a vertical fluid pocket <2 cm or an amniotic fluid index <5 cm), and the absence of fetal bladder, polyhydramnios (defined by a vertical pocket >8 cm or an amniotic fluid index >20 cm) in the recipient and signs of significant fetal cardiac decompensation, cardiac hypertrophy, tricuspid insufficiency and hydrops. Using the above criteria, TTTS was diagnosed in 0.018% of all births >20 weeks, gestation, 1.6% of all twins, and 5.8% of monochorionic twins (Table 2.4).

TWIN–TWIN TRANSFUSION SYNDROME IN MONOCHORIONIC–MONOAMNIOTIC TWINS

The incidence of monochorionic–monoamniotic twins ranges between 1% and 3% of twin births.[18,30] Aside from few case reports,[31] TTTS has rarely been documented in monochorionic–monoamniotic twins, despite the presence of extensive vascular anastomoses similar to those found in monochorionic–diamniotic twins. Benirschke and Driscoll[32] attribute the absence of the syndrome in the monoamniotic twin category to either a lack of the arteriovenous anastomoses between twins or a more extensive anastomoses connection that may balance the

net volume between twins. Similarly, Umur et al[33] have found a significantly higher arterioarterial anastomoses in monochorionic–monoamniotic twin placentas compared to monochorionic–diamniotic twin placentae (100% vs 80%), and significantly lower arteriovenous anastomoses (50% vs 83%). This may imply that placentas of monoamniotic twins are more likely to have extensive and balanced anastomosis than those of diamniotic twins. By correlating the percentage of the TTTS in monochorionic–diamniotic twins with arterioarterial anastomoses, the authors were able to draw a parallel to extrapolate an incidence rate of developing TTTS in monochorionic–monoamniotic twins to be 3.8% (2.6 times lower than the incidence in monochorionic–diamniotic twins). Suzuki et al[31] (hospital-based cohort) had estimated 9.6% of their monochorionic–monoamniotic twins to have TTTS. Obstetrical criteria such as amniotic fluid discordance in monoamniotic twins is not useful for the diagnosis of TTTS. The higher mortality associated with cord entanglement in monoamniotic twins may affect the incidence of TTTS in liveborn twins. Lutfi showed no TTTS in 48 monochorionic–monamniotic twin pregnancies.[18]

TWIN–TWIN TRANSFUSION SYNDROME IN HIGHER MULTIPLE BIRTHS

Triplets and higher multiple births constitute 1–6% of multiple births.[5,6] TTTS may be noted in pregnancies carrying three or more fetuses.[34] Triplet pregnancy may be trichorionic (40%), dichorionic (47%), or monochorionic (13%).[35] With monochorionic triplets, either two or all three fetuses may be affected with TTTS.[36–39] Chasen et al[40] studied TTTS in a cohort of

Table 2.4 Incidence of TTTS per monochorionic twin birth

Author	Study type	Proportion of monochorionic twins (%)	Criteria used for diagnosis of TTTS	Incidence of TTTS
Lutfi[18]	Population-based study	452 (28%)	Obstetrical diagnostic criteria	5.8%
Rausen[27]	Hospital-based cohort	128 (21%)	Neonatal diagnostic criteria	14.8%

151 triplets. Only three pregnancies identified with severe antenatal features of TTTS, including 'stuck twin', were noted, resulting in an incidence of 2% in all triplets.

PREDICTORS OF TWIN–TWIN TRANSFUSION SYNDROME

Hemodynamic changes in severe twin-to-twin transfusion may be seen as early as 11–14 weeks as an increased nuchal translucency thickness,[41,42] representing a 3.5–4.4-fold increased risk for developing TTTS.[43] Intertwin membrane folding represents a 4.2-fold increased risk for developing TTTS.[43] Abnormal flow patterns in the ductus venosus in monochorionic twin pregnancies has also been proposed as a prediction of TTTS.[44]

PROGNOSTIC FACTORS FOR ADVERSE OUTCOME

Absent or reversed end-diastolic flow in the donor umbilical artery, abnormal pulsatility of the venous system in the recipient, and absence of an arterioarterial anastomosis are predictive of fetal mortality.[45] Preoperative absent or reversed end-diastolic velocity in the umbilical Doppler, but not other Doppler studies, may predict demise in the donor twin following laser therapy.[46] Short cervical length, parity, and intrauterine demise of one twin have been shown to be predictors of preterm delivery in pregnancies identified with TTTS following laser coagulation of vascular anastomoses.[47]

SUMMARY

Evaluation of the incidence of TTTS is limited by the continuum of mild to severe disease and by the assessment in select populations, including referral centers and population-based studies. By current diagnostic criteria, less than 2% of twins or higher multiple births born >20 weeks' gestation may develop TTTS. This incidence is likely to change with increasing rates of multiple births worldwide. Predicting TTTS in early pregnancy may be more valuable than the diagnosis of clinically overt disease. In addition to its prognostic value, Doppler ultrasound studies may

play a bigger role in diagnosing TTTS in the future. The true incidence of TTTS may fall somewhere in between the percent of histopathologically abnormal monochorionic placentas and the yet immeasurable subtle manifestations of the syndrome.

ACKNOWLEDGMENT

We are grateful to the co-authors of our primary work, John Fahey, Colleen M O'Connell, and Dr Michael J Vincer, for their contributions that have made this work possible. We also thank Dr Badreldeen Ahmed and Dr Khalil Salameh for sharing some of their data records utilized in this chapter.

REFERENCES

1. Seski AG, Miller LA. Plural pregnancies – the cause of plural problems. Obstet Gynecol 1963; 21:227–33.
2. Hall JG. Twinning. Lancet 2003; 362:735–43.
3. Elster N. Less is more: the risks of multiple births. The Institute for Science, Law, and Technology Working Group on Reproductive Technology. Fertil Steril 2000; 74(4):617–23.
4. Campbell D, van Teijlingen ER, Yip L. Economic and social implications of multiple birth. Best Pract Res Clin Obstet Gynaecol 2004; 18:657–68.
5. Martin JA, Park MM. National Center For Health Statistics. Trends in Twin and Triplet Births: 1980–97. Natl Vital Stat Rep 1999; 47:1–16.
6. Millar WJ, Wadhera S, Nimrod C. Multiple births: trends and patterns in Canada, 1974–1990. Health Rep 1992; 4:223–50.
7. Nylander PP. Biosocial aspects of multiple births. J Biosoc Sci Suppl 1971; 3:29–38.
8. Imaizumi Y, Nonaka K. The twinning rates by zygosity in Japan, 1975–1994. Acta Genet Med Gemellol (Roma) 1997; 46:9–22.
9. Milki AA, Jun SH, Hinckley MD et al. Incidence of monozygotic twinning with blastocyst transfer compared to cleavage stage transfer. Fertil Steril 2003; 79:503–6.
10. Sebire NJ, Snijders RJ, Hughes K et al. The hidden mortality of monochorionic twin pregnancies. Br J Obstet Gynaecol 1997; 104:1203–7.
11. Dube J, Dodds L, Armson BA. Does chorionicity or zygosity predict adverse perinatal outcomes in twins? Am J Obstet Gynecol 2002; 186:579–83.
12. Imaizumi Y. A comparative study of zygotic twinning and triplet rates in eight countries, 1972–1999. J Biosoc Sci 2003; 35:287–302.

13. Miura K, Niikawa N. Do monochorionic dizygotic twins increase after pregnancy by assisted reproductive technology? J Hum Genet 2005; 50:1–6.

14. Ginsberg NA, Ginsberg S, Rechitsky S et al. Fusion as the etiology of chimerism in monochorionic dizygotic twins. Fetal Diagn Ther 2005; 20:20–2.

15. Quintero RA, Mueller OT, Martinez JM et al. Twin–twin transfusion syndrome in a dizygotic monochorionic-diamniotic twin pregnancy. J Matern Fetal Neonatal Med 2003; 14:279–81.

16. Schachter M, Raziel A, Friedler S et al. Monozygotic twinning after assisted reproductive techniques: a phenomenon independent of micromanipulation. Human Reprod 2001; 16:1264–9.

17. Naeye RL. Human intrauterine parabiotic syndrome and its complications. N Engl J Med 1963; 268:804–9.

18. Lutfi S, Allen VM, Fahey J et al. Twin–twin transfusion syndrome: a population-based study. Obstet Gynecol 2004; 104:1289–97.

19. Dickinson JE, Evans SF. Obstetric and perinatal outcomes from the Australian and New Zealand twin–twin transfusion syndrome registry. Am J Obstet Gynecol 2000; 182:706–12.

20. Seng YC, Rajadurai VS. Twin–twin transfusion syndrome: a five year review. Arch Dis Child Fetal Neonatal Ed 2000; 83:F168–70.

21. Cincotta RB, Gray PH, Phythian G et al. Long term outcome of twin–twin transfusion syndrome. Arch Dis Child Fetal Neonatal Ed 2000; 83:F171–6.

22. Strong SJ, Corney G. The placenta in twin pregnancy. Oxford: Pergamon Press; 1967.

23. Bajoria R, Wigglesworth J, Fisk NM. Angioarchitecture of monochorionic placentas in relation to the twin–twin transfusion syndrome. Am J Obstet Gynecol 1995; 172:856–63.

24. Herlitz G. Zur Kenntnis der anamischen und polyzytamischen Zustande bei Neugeborenen, Sowie des Icterus gravis neonatorum. Acta Paediatr 1941; 29:211–14.

25. Tan KL, Tan R, Tan SH et al. The twin transfusion syndrome. Clinical observations on 35 affected pairs. Clin Pediatr (Phila) 1979; 18:111–14.

26. Shah DM, Chaffin D. Perinatal outcome in very preterm births with twin–twin transfusion syndrome. Am J Obstet Gynecol 1989; 161:1111–13.

27. Rausen AR, Sekim M, Strauss L. Twin transfusion syndrome. A review of 19 cases studied at one institution. J Pediatr 1965; 66:613–28.

28. Brennan JN, Diwan RV, Rosen MG et al. Radiology 1982; 143:535–6.

29. Quintero RA, Morales WJ, Allen MH et al. Staging of twin–twin transfusion syndrome. J Perinatol 1999; 19:550–5.

30. Benirschke K, Koufmann P. Pathology of the human placenta, 3rd edn. New York: Springer Verlag; 1995:742.

31. Suzuki S, Kaneko K, Shin S et al. Incidence of intrauterine complications in monoamniotic twin gestation. Arch Gynecol Obstet 2001; 265:57–9.

32. Benirschke K, Driscoll SG. The pathology of the human placenta. Berlin: Springer Verlag, 1967.

33. Umur A, van Gemert MJ, Nikkels PG. Monoamniotic-versus diamniotic-monochorionic twin placentas: anastomoses and twin–twin transfusion syndrome. Am J Obstet Gynecol 2003; 189:1325–9.

34. Sepulveda W, Surerus E, Vandecruys H et al. Fetofetal transfusion syndrome in triplet pregnancies: outcome after endoscopic laser surgery. Am J Obstet Gynecol 2005; 192:161–4.

35. Machin GA, Bamforth F. Zygosity and placental anatomy in 15 consecutive sets of spontaneously conceived triplets. Am J Med Genet 1996 22; 61:247–52.

36. Rehan VK, Menticoglou SM, Seshia MM et al. Fetofetal transfusion in triplets. Arch Dis Child Fetal Neonatal Ed 1995; 73:F41–3.

37. Pons JC, Olivennes F, Fernandez H et al. Transfusion syndrome in a triplet pregnancy. Acta Genet Med Gemellol (Roma) 1990; 39:389–93.

38. Leung WC, Wong KY, Leung KY et al. Successful outcome after serial amnioreductions in triplet fetofetal transfusion syndrome. Obstet Gynecol 2003; 101:1107–10.

39. Entezami M, Runkel S, Becker R et al. Feto-feto-fetal triplet transfusion syndrome (FFFTTS). J Matern Fetal Med 1997; 6:334–7.

40. Chasen ST, Al-Kouatly HB, Ballabh P et al. Outcomes of dichorionic triplet pregnancies. Am J Obstet Gynecol 2002; 186:765–7.

41. Sebire NJ, D'Ercole C, Hughes K et al. Increased nuchal translucency thickness at 10–14 weeks gestation as a predictor of severe twin-to-twin transfusion syndrome. Ultrasound Obstet Gynecol 1997; 10:86–9.

42. Nicolaides KH, Heath V, Cicero S. Increased fetal nuchal translucency at 11–14 weeks. Prenat Diagn 2002; 22:308–15.

43. Sebire NJ, Souka A, Skentou H et al. Early prediction of severe twin-to-twin transfusion syndrome. Hum Reprod 2000; 15:2008–10.

44. Germer U, Kohl T, Smercek JM et al. Comparison of ductus venosus blood flow indices of 607 singletons with 133 multiples at 10–14 weeks gestation. An evaluation in uncomplicated pregnancies. Arch Gynecol Obstet 2002; 266:187–192.

45. Taylor MJO, Denbow ML, Duncan KR et al. Antenatal factors at diagnosis that predict outcome in twin–twin transfusion syndrome. Am J Obstet Gynecol 2000; 183:1023–8.

46. Martinez JM, Bermudez C, Becerra C et al. The role of Doppler studies in predicting individual intrauterine fetal demise after laser therapy for twin–twin transfusion syndrome. Ultrasound Obstet Gynecol 2003; 22:246–51.

47. Robyr R, Boulvain M, Lewi L et al. Cervical length as a prognostic factor for preterm delivery in a twin-to-twin transfusion syndrome treated by fetoscopic laser coagulation of chorionic plate anastomoses. Ultrasound Obstet Gynecol 2005; 25:37–41.

48. Assisted Reproductive Technology in the United States: 2000 results generated from the American Society for Reproductive Medicine/Society for Assisted Reproductive Technology (ASRM/SART) Registry. Fertil Steril 2004; 81:1207–20.

49. Anderson AN, Gianaroli L, Nygren KG. Assisted reproductive technology in Europe, 2000. Results generated from European registers by the ESHRE. Hum Reprod 2004; 19:490–503.

50. http://www.cfas.ca/english/news/dec5_2005.asp

3

Pathophysiology

Rubén A Quintero

Introduction • Etiology of twin–twin syndrome • Consequences of the unbalanced net blood flow exchange • Summary of the pathophysiology of twin–twin transfusion syndrome

INTRODUCTION

Twin–twin transfusion syndrome (TTTS) is thought to result from an unbalanced sharing of blood between two fetuses via placental vascular anastomoses. The negative corollary is evident from the fact that the disease does not occur in dichorionic pregnancies, as vascular anastomoses do not develop in such placentas. As a result of the unbalanced blood exchange, one fetus receives too much blood (the recipient twin, or recipient), and one fetus loses too much blood (the donor twin, or donor). The unbalanced blood sharing triggers a series of pathophysiological changes that characterize the natural history and outcome of the disease.

Most monochorionic placentas have vascular anastomoses,[1] but only 5–10% of monochorionic pregnancies develop TTTS.[2] What determines then the development of the disease in these patients? Two theories have evolved over the years in our laboratory regarding the etiology of TTTS and, analogous to the microbiology terminology, we have termed them 'obligatory' and 'facultative.'

ETIOLOGY OF TWIN–TWIN SYNDROME

Obligatory etiology

In obligatory TTTS, the placental vascular design is deterministic or fatalistic. The faulty placental vascular design consists of the presence of either more numerous or larger arteriovenous (AV) anastomoses from donor to recipient. As a result,

more blood flows from donor to recipient. To investigate this hypothesis, we assessed the size, number, and direction of arteriovenous anastomoses.

Demonstration of faulty placental vascular design: The DR score[3]

Detailed endoscopic analysis of the size, number, and direction of AV anastomoses in TTTS placentas indeed suggests larger or more numerous AV anastomoses from donor to recipient. In a study we conducted on 20 TTTS patients with pure AV anastomoses identified endoscopically during laser surgery, the number of vascular communications was established in two ways:

- as a single communication, if only an artery and a vein participated
- as multiple communications, if prolific branching precluded an accurate estimate of the number of vessels.

For single communications, the vessel size used for the calculations was that of the largest participating vessel. For areas with multiple communications, the vessel size used was that of the largest vessel immediately prior to the branching. Vessel size was subjectively classified as hair, small, medium, or large (Figure 3.1). A relative weight of ×1 (small), ×1.4 (medium), or ×1.9 (large) was assigned for the different vessel sizes, based on visual observations. The direction of flow of AV communications, whether from donor (AVDR) or from recipient (AVRD) was established by tracing back the artery to the

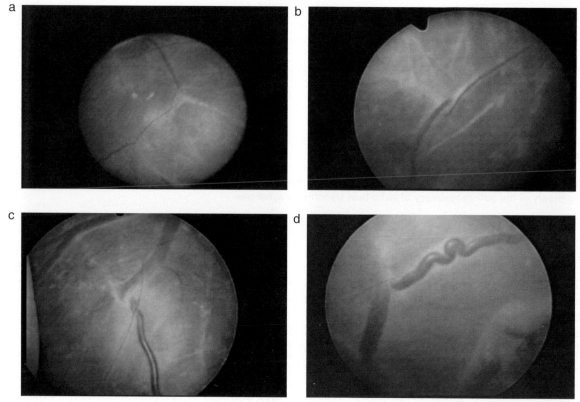

Figure 3.1 (a) Hair anastomosis. (b) Small anastomosis. (c) Medium anastomosis. (d) Large anastomosis. (See also color plate section, page xiii.)

corresponding fetus of origin, knowing that arteries cross over veins. Four additional patients had superficial arterioarterial (AA) or venovenous (VV) anastomoses. Because the direction of flow in AA or VV communications could not be established, these patients were excluded from the analysis. The net direction of blood flow in each case was determined by performing an algebraic sum of the AV communications using Poiseuille's law for capillary flow:[4]

$$q = C \frac{\pi r^4 (p_1 - p_2)}{B\mu L}$$

where q is flow rate, C is a constant to account for unit conversion, r is the radius of the capillary, p is pressure, B is the volume factor of the fluid, μ is viscosity, and L is the length of the capillary. Although differences in blood pressure, fluid viscosity, and vessel length could be present, the prevailing factor in the equation is the radius of

the blood vessel, elevated to the 4th power. An algebraic sum of the weighted flow in each case (ΣAVRDs – ΣAVDRs) yielded a donor recipient (DR) score (Figure 3.2).

Table 3.1 shows the number, size, and direction of the communications and the corresponding DR score for each individual case in the 20 patients studied. The mean number of communications was 4.1 (range 1–8). Communications were bidirectional (i.e. both AVDRs and AVRDs were present in the same placenta) in 18/20 (90%) of cases. In 2 patients, a single unidirectional AVDR was found. Eighty percent of cases had a negative DR score, suggesting indeed a net exchange of blood from donor to recipient. Two patients had a positive DR score, suggesting an apparent net flow of blood from recipient to donor. This most likely represents the relative imprecision of vessel size assessment.

To test the validity of the conclusion with regard to the sensitivity of the measurement, we

$$DR\ Score =$$
$$[(n_1 S_D)^4 + [(n_2 M_D)^4 + [(n_3 L_D)^4] -$$
$$[(n_4 S_R)^4 + [(n_5 M_R)^4 + [(n_6 L_R)^4]$$

Figure 3.2 Calculation of net blood flow: DR score. n, number of vessels; S, small; M, medium; L, large; D, donor; R, recipient.

tabulated the DR score for varying ranges of relative vessel size. Table 3.2 shows different scenarios for the medium- and large-sized vessels considered (1.2–1.6 for the medium, and 1.7–2.1 for the large; Figure 3.3). As can be seen, the minimum percent of negative DRs in the worst scenario is 75%. Actually, even if with extreme relative sizes, such as ×1, ×10, and ×100 for small, medium, and large vessels, the results of the DR score remain unchanged. This means that the key element in the assessment of the size of the anastomosis is the subjective qualification of the vessel as small, medium, or large. Misjudgment of the relative vessel sizes within the same patient

is unlikely, as one can continuously compare their sizes during surgery. Differences in size assignment between patients do not alter the results, since the DR score is performed individually.

Our subsequent assessment of the size, number, and direction of AV anastomoses in a total of 400 TTTS patients has shown the presence of at least one AVDR in all cases. In no instance were there communications only from recipient to donor (AVRDs). Sixteen cases (4%) had communications only from donor to recipient (AVDRs).

The endoscopic analysis of the number, size, and direction of AV anastomoses suggests that a vascular anatomical basis may indeed be responsible for the development of TTTS in a subset of patients. Although the actual amount of blood exchange can only be estimated from this assessment, a larger number or larger size of AVDRs suggests that, indeed, a net flow of blood may take place from donor to recipient twin and be responsible for the syndrome.

Table 3.1 Number, size, and direction of the communications and the corresponding DR score for the 20 patients

Case	Donor Small	Donor Medium	Donor Large	Recipient Small	Recipient Medium	Recipient Large	DR score	No. of anastomoses
1	0	1	0	0	1	0	0.0	2
2	1	0	2	1	2	0	−18.4	6
3	0	1	0	1	0	0	−2.8	2
4	1	2	0	0	1	1	−8.2	5
5	0	1	0	0	0	0	−3.8	1
6	1	1	0	1	0	0	−3.8	3
7	0	0	1	2	2	0	−3.3	5
8	0	3	1	2	2	0	−14.9	8
9	0	2	0	1	0	0	−6.7	3
10	0	1	0	0	0	0	−3.8	1
11	0	0	1	0	1	0	−9.2	2
12	0	3	1	1	1	0	−19.7	6
13	0	4	0	0	2	0	−7.7	6
14	3	0	0	1	0	0	−2.0	4
15	0	1	1	1	1	0	−12.0	4
16	0	3	0	0	2	1	9.2	6
17	0	2	0	0	1	0	−3.8	3
18	0	0	1	0	0	1	0.0	2
19	0	3	0	2	2	0	−1.8	7
20	4	0	0	2	0	0	−2.0	6
					% negative	80%		
					Average		−4.9	4.1

Table 3.2 Different scenarios for medium- and large-sized vessels. (Reproduced with permission from[3].)

	Scenarios							
Case	M(lo),L(lo) DR	M(lo),L DR	M(lo),L(hi) DR	M,L(lo) DR	M,L(hi) DR	M(hi),L(lo) DR	M(hi),L DR	M(hi),L(hi) DR
1	0.0	0.0	0.0	0.0	0.0	0.0	0.0	0.0
2	−121.7	−320.0	−680.6	−98.7	−657.7	−56.9	−255.3	−615.9
3	−7.0	−7.0	−7.0	−18.4	−18.4	−39.3	−39.3	−39.3
4	59.8	159.0	339.3	48.3	327.8	27.5	126.6	307.0
5	−8.0	−8.0	−8.0	−19.4	−19.4	−40.3	−40.3	−40.3
6	−8.0	−8.0	−8.0	−19.4	−19.4	−40.3	−40.3	−40.3
7	−50.9	−150.0	−330.4	−27.9	−307.4	13.9	−85.3	−265.6
8	−74.8	−173.9	−354.3	−86.2	−365.7	−107.1	−206.3	−386.6
9	−14.9	−14.9	−14.9	−37.9	−37.9	−79.7	−79.7	−79.7
10	−8.0	−8.0	−8.0	−19.4	−19.4	−40.3	−40.3	−40.3
11	−60.8	−160.0	−340.3	−49.3	−328.8	−28.5	−127.6	−308.0
12	−83.7	−182.9	−363.2	−106.7	−386.2	−148.5	−247.6	−427.9
13	−15.9	−15.9	−15.9	−38.9	−38.9	−80.7	−80.7	−80.7
14	−2.0	−2.0	−2.0	−2.0	−2.0	−2.0	−2.0	−2.0
15	−67.8	−167.0	−347.3	−67.8	−347.3	−67.8	−167.0	−347.3
16	60.8	160.0	340.3	49.3	328.8	28.5	127.6	308.0
17	−8.0	−8.0	−8.0	−19.4	−19.4	−40.3	−40.3	−40.3
18	0.0	0.0	0.0	0.0	0.0	0.0	0.0	0.0
19	−6.0	−6.0	−6.0	−17.4	−17.4	−38.3	−38.3	−38.3
20	−2.0	−2.0	−2.0	−2.0	−2.0	−2.0	−2.0	−2.0
% Negative	80%	80%	80%	80%	80%	75%	80%	80%

M, medium size vessel; lo, lower size estimate; DR, DR score; L, large size vessel; hi, higher size estimate.

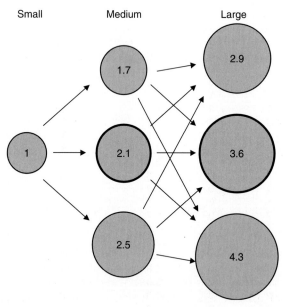

Figure 3.3 The medium- and the large-sized vessels. Relative vessel sizes compared to small vessel (1) used for different DR score scenarios.

Persistent or reverse twin–twin transfusion syndrome as further evidence of the obligatory etiology

Persistent or reverse TTTS may result from patent anastomoses left after laser therapy for TTTS. The anastomoses may have been over-looked altogether, or, as in most cases, sub-lasered. Patients with persistent TTTS will show one or more patent AVDRs. Patients with reverse TTTS will show one or more patent AVRDs. If the opportunity permits, a second laser procedure will allow identification and lasering of the patent anastomosis. Resolution of the syndrome occurs invariably. Thus, cases where a single anastomosis, AVDR or AVRD has been left patent, constitute an unintended iatrogenic experimental demonstration of the obligatory pathophysiological mechanism for TTTS. The following case illustrates the point.

Case report

The patient was a gravida-2, para-1 at 17.6 weeks' gestation referred with the diagnosis of TTTS. She had not undergone genetic or therapeutic amniocentesis. Ultrasound confirmed the presence of a monochorionic, diamniotic twins with a posterior placenta. The maximum vertical pocket (MVP) in the recipient was 8.6 cm, and 0.9 cm in the donor. The bladder of the donor twin was visible and Doppler studies were not critically abnormal, making it a stage II disease (see Chapter 7). During surgery, 4 AV anastomoses were identified and photocoagulated: from donor to recipient, 1 large, 1 medium, from recipient to donor; 1 large and 1 small. A follow-up ultrasound on the first post-op day revealed a normal fetal heart rate for both twins. The patient returned with reverse TTTS at 24.3 weeks' gestation. The MVP in the former recipient sac was 1.4 cm and 12.8 cm in the sac of the former donor. The patient underwent a second procedure during which two small AV communications were ablated (one from donor to recipient, one from recipient to donor). Symptoms of TTTS did not recur. The patient delivered two viable female infants at 34 weeks' gestation. Surgical pathology revealed no residual patent anastomosis.

Facultative etiology

Monochorionic twins may be viewed hemodynamically as two pumps connected in parallel via placental vascular anastomoses. The hemodynamic equilibrium is maintained as long as both fetuses pump the same amount of blood in opposite directions. Selective pump failure may occur in one of the twins from cardiac dysfunction secondary congenital heart disease, myocarditis or obstruction at the level of the umbilical cord. The affected fetus may not be able to tolerate the additional amount of blood coming from the other twin. As a result, the affected fetus becomes the recipient and the other twin the donor. The sonographic characteristics of the syndrome in this twin pair may show two important features:

1. The recipient twin may be affected out of proportion to the degree of involvement of the donor twin. For example, the recipient twin may show hydrops, while the donor twin may still show a visible bladder (atypical stage IV disease; see Chapter 7).

2. Further failure of the recipient twin may actually show improvement of the disease, as increased impedance to the flow of blood from the donor to the recipient twin may hinder further blood loss from the donor.

Indirect evidence in support of the facultative etiology comes from a selected group of cases in which the diagnosis of congenital heart disease is made in one of the fetuses. Almost invariably, the affected twin would be the recipient. Of 615 patients assessed at our institution, congenital heart disease was diagnosed in 6 fetuses (0.9%), mostly pulmonary artery stenosis (Table 3.3). An additional 3 patients had abnormalities of the umbilical cord, which presumably could also hinder blood return to the donor, or impair oxygenation in the recipient from obstruction of the umbilical vein, resulting in congestive heart failure of the recipient. One of the patients with cord abnormalities had a double tight knot (Figure 3.4). The other two patients had an umbilical cord kink. In all but one case, the fetus with either congenital heart disease or umbilical cord obstruction was the recipient.

Facultative etiology could also result from a donor twin with increased placental impedance as a result of decreased placental mass. Initial elevation of the blood pressure in the donor to improve perfusion of the reduced placental mass could result in an excessive amount of blood being forced through the vascular anastomoses to the recipient twin. Excessive blood loss to the recipient would perpetuate the cycle.

Estimation of the net blood volume exchange

Direct assessment of the net blood flow exchange between the donor and the recipient twins has not been possible thus far. Although our endoscopic study for the DR score showed an apparent greater size or number of AV anastomoses from donor to recipient, this approach cannot be used to quantify the actual amount of blood flow exchange.

Table 3.3 Incidence of prenatally diagnosed cardiovascular system anomalies in TTTS population

Case	Stage	GA at procedure	Additional diagnosis
1	II	20.0	True knot
2	IV – Recipient	21.9	Pseudo knot
3	IV – Recipient	23.3	Pseudo knot
4	III – Donor	21.9	Recipient – mild pulmonic stenosis
5	IV – Recipient	19.3	Recipient – possible pulmonic stenosis
6	IV – Recipient	21.1	Recipient – pulmonic stenosis
7	IV – Recipient	25.9	Recipient – aorta and pulmonary artery calcified
8	II	22.4	Recipient – possible pulmonic stenosis
9	IV – Recipient	23.0	Recipient – small right ventricle, narrow aortic root

GA, gestational age in weeks.

Blood returning through the umbilical vein represents the sum of blood sent by one fetus to the placenta plus the amount of blood received from its co-twin minus the blood lost to the co-twin. Assessment of the net blood flow exchange could be addressed in two different ways:

- comparing umbilical venous blood flow before and after complete laser obliteration of the vascular anastomoses
- estimating the blood flow exchange at the level of the anastomoses themselves.

The combined cardiac output of the right and left ventricle is 100–500 ml/min for 20–28 weeks'
gestation.[5] Of that, 40–45% is directed into the placenta. There are approximately 12–30 individually perfused cotyledons.[1] Thus, the amount of blood flow in the umbilical vein ranges between 40 and 200 ml/min, and the amount of blood flow through each cotyledon approximately 1.3–16.6 ml/min. In addition, there are approximately 50–60 main stem villi present in the placenta.[1] Thus, the blood flow volume through each main stem is approximately 0.3–3 ml/min. These figures serve as a reference to understand the results of sonographic estimates of blood flow exchange between the fetuses.

Assessment of umbilical venous blood flow before and after laser obliteration of all vascular anastomoses

We conducted a study to evaluate total umbilical venous flow (TUVF) before and after SLPCV.[6] Forty-one TTTS patients were assessed sonographically before and 24 hours after surgery. The umbilical vein was sampled in a free loop close to the abdominal wall insertion. The diameter of the umbilical vein was measured from 'inner to inner' in a section of the vessel perpendicular to the ultrasound beam. Measurement of the time-averaged velocity was done with an angle of insonation as close to 0 degrees as possible. All measurements were made in the absence of fetal movements or breathing. Angle correction

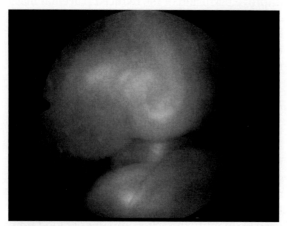

Figure 3.4 Double tight knot. (See also color plate section, page xiii.)

for measurements was performed where necessary. TUVF was calculated as follows:

$$\text{TUVF (ml/min)} = \text{mean venous time-averaged velocity (cm/s)} \times \text{mean cross-sectional area (cm}^2) \times 60\ \text{s.}$$

TUVF was significantly higher in the recipient (111.2 ml/min) than in the donor twin (44.8 ml/min) before SLPCV ($p < 0.0001$). However, TUVF was no different between recipient and donor twin after SLPCV (93.1 ml/min vs 70.7 ml/min, recipient and donor twin, respectively ($p = 0.11$). The donor's TUVF increased after surgery ($p < 0.0001$), while the recipient's TUVF decreased ($p = 0.041$) (Figure 3.5). The median postoperative increase in the donor's TUVF 25.9 ml/min had a corresponding decrease of TUVF in the recipient twin 18.1 ml/min ($p = 0.27$). Assuming an average of 4–5 vascular anastomoses in each placenta, the blood flow through each anastomosis would be approximately 4.4 ml/min. These estimates are in agreement with classic physiology and surgical pathology data, as noted above.

Assessment of net blood flow exchange by ultrasound interrogation of the individual vascular anastomoses via intra-amniotic ultrasound

The net blood flow exchange between the fetuses can also be estimated from the algebraic sum of the individual vascular anastomoses. To do this, insonation of each anastomosis is required. Because transabdominal ultrasound lacks the necessary resolution to identify each and every vascular anastomosis, we conducted a study using direct sonographic assessment of the vessels via intra-amniotic ultrasound.[7] Patients with TTTS, an anterior placenta, and without superficial placental vascular anastomoses undergoing laser therapy for TTTS were considered eligible for the study. After adequate endoscopic documentation of all vascular anastomoses, an 8.5 MHz diagnostic ultrasound catheter (ACUSON AcuNav, Siemens Medical Solutions, Inc., Mountainview, CA) was inserted into the amniotic cavity through a separate 2 mm port. Under endoscopic guidance, the catheter was placed directly beneath each arteriovenous

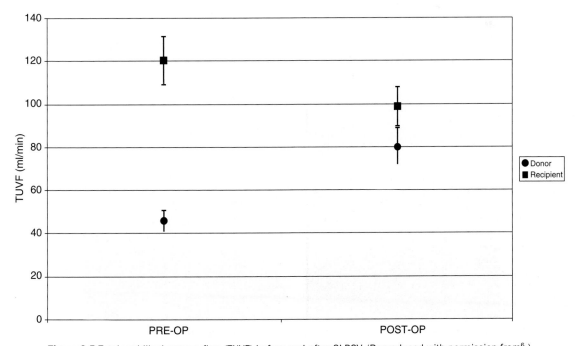

Figure 3.5 Total umbilical venous flow (TUVF) before and after SLPCV. (Reproduced with permission from[6].)

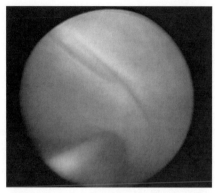

Figure 3.6 Placement of catheter. (Reproduced with permission from[7].) (See also color plate section, page xv.)

(AV) anastomosis (from donor to recipient, AVDR, and from recipient to donor, AVRD) (Figure 3.6). Color flow images and pulsed Doppler waveforms of the arterial component of the AV anastomoses were obtained (Figure 3.7). The diameter of the artery was measured from the color flow mapping image. Arterial blood flow volume was calculated offline. Net blood flow exchange was calculated as:

Total AVDR flow – Total AVRD flow

The protocol was approved by the Institutional Review Board of St. Joseph's Hospital in Tampa, FL, USA and all patients gave written informed consent.

Three patients agreed to participate in this study. Complete measurements could be obtained in two of them. Table 3.4 shows the individual blood flow values in each of the assessed anastomoses. The net blood flow was 1.6 ml/min and 11.6 ml/min in the two patients measured. However, contrary to expectations, the calculated net blood flow was from recipient to donor in both cases. Although the study was significantly limited by the focal length of the ultrasound transducer, the orders of magnitude were again within those expected.

Ultrasound estimate of the net blood flow exchange using TUVF agreed with the fundamental hypothesis of TTTS, with estimates of the exchange consistent with classic physiology and surgical pathology data. Estimates using intra-amniotic ultrasound were limited by technical reasons, perhaps explaining the contradictory results, but were also within the same order of magnitude. Future work in this area will probably be geared to improving the accuracy of blood

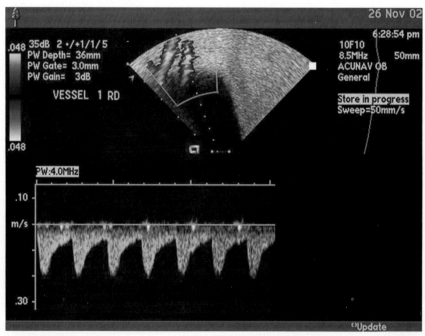

Figure 3.7 Color flow images and pulsed Doppler waveforms of the arterial component of the AV anastomoses. (Reproduced with permission from[7].) (See also color plate section, page xiv.)

Table 3.4 Calculation of blood flow exchange through placental anastomosis as measured by intra-amniotic ultrasound. (Reproduced with permission from[7].)

| | Type of placental anastomosis | | | |
	AVDR1	AVRD1	AVRD2	Net balance (ml/min)
Case 1	2.0	0.7	2.9	−1.6
Case 2	13.7	25.3	–	−11.6

AVDR, arteriovenous anastomosis from donor to recipient;
AVRD, arteriovenous anastomosis from recipient to donor

flow estimates at the level of the individual anastomoses with better technology.

CONSEQUENCES OF THE UNBALANCED NET BLOOD FLOW EXCHANGE

Uneven blood volume exchange is handled differently by the donor and the recipient twin.

Consequences in the donor twin

Net blood loss in the donor twin presumably actives the renin–angiotensin system (RAS). Mahieu-Caputo et al have performed immuno-histochemical studies with renin antiserum and with in-situ hybridization using riboprobes complementary to renin mRNA, and renin-secreting cells (RSCs) to assess the renin production in twin pairs affected by transfusion syndrome.[8] The overall maturation of the renal cortex, as determined by the percentage of immature glomeruli, was simultaneously assessed. Although donor twin kidneys were smaller than those of recipients, the maturation of the renal cortex was not significantly different (28.2% immature glomeruli in the donor and 24.4% in the recipient kidney). The donor kidney showed increased renin gene expression with hyperplastic juxtaglomerular apparatuses (JGAs) that contained excess RSCs (median 20.02 [25th–75th centiles, 5.4, 25.1 RSCs per 100 glomeruli]). In contrast, the recipient kidney is virtually devoid of these cells (0.04 [0, 0.36] RSCs per 100 glomeruli; $p < 0.05$).

Increased renin release in the kidney of the donor may act locally and result in renal vasoconstriction and oliguria. As a consequence, the fetal bladder is either small or nonvisible on ultrasound, and the fetus develops oligoanhydramnios.

The donor twin is presumably hypotensive in utero as a result of the net blood loss to the recipient. Postnatally, it is not uncommon for the donor twin to require inotropic support. In-utero hypotension of the donor, however, has never been documented.

Spontaneous in-utero demise of the donor twin may result from hypotension, chronic hypoxia, severe growth restriction, or anemia.

Effect of unbalanced blood exchange in the recipient twin

The excessive blood volume in the recipient twin presumably results in an increased production of atrial natriuretic factor, or ANF.[9] Wieacker et al studied three cases of severe twin transfusion syndrome and demonstrated that the concentration of ANF in the cord blood of recipient twins is significantly elevated compared to that of donor twins. Increased ANF results in increased fetal urine production, bladder distention, and polyhydramnios. The discrepancy between recipient and donor concentration correlated with the volume of transfusion. They proposed the following pathophysiological mechanism to explain the development of polyhydramnios in recipient twins: chronic blood volume overload in twins causes enhanced release of ANF from the fetal heart; increased fetal urine production leads to polyhydramnios, which is additionally enhanced by inhibition of antidiuretic hormone (ADH) release.

Hypertension may also develop in the recipient twin, both as a result of hypervolemia as well as from transfer of angiotensin II and paradoxical activation of the RAS system from the donor twin. Hypertension in the recipient twin results in thickened myocardial walls and potential myocardial dysfunction. Hypertension may be severe enough to cause myocardial infarction in the recipient. Hypertension in the recipient twin may be assessed with pulsed

Doppler assessment of the tricuspid regurgitant jet using the modified Bernoulli equation:

$$\Delta P = 4 \times V_{max}^2$$

We have noted tricuspid regurgitation in approximately 27% of recipients (138/498). The incidence of tricuspid regurgitation increased with stage (Figure 3.8), but has no prognostic value.

Transplacental passage of renin and/or angiotensin II from the donor to the recipient may suppress renin synthesis by the recipient kidney. This would result in increased renal blood flow, polyuria, and polyhydramnios.

Spontaneous demise of the recipient twin may result from hypertension, heart failure with hydrops, hemorrhage, or thrombosis from hyperviscosity.

Cause versus effect

The endocrine findings in TTTS are commonly viewed as the effect of the uneven blood exchange. Increased renin in the donor and increased ANF in the recipient, with their hemodynamic and renal consequences, follow the uneven exchange of blood. This view would be in accordance with the obligatory etiology as described above. Alternatively, increased renin, increased ADH, and a tendency to raise the blood pressure in the donor could result from placental insufficiency. The increased blood pressure in the donor would in turn force more blood through placental vascular anastomoses into the recipient twin, setting off the vicious cycle. This alternative

pathophysiological mechanism could operate in the facultative etiology theory discussed above. Potential circumstantial evidence of this mechanism could be seen in post-laser donors that develop hypertension. Baud et al recently reported on a hypertensive ex-donor after laser therapy, with right ventricular pressures of 60 mmHg.[10] The authors speculated that the development of hypertension in this fetus may have been due to increased placental resistance or reverse TTTS. In our series, eight donors out of 438 (1.8%) surgeries showed new onset of post-operative TR.

Pulmonic stenosis has also been viewed as an acquired disease in patients with TTTS.[11] As shown in Table 3.3, pulmonic stenosis is a rather rare event (4/615, 0.6%). The low incidence of this complication would suggest it as a cause rather than a consequence of TTTS (facultative etiology). At least two of these fetuses underwent postnatal balloon valvuloplasty, suggesting a permanent rather than a circumstantial change to the pulmonic valve. The issue is not clear, however, and will need further investigation.

SUMMARY OF THE PATHOPHYSIOLOGY OF TWIN–TWIN TRANSFUSION SYNDROME

TTTS presumably results from an unbalanced exchange of blood between two or more fetuses via placental vascular anastomoses. While this fundamental hypothesis has not been proven, circumstantial evidence suggests that this indeed may be the main operating pathophysiological mechanism. The etiology of the unbalanced blood

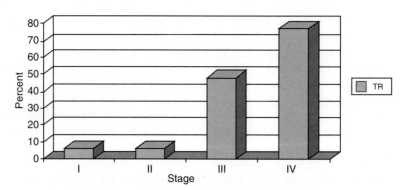

Figure 3.8 Tricuspid regurgitation (TR) by stage.

exchange can be traced back to either an abnormal design of the placental vascular anastomoses (obligatory etiology), or, less often, to primary hemodynamic differences between the fetuses. Hypovolemia in the donor twin elicits the RAS and increased ADH, causing local vasoconstriction, oliguria, oligohydramnios, and renal tubular dysgenesis. Hypervolemia in the recipient twin results in increased ANF secretion, polyuria, polyhydramnios, and hypertension. Hypertension in the recipient twin may also result from passive transfer of angiotensin II, and lead to cardiac hypertrophy, dysfunction, and eventually failure and or death. The degree of polyuria in the recipient twin seems to be out of proportion to the presumed amount of excessive blood transfer, consistent with an endocrine effect on the recipient's vascular system. The resulting vicious cycle may lead to death of one or both fetuses, or to miscarriage from polyhydramnios and incompetent cervix in 95% of cases. Therapy is therefore indicated, to avert the natural history of the disease.

REFERENCES

1. Benirschke K, Kaufmann P. Pathology of the human placenta. New York: Springer-Verlang; 1990.
2. Lutfi S, Allen VM, Fahey J, O'Connell CM, Vincer MJ. Twin–twin transfusion syndrome: a population-based study. Obstet Gynecol 2004; 104:1289–97.
3. Quintero R, Quintero L, Pivatelli A et al. The donor–recipient (D-R) score: in vivo endoscopic evidence to support the hypothesis of a net transfer of blood from donor to recipient in twin–twin transfusion syndrome. Prenat Neonat Med 2000; 5:84–91.
4. Powis R, Schwartz R. Practical Doppler ultrasound for the clinician. Baltimore: Williams & Wilkins; 1991.
5. Mielke G, Benda N. Cardiac output and central distribution of blood flow in the human fetus. Circulation 2001; 103:1662–8.
6. Ishii K, Chmait RH, Martinez JM, Nakata M, Quintero RA. Ultrasound assessment of venous blood flow before and after laser therapy: approach to understanding the pathophysiology of twin–twin transfusion syndrome. Ultrasound Obstet Gynecol 2004; 24:164–8.
7. Nakata M, Martinez JM, Diaz C, Chmait R, Quintero RA. Intra-amniotic Doppler measurement of blood flow in placental vascular anastomoses in twin–twin transfusion syndrome. Ultrasound Obstet Gynecol 2004; 24:102–3.
8. Mahieu-Caputo D, Meulemans A, Martinovic J et al. Paradoxic activation of the renin–angiotensin system in twin–twin transfusion syndrome: an explanation for cardiovascular disturbances in the recipient. Pediatr Res 2005; 58:685–8.
9. Wieacker P, Wilhelm C, Prompeler H et al. Pathophysiology of polyhydramnios in twin transfusion syndrome. Fetal Diagn Ther 1992; 7:87–92.
10. Baud O, Lebidois J, Van Peborgh P, Ville Y. Fetal and neonatal hypertension in twin–twin transfusion syndrome: a case report. Fetal Diagn Ther 1998; 13:223–6.
11. Nizard J, Bonnet D, Fermont L, Ville Y. Acquired right heart outflow tract anomaly without systemic hypertension in recipient twins in twin–twin transfusion syndrome. Ultrasound Obstet Gynecol 2001; 18:669–72.

4

Evidence on physiopathology

Masami Yamamoto and Yves H Ville

Introduction • The case definition problem • Placenta • Evidence from fetal blood sampling • Ultrasound staging of twin–twin transfusion syndrome • Mathematical modeling • Case reports • Conclusions

INTRODUCTION

The twin–twin transfusion syndrome (TTTS) (Figure 4.1) occurs in 15% of monochorionic–diamniotic pregnancies,[1] with a high perinatal mortality rate.[2] These are morphologically normal fetuses, in which the vascular communications in the placenta are thought to be responsible for the development of the disease. Besides the primary phenomenon, the disease may lead to disruptive lesions in both twins. This chapter will review the evidence for the development of the disease, its complications, and implications in therapeutical approaches. The chapter focuses at defining the clinical problem, the histopathology correlation of the clinical condition, and the ultrasonographic features that support or reject the pathophysiology of the disease. Some particular conditions that lead to TTTS are mentioned in order to understand the disease better.

THE CASE DEFINITION PROBLEM

Before the use of ultrasound, TTTS was diagnosed by a 20% discordance in the weights and at least 5 g/dl difference in the hemoglobin concentration at birth of two twins of the same sex.[3] These criteria were left aside because they were not always possible to demonstrate antenatally by ultrasound and because it is frequent in diamniotic twins as much as in monochorionic twins. Besides, these were used for surviving twins but not in cases of double- or single-fetal demise, which were more possibly affected by severe TTTS. With the development of ultrasound,

new antenatal findings were correlated to adverse outcome. The polyhydramnios/oligohydramnios sequence has been found to be the condition with one of the highest mortalities in obstetrics, with 90% mortality without treatment. Recently, growth discordance with abnormal umbilical Doppler has been considered a new indication for laser photocoagulation of anastomoses on the chorionic plate. There are cases that led to anemia of one twin and polycythemia of the other, outside the polyhydramnios/oligohydramnios sequence. These scenarios suggest that the presence of vascular communications are variable in number and type, producing pathophysiologically different problems, and that the TTTS is a complex situation in which fetal growth, fetal volemia, amniotic fluid discordance, and anemia are conjugated to produce a specific condition. Mortality and morbidity may be related to these complications in different ways. Comprehension of the mechanisms leading to complications and death is important to plan diagnostic and treatment strategies. With the use of Doppler and high-resolution two-dimensional (2D) imaging, new data on fetal anemia, hypervolemia, and fetal diuresis have been identified.

TTTS is now defined on ultrasound as oligohydramnios and polyhydramnios in the donor and recipient, respectively. The demonstration of the effectiveness of laser photocoagulation in these cases[4] has largely oriented the investigation of the anastomoses on the pathophysiology of this condition.

The mechanisms by which TTTS may produce death and sequealae are multiple. The study of

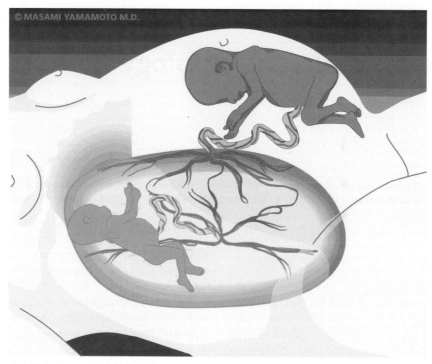

Figure 4.1 Characteristic features of polyhydramnios and oligohydramnios are due to hypervolemia and hypovolemia in recipient and donor twins, respectively.

these complications, as well as the possibility of treating them independently, will increase the chances of survival and the global rate of success of the different treatment modalities. TTTS may lead to fetal demise in utero through cardiac overload or severe intrauterine growth restriction. It may lead to extreme preterm delivery because of the effect of polyhydraminios on the cervix that mimics cervical incompetence, may produce extreme premature fetuses, and may provoke vascular disruptive consequences.

PLACENTA

The normal fetoplacental circulation consists of two arteries and one vein, which divide progressively in the chorionic plate (fetal surface of the placenta), and irrigate each cotyledon in a separate way. This means that normal vascularization of the placentas may be clearly recognized by the naked eye, until it reaches the corresponding cotyledon.

All monochorionic placentas have vascular communications between the cords,[5] which was

demonstrated in 278 placentas from twin pregnancies. Monochorionic placentas always have vascular communications, in comparison with dichorionic fused placentas. Despite this finding, TTTS only occurs in 15% of monochorionic pregnancies. The pattern of the anastomoses is therefore determinant in the occurrence of TTTS.

The anastomoses are classified into superficial arterioarterial (AA), superficial venovenous (VV), and deep arteriovenous (AV). Superficial anastomoses are direct vascular communications between vessels that come from each cord insertion. They may connect arteries (AA) or veins (VV) directly, and are called superficial because they are visible in the surface. Their main particularity is that they can compensate for higher volumes of blood in a rapid manner, in both directions, depending on arterial system or venous system blood pressure differences between the fetuses. Superficial arteriovenous anastomoses do not exist because they would produce a rapid exanguination of one fetus into the other. On the other hand, deep anastomoses are not real direct vascular communications, but cotyledons that

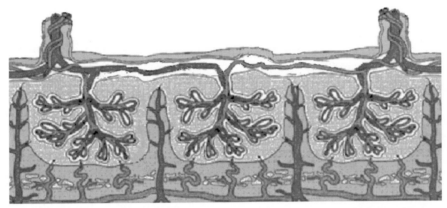

Figure 4.2 A monochorionic placenta is represented. The red vessels correspond to arteries and blue vessels to veins. One artery from the right cord irrigates a cotyledon that is drained by a vein from the left cord. This is a deep arteriovenous anastomosis.

are irrigated by a chorionic artery of one fetus that is drained by a chorionic vein of the other. They function in a much slower manner, and they are unidirectional (Figures 4.2, 4.3, 4.4, 4.5, and 4.6).

The vascular anatomy of monochorionic placentas was first described at the beginning of the century.[6] It is only in the 1990s that larger series were published to review the evidence of its role in TTTS.

The study of placentas require a standardized technique and a clear clinical diagnosis, with inclusion and exclusion criteria, to avoid selection bias.

The methods for ex-vivo evaluations described in the literature are colored ink injection, milk injection, air injection, ex-vivo angiography, and direct visualization of the placenta. In most

Figure 4.3 A monochorionic–diamniotic placenta with TTTS diagnosed at 25 weeks and delivered at 28 weeks treated only with amniodrainage. The intertwin membrane and amnios has been removed. Direct visualization of the chorionic plate after delivery shows the cord insertions of the donor (right) and the recipient (left). Three deep arteriovenous anastomoses were identified in this part of the chorionic plate, all directed from the donor to the recipient (white arrows). It is demonstrated that it comes from the donor's artery because it is directly connected to one of the thinner vessels in the cord (red arrow).

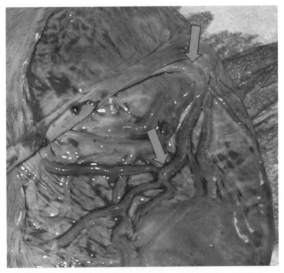

Figure 4.4 The same monochorionic–diamniotic placenta in the side of the donor with greater augmentation. The direct continuation of the anastomotic vessels with the artery in the cord is showed with the red arrows. The intertwin membrane is still in the placenta.

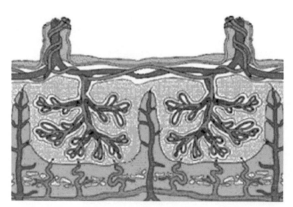

Figure 4.5 A monochorionic placenta with arterioarterial (red) and venovenous (blue) anastomoses. These correspond to direct communications between both cords, in which blood flow may be bidirectional. They may be present together or independently in monochorionic placentas.

techniques, veins and arteries catheterization is necessary, in order to identify the communicating vessels more easily and to be able to observe clear images of the vessels. In our experience, direct visualization is an excellent technique, with a good quality of vessel identification. The

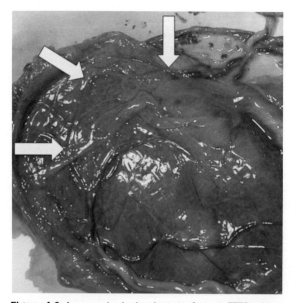

Figure 4.6 A monochorionic placenta from a TTTS with a superficial arterioarterial anastomosis. The white arrows show the passage of the vessel from one cord to the other. The donor (higher in the image) had a velamental insertion of the cord.

benefit of colored ink injection is that it can be easily photographed, so that post-hoc evaluations can be performed. There are no studies that compare direct visualization, air injection, or ink injection in terms of sensitivity. Injection studies have the problem of the dye viscosity and vascular thrombosis. This affects the perfusion of terminal circulation, and may give false-negative results. Normally, all vessels well seen by direct visualization will be well seen in ink injection studies. Rarely, a vessel not seen by the naked eye can be discovered by an ink injection. Air injection may aid in the identification of patent anastomoses after laser therapy. Finally, the death of one twin will produce an obliteration of the arteries and veins of the dead twin, making difficulty for an injection study later after delivery. The best cases for evaluation are those delivered before laser treatment of those with double-fetal demise in which delivery was induced soon after.

The differences in etiology, natural history, and treatment options are still debatable, and are related to the differences in the studies published.[7] The following studies correlate the placental findings with clinical data.

A study of monochorionic placentas by Machin et al[8] examined 69 placentas consecutively from monochorionic twin pregnancies that presented in their center. They studied the presence of vascular anastomoses, placental sharing, and their correlation with perinatal mortality, growth discordance, gestational age at delivery, and polyhydramnios. They provided a good classification of the 13 patterns of anastomoses. In their study, the worst clinical outcomes were the cases of unequal placental sharing, with the presence of deep AV anastomoses and paucity of superficial anastomoses (60% of TTTS within this group). They had 23% of placentas without anastomoses.

Bajoria et al published an interesting work of 10 placentas from TTTS and 10 from normal monochorionic pregnancies.[9] Exclusion criteria were the death of one or both twins and laser therapy, although the number of excluded placentas is not mentioned. They described a technique with room temperature and humidity control, right after delivery with a perfusion protocol of dextran, heparin, and procaine as vasodilator. Pressure, time intervals, and pH were controlled in the perfusion. A minimum of 25 cycles of 15 minutes each were performed for a blood-free outflow. Later, a dye injection procedure was described to ascertain the anastomoses pattern of the placenta. They found globally less anastomoses in the TTTS group (median 1 [0–2] vs 6 [4–8], p <0.001, Mann–Whitney). They found that TTTS placentas had fewer AA anastomoses (median 0 vs 2, p <0.0001), less VV anastomoses (median 0 vs 2, p <0.0001), and less deep AV anastomoses (median 1 vs 2.5, p <0.001). TTTS placentas had the particularity that they usually had one anastomosis, except in one case that had two anastomoses, in comparison to non-TTTS that presented with multiple anastomoses. The type of anastomosis was also different: whereas TTTS placentas had deep AV in 80% of the cases, non-TTTS presented them in only 36% of the cases. The deep AV in TTTS cases were always donor to recipient, in comparison to non-TTTS cases. All control cases had both AA and VV anastomoses. The authors conclude that is that TTTS placentas have generally one anastomosis, and that the anastomoses are deep AV without superficial ones. In controls, multiple anastomoses were present, with deep AV and superficial ones.

Denbow et al[10] studied 71 placentas from consecutive monochorionic–diamniotic pregnancies using a simpler technique: 82 patients were initially recruited, but exclusion criteria were applied for TRAP sequence (2), selective feticide (2), placental destruction at delivery (2), conjoined twins (2), and lost on follow-up (3). Four monoamniotic cases were included. This is the only study blinded to the perinatal outcome in which the ink injection was performed by a senior perinatal pathologist. The article explains clearly that in three cases only a limited assessment was possible, because of autolysis after fetal demise or damage at delivery. They found that TTTS placentas have fewer AA anastomoses (median 0 [0–1] vs 1 [0–1], p <0.0001), with similar frequency of AV and VV anastomoses. The highest rate of TTTS was found in placentas with one AV and no AA anastomoses (78%). All TTTS placentas had deep AV anastomoses, in comparison to 84% of non-TTTS placentas. The direction of AV anastomoses is not described in the study.

TTTS cases with death of one twin were no different than those in which both survived. The authors do not describe difficulties in catheterizing the umbilical cord in the dead twin's side.

Bermudez et al published the last series on placental studies in TTTS.[11] They included placentas from 26 non-complicated monochorionic–diamniotic pregnancies and from 105 TTTS cases treated by laser. They correlated the fetoscopy findings with an air injection test in order to analyze the photocoagulated areas. The placentas were classified according to the presence of anastomoses in four groups:

- absence (A)
- presence of only AV anastomoses (B)
- presence of only superficial anastomoses (C)
- presence of both superficial and deep anastomoses (D).

The highest rate of TTTS was found in group B (85/85). The overall number of anastomoses in TTTS placentas was higher than in non-complicated monochorionic pregnancies, (4.7 ± 2.48 vs 1.77 ± 1.27, p = 0.000). This study found that deep AV anastomoses were more frequent in TTTS (4.6 ± 2.22 vs 1.4 ± 0.5, p = 0.02), whereas superficial anastomoses were equally similar in both groups (1.6 ± 0.61 vs 1.7 ± 0.96, p = 0.69). The study does not inform which were the number of anastomoses that had to be considered AV or superficial by fetoscopical means.

This study contradicted previous studies and has been critically evaluated.[12] Laser treatment may alter postnatal injection studies. A referral bias has been mentioned because control placentas were less than one-fifth in number of TTTS placentas. Even though there are technical differences in the method, the main conclusion is that the presence of deep AV in the absence of superficial anastomoses are more frequent in TTTS cases.

Ex-vivo placental studies are not uniform in selection criteria, and a greater effort should be made in order to select clinically valuable data (Table 4.1). The technique has yet to be uniformly standardized. The findings of different studies are not completely concordant, since one supports the absence of superficial anastomoses as the main conclusion and another supports the absence of superficial AA anastomoses as the main pathological factor. Bajoria and Denbow disagree on the main concept that AV is a critical condition for the occurrence of TTTS. Despite this difference, all workers support the idea that the lack in AA or both AA and VV may generate a circulation system that favors the hypervolemic state of one twin.[13]

In-vivo studies

The description of placental vascular anastomoses from fetoscopies during laser photocoagulation of the chorionic plate may be used to study the placental architecture. This method is sensitive because of the endoscopic magnification of the image and is controlled because the placental surface remains with a white scar at the coagulation point. The problem is that technically difficult fetoscopies as anterior placentas or turbid amniotic fluid may give false negative for anastomoses detection.

De Lia et al[14] described ablating 8–10 communicating vessels per placenta in TTTS.

In a recent study from Hamburg[15] of 126 fetoscopies for laser photocoagulation of the chorionic plate vessels, the median number of anastomoses found was 5 (range 1–14), with 74% cases showing a higher number of AV anastomoses from donor to recipient. They always found at least one AV donor to recipient anastomoses. The postnatal correlation of the placenta was not possible in this study; 31% of the placentas had AA anastomoses and this was concordant with ex-vivo studies.

Doppler diagnosis of arteriovenous anastomoses has been reported with a sensitivity of 33%.[16] The only TTTS case presented in this paper was found to have one AV anastomosis at Doppler but five at placental dye injection.

Histological evidence

An interesting study on placental histology was performed in 1998.[17] Tertiary villi were studied and the number of muscular arteries was counted in a subset of 9 consecutive TTTS diagnosed by ultrasound, with 20% growth discordance and oligo–polyhydramnios sequence. The placenta

near the cord insertion of the donor and the recipient was studied blinded for the pathologist. They found significantly less muscular arteries in the donors (5.81 ± 0.55 vs 6.66 ± 0.24; $p = 0.017$). Concomitantly, the umbilical artery S/D Doppler index was higher in the donors than in the recipients. In a previous publication of the same cases, they found that 66% of the pairs had feto–fetal transfusion, and only 25% of them had anemia/polycythemia. The authors sustain the hypothesis that the primary factor is the vascular resistance in the donor's placenta, which increases until a threshold at which it becomes higher than the pressure in the anastomoses and provokes the perfusion of the recipient.[18]

This interesting theory supposes that fetal hypertension in the donor is a condition for the feto–fetal transfusion.

An interesting study was performed in 21 TTTS cases with death of both twins, with striking differences in kidney changes between the donors and recipients.[19] Most donors had renal tubular dysgenesis, characterized by nearly complete absence of identifiable proximal tubules and the ischemic appearance of the glomeruli. Donor twins are thought to suffer from chronic hypovolemia, so it may be assumed that the renal tubular disgenesis (RTD) lesions of these fetuses result from chronic hypoperfusion of the kidney, as it has also been observed as a congenital autosomal, recessive disorder responsible for oligohydramnios and in fetuses exposed in utero to angiotensin-converting enzyme inhibitors. This hypothesis is also supported by the observation of similar tubular changes in children with postnatal renal ischemia. Up-regulation of renin synthesis was also demonstrated using immunohistochemistry and in-situ hybridization, with a strong increase in renin protein and mRNA content in the donor kidneys. The recipient kidneys were large and congested, showing various degrees of hemorrhagic infarction and glomeruli. Renin was not detected in 20/21 recipient fetuses. Plasma renin concentration or activity was not measured in this series. However, it was speculated that circulating renin from the donor is transferred to the recipient through placental vascular anastomoses. Indeed, renin activity was previously detected in both twins in three cases

Table 4.1 Ex-vivo placental studies

Author, year (number of TTTS/non-TTTS placentas)	TTTS Superficial Placentas with AA	Superficial Placentas with VV	Deep Placentas with AV	Non-TTTS Superficial Placentas with AA	Superficial Placentas with VV	Deep Placentas with AV	Comments
Machin Four years before 1996 (14/55)	21% (3)	14% (2)	93% (13)	56% (31)	13% (7)	56% (31)	The case definition of TTTS was polyhydramnios of one but not the poly/oligohydramnios sequence
Bajoria 1992–1993 (10/10)	10% (1)	10% (1)	80% (8)	100% (10)	100% (10)	100% (10)	Selection bias is possible because excluded placentas are not mentioned and no dead fetuses were included
Denbow 1995–1998 (21/49)	24% (5)	100% (21)	100% (21)	16% (8)	16% (8)	84% (41)	Well-described selection criteria but ink injection protocol is lacking. Fetal demise cases were included but considered together
Bermudez 1997–2000 (105/26)	21%* (20)		99% 104	84%* (22)		19% (5)	Possible selection bias because no selection criteria were included for controls. Placentas were treated by laser and air injection techniques have not been compared with ink injection

*AA and VV were considered together.

of TTTS.[20] This inappropriate presence of renin in hypervolemic fetuses, with the eventual increase of angiotensin II generation and aldosterone synthesis, represents a potential factor in aggravating hypervolemia and its renal and extrarenal consequences for the recipient, including systemic hypertension. The hypothesis of the investigators was that adaptation of the donor by renin–angiotensin up-regulation may finally become deleterious to both twins, because in donors it may aggravate renal vasoconstriction and perfusion, and in recipients it may increase diuresis.

EVIDENCE FROM FETAL BLOOD SAMPLING

The neonatal criterion of a difference in 5 g/dl of hemoglobin has shown to be unsuitable in utero, because of its lack of correlation with the ultrasonographic criteria and because neonatal cases select those TTTS cases with better outcome. Bruner and Rosemond[18] found a difference of more than 5 g/dl by cordocentesis in only 1 of 6 cases with TTTS. This study aimed to demonstrate donor–recipient passage of blood by a positive Kleihauer–Betke test in the recipient after in-utero tranfusion of the donor with adult O Rh– red cells. In 6 cases in which the procedure could be performed, Kleihauer–Betke was positive in 4 recipients 5–19 minutes following transfusion in the donor. The conclusion of the authors was that 4/6 of TTTS diagnosed by ultrasound had a real donor to recipient transfusion (1–17%), and that perhaps the ultrasonographic criteria should be reviewed since in 2 out of 6 cases no transfusion could be demonstrated. The major criticism of that study is that perhaps 5 minutes is not enough time for the donor to replace 1% of the recipient's volemia. Therefore this method may be insensitive for the diagnosis of feto–fetal transfusion.

In a later report from Detroit,[21] cordocentesis was performed in 8 cases of TTTS. Hemoglobin values were significantly lower in donors vs recipients, but were over 5 g/dl in only 3 cases. It was suggested that the tranfusion syndrome did not exist in 5 cases because the hemoglobin level was normal.

An interesting study was performed to assess the difference in erythropoietin in fetuses with TTTS.[22] In 15 TTTS pregnancies, erythropoietin was similar between donors and recipients, despite an important difference in fetal hemoglobin. In 6 monochorionic–diamniotic pregnancies used as controls, erythropoietin was found to be similar between the twins, but lower than in TTTS. The study was completed with immunohistology, in which the kidneys of donors and recipients stained similarly for erythropoietin antibodies, supporting the idea that both fetuses are synthethizing the hormone and that the similar concentration is not by the passage from the donor to the recipient.

Ferritin and iron was studied by the same authors.[23] A higher concentration of ferritin was found in the recipient, although it was well below that found in cases of iron overload. Ferritin was similar between donors and controls (non-TTTS monochorionic–diamniotic fetuses) and iron was similar in all groups. After these two studies, the authors conclude that anemia/polycythemia is not a constant characteristic of TTTS, because erythropoiesis is similar in both fetuses and no signs of iron overload have been confirmed in the recipient, despite some differences in fetal hemoglobins.

The study on fetal hormones and differences between donors and recipients in TTTS has contributed to the understanding of the pathophysiology. Although vascular anastomoses may equilibrate hormone concentrations on both sides, some substances have been found to have similar concentrations in both fetuses but others do not. Differences in the half-life of the hormones may also explain the results found.

Cordocentesis was performed in 14 TTTS and 6 normal monochorionic–diamniotic pregnancies. Atrial natriuretic peptide and brain natriuretic peptides were higher in recipients than donors, and donors had similar concentrations with non-TTTS monochorionic twins.[24]

Vasopressin was measured in 44 non-TTTS monochorionic twins, 17 TTTS twins, and their mothers. Vasopressin was found to be three times higher in the donors than in recipients with TTTS. The normal fetuses had concentrations lower than that in donors but higher than in recipients, and the mothers had similar concentrations, whereas the condition of their fetuses.[25] This suggests that the vasoconstriction in the donor is an important factor in the development of TTTS.

ULTRASOUND STAGING OF TWIN–TWIN TRANSFUSION SYNDROME

TTTS staging was introduced by Quintero et al in 1999.[26] This is based on ultrasound features:

- stage 1 – oligo/polyhydramnios sequence only with bladder visualized in the donor twin
- stage 2 – bladder not visualized in the donor twin
- stage 3 – critically abnormal Dopplers (absent or reversed diastolic flow) in the donor umbilical artery, pulsitile venous or reverse flow in the ductus venosus
- stage 4 – hydrops in either twin
- stage 5 – demise of one or both twins.

A retrospective study of 50 TTTS cases treated by amnioreduction in Australia[27] between 1993 and 2002, classified patients into stages at presentation. Overall, 22% of the cases improved after one amnioreduction, 40% remained with the same stage, and 38% progressed. It was found that the less severe TTTS was at presentation, the higher the chance to improve.

A prospective study of 52 cases from London[28] showed that 15–60% of the cases can improve in stage, and that mortality was similar regardless of improvement. The gestational age at presentation was 24, 20, 20, 21, and 16 weeks for stages I–V, respectively.

Data from our center with 175 cases of TTTS treated by laser is shown in (Figure 4.7). We found that gestational age between groups was not different.

This information suggests that stages may not represent different times during the natural history of the disease, but rather different forms of presentation with possibly different prognosis. In Quintero et al's paper[30] where the stage system is analyzed as a prognostic factor for outcome, laser photocoagulation appeared to be better than amnioreduction in stages III or IV, whereas the outcome in stages I and II was similar in both groups. However, in the Eurofetus randomized trial,[31] 72 TTTS treated by laser were compared with 70 TTTS treated by amnioreduction. At least one survivor was obtained in 86% and 58% of the cases treated by laser and amnioreduction in TTTS stages I or II. This difference persisted in stages III and IV (66% vs 44%).

Doppler

Doppler studies in TTTS were first reported in 20 consecutive cases in 1995.[32] This cross-sectional study investigated the circulatory profile of the donor and recipient fetuses in 20 pregnancies with twin–twin transfusion syndrome presenting with acute polyhydramnios at 17–27 (mean 22) weeks' gestation. Doppler investigations of the

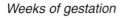

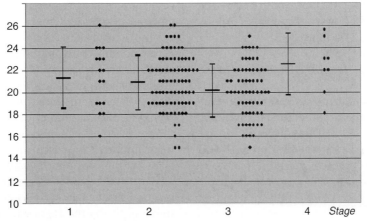

Figure 4.7 Gestational age at presentation of 175 cases of TTTS. Median and standard deviations are represented. No difference was found (Anova $p = 0.06$).[29]

arterial vessels and ductus venosus, inferior vena cava, right hepatic vein, tricuspid, and mitral ventricular inflow were performed in both fetuses. The most significant findings on the arterial side were an increased mean umbilical artery pulsatility index and a decreased mean value for aortic blood flow velocity in both groups of fetuses. Five recipients and 4 donors had absence or reversal of blood flow during atrial contraction in the ductus venosus. All these fetuses showed pulsations in the umbilical vein. Tricuspid regurgitation was present in 8 recipients. Absence or reversal of end-diastolic velocities in the umbilical artery was found in 4 donors. The recipient's circulation showed characteristics of congestive heart failure due to hypervolemia. Alterations in the donor's circulation were consistent with decreased venous return due to hypovolemia and increased cardiac afterload due to increased placental resistance.

Intra-amniotic Doppler measurements were performed by Nakata et al.[33] A 2 mm probe was introduced in the amniotic cavity and Doppler measurements were performed in the anastomoses, directly visualized by the endoscope. Two cases were included in this study and the flow was calculated by the diameter of the vessel by Doppler and the mean velocity. The net flow in both cases was from recipient to donor.

Recently, venous flow measurements have been introduced in the evaluation of TTTS. The umbilical vein flow calculated as a flow per fetal weight has been measured in recipients and donors before and after laser in 32 cases, with a significative difference between both twins and an increase of 50% in donors after laser.[34] A later report confirmed the findings.[35]

MATHEMATICAL MODELING

Animal models of monochorionic multiple pregnancies are lacking, so mathematical modeling has become an interesting way of studying the pathophysiology of TTTS. The first model[36] was based on two circulations in which a communication was produced at 28 weeks of pregnancy, reproducing the oligo/polyhydramnios sequence.

An important pathophysiological consideration is the timing on the development of TTTS relative to existence of the vascular anastomoses. Since TTTS develops in the midtrimester, despite the existence of vascular anastomoses since the beginning of the pregnancy. Later mathematical models suggested that the growth of the vessels diminish the vascular resistance faster than the growth of the fetus, which in turn the existent anastomoses into functional low resistance anastomoses.[37] The models are explained in detail in Chapter 6.

CASE REPORTS

Some pathophysiological arguments come from particular cases. Acute TTTS developed at 32 weeks with previously normal amniotic fluid and non-discordant monochorionic twins.[38] After delivery, a recent thrombosis of a superficial arterioarterial anastomosis was found. In addition, the placenta had 5 donor-to-recipient deep AV anastomoses, and 2 recipient-to-donor deep AV anastomoses.

CONCLUSIONS

The pathophysiology of TTTS is still poorly understood. It is generally accepted that neonatal criteria are inadequate for the diagnosis, and have been replaced by ultrasonographic criteria of amniotic fluid discordance. Most authors agree that the placental vascular connections are the main basis for the development of the condition. The TTTS stages may represent natural history or different presentations of TTTS, rather than progressive stages. Data from cordocentesis has concluded that the ultrasonographic diagnosis of TTTS (oligo/polyhydramnios) has rarely anemia/polycythemia, with similar iron/ferritin profile in both fetuses. The renin–angiotensin system is unbalanced, with overfuncion in the donor and down-regulation in the recipient, but the effect of the oversecretion in the recipient may be part of the passage of blood from donor to recipient, aggravating the condition. Arterial Doppler measurements are not different between twins in general, even in middle cerebral artery territory. Venous flow measurement supports the theory that the main disturbance is volume overload in one fetus and depletion in the other.

REFERENCES

1. Sebire NJ, Snijders RJ, Hughes K et al. The hidden mortality of monochorionic twin pregnancies. Br J Obstet Gynecol 1997; 104(10):1203–7.

2. Patten RM, Mack LA, Harvey D, Cyr DR, Pretorius DH. Disparity of amniotic fluid volume and fetal size: problem of the stuck twin – US studies. Radiology 1989; 172:153–7.

3. Danskin FH, Neilson JP. Twin-to-twin transfusion syndrome: What are appropriate diagnostic criteria? Am J Obstet Gynecol 1989; 161:365–9.

4. Senat MV, Deprest J, Boulrain M, et al. Endoscopic laser surgery vs serial amnioreduction for severe twin-to-twin transfusion syndrome. NEJM 2004; 351:136–44.

5. Robertson EG, Neer KJ. Placental injection studies in twin gestation. Am J Obstet Gynecol 1983; 147:170–4.

6. Schatz F. Klinische Beitrage zur Physiologie des Fotus. Berlin: Hirschwald; 1900.

7. Campbell S. Twin-to-twin transfusion syndrome – debates on the etiology, natural history and management. Ultrasound Obstet Gynecol 2000; 16:210–13.

8. Machin G, Still K, Lalani T. Correlations of placental vascular anatomy and clinical outcomes in 69 monochorionic twin pregnancies Am J Med Genet 1996; 61:229–36.

9. Bajoria R, Wigglesworth J, Fisk N. Fetus-placenta-newborn: angioarchitecture of monochorionic placentas in relation to the twin–twin transfusion syndrome. Am J Obstet Gynecol 1995; 172(3):856–63.

10. Denbow M, Cox P, Taylor M et al. Placental angioarchitecture in monochorionic twin pregnancies: relationship to fetal growth, fetofetal transfusion syndrome, and pregnancy outcome. Am J Obstet Gynecol 2000; 182(2): 417–26.

11. Bermudez C, Becerra C, Bornick P et al. Placental types and twin–twin transfusion syndrome. Ultrasound Obstet Gynecol 2002; 187:489–94.

12. Taylor M, Wee L, Fisk N. Placental types and twin–twin transfusion syndrome. Am J Obstet Gynecol 2003; 188(4):1119.

13. Machin G. The monochorionic twin placenta in vivo is not a black box. Ultrasound Obstet Gynecol 2001; 17:4–6.

14. De Lia JE, Cruikshank DP, Keye W Jr. Fetoscopic neodymium:YAG laser occlusion of placental vessels in severe twin–twin transfusion syndrome. Obstet Gynecol 1990; 75:1046–53.

15. Diehl W, Hecher K, Vetter M et al. Placental vascular anastomoses visualized during fetoscopic laser surgery in severe mid-trimester twin–twin transfusion syndrome. Placenta 2001; 22:876–81.

16. Taylor MJO, Farquharson D, Cox PM, Fisk NM. Identification of arterio-venous anastomoses in vivo in monochorionic twin pregnancies: preliminary report. Ultrasound Obstet Gynecol 2000; 16:218–22.

17. Bruner JP, Anderson L, Rosemond RL. Placental pathophysiology of the twin oligohydramnios–polyhydramnios sequence and the twin–twin transfusion syndrome. Placenta 1998; 19:81–6.

18. Bruner JP, Rosemond RL. Twin-to-twin transfusion syndrome: a subset of the twin oligohydramnios–polyhydramnios sequence. Am J Obstet Gynecol 1993; 169(4):925–30.

19. Mahieu-Caputo D, Dommergues M, Delezoide AL et al. Twin-to-twin transfusion syndrome. Role of the fetal renin–angiotensin system. Am J Pathol 2000; 156: 629–36.

20. Wiecaker P, Wilhelm C, Prompeler H et al. Pathophysiology of polyhydramnios in twin transfusion syndrome. Fetal Diag Ther 1992; 7:87–92.

21. Berry S, Puder K, Bottoms S et al. Comparison of intrauterine hematologic and biochemical values between twin pairs with and without stuck twin syndrome. Am J Obstet Gynecol 1995; 172:1403–1410.

22. Bajoria R, Ward S, Sooranna S. Erythropoietin in monochorionic twin pregnancies in relation to twin–twin transfusion syndrome. Hum Reprod 2001; 16(3): 574–580.

23. Baroia R, Lazda EJ, Ward S et al. Iron metabolism in monochorionic twin pregnanicies in relation to twin–twin transfusion syndrome. Hum Reprod 2001; 16 (3):567–73.

24. Bajoria R, Ward S, Chatterjee R. Natriuretic peptides in the pathogenesis of cardiac dysfunction in the recipient fetus of twin–twin transfusion syndrome. Am J Obstet Gynecol 2002; 186:121–7.

25. Bajoria R, Ward S, Sooranna S. Influence of vasopressin in the pathogenesis of oligohydramnios–polyhydramnios in monochorionic twins. Eur J Obstet Gynecol 2004; 113:49–55.

26. Quintero RA, Morales WJ, Allen MH. Staging twin–twin transfusion syndrome. J Perinatol 1999; 19:550–5.

27. Cincotta R, Chan FY, Cuncombe G et al. A staged assessment of the progression of twin–twin transfusion syndrome (TTTS). Am J Obstet Gynecol 2003; S224:604.

28. Taylor MJ, Govender L, Wee L et al. Validation of the Quintero staging system for twin–twin transfusion syndrome. Obstet Gynecol 2002; 100(6):1257–65.

29. Yamamoto M, El Murr L, Robyr R, et al. Incidence and impact of perioperative complications in 175 fetoscopy-guided laser coagulation of chorionic plate anastomoses in fetal–fetal transfusion syndrome before 26 weeks of gestation. Am J Obstet Gynecol 2005; 193 (3 pt 2):1110–16.

30. Quintero R, Dickinson J, Morales W et al. Stage-based treatment of twin–twin transfusion syndrome. Am J Obstet Gynecol 2003; 188:1333–40.

31. Senat MV, Deprest J, Boulvain M et al. Endoscopic laser surgery vs serial amnioreduction for severe twin-to-twin transfusion syndrome. N Engl J Med 2004; 351:136–44.

32. Hecher K, Ville Y, Snijders R et al. Doppler studies of the fetal circulation in twin–twin transfusion syndrome. Ultrasound Obstet Gynecol 1995; 5:318–24.

33. Nakata M, Martinez JM, Diaz CM et al. Intra-amniotic Doppler measurement of blood flow in placental vascular anastomoses in twin–twin transfusion syndrome. Ultrasound Obstet Gynecol 2004. 24:102–3.

34. Gratacos E, Van Schoubroeck D, Carreras E et al. Impact of laser coagulation in severe twin–twin transfusion syndrome on fetal Doppler indices and venous blood flow volume. Ultrasound Obstet Gynecol 2002; 20:125–30.

35. Ishii K, Chmait RH, Martinez JM et al. Ultrasound assessment of venous blood flow before and after laser therapy: approach to understanding the pathophysiology of twin–twin transfusion syndrome. Ultrasound Obstet Gynecol 2004; 24:164–8.

36. Talbert DG, Bajoria R, Sepulveda W et al. Hydrostatic and osmotic pressure gradients produce manifestations of fetofetal transfusion syndrome in a computerized model of monochorial twin pregnancy. Am J Obstet Gynecol 1996; 174:598–608.

37. Van Gemert M, Sterengborg HJ. Haemodynamic model of twin–twin transfusion syndrome in monochorionic twin pregnancies. Placenta 1998; 19:195–208.

38. Tan TY, Denbow ML, Cox PM et al. Occlusion of arterio-arterial anastomoses manifesting as acute twin–twin transfusion syndrome. Placenta 2004; 25:238–42.

5

Placental pathology and twin–twin transfusion syndrome

Ramen H Chmait, Carlos Bermúdez, Enrico Lopriore and Kurt Benirschke

INTRODUCTION

Twin–twin transfusion syndrome (TTTS) was initially characterized by Friedrich Schatz in the late 1800s. This body of work included a case of a monochorionic twin pregnancy that was complicated by marked discordance of infant size at birth.[1-5] The larger twin was noted to be edematous and found to have micturated frequently prior to death at 12 hours of age, while the smaller co-twin never urinated and died at 53 hours of age with an empty bladder. From detailed study of monochorionic placentas, Schatz suggested that anastomotic vessels linked the circulations of monochorionic twins. The presence of these vascular anastomoses served as a conduit for the unbalanced exchange of blood between the twins, thus setting up the circumstances for the development of TTTS.

To better understand the etiology and management of TTTS, a detailed understanding of the placenta is required. The aim of this chapter is to review placental anatomy and related pathophysiology as it pertains to TTTS.

ZYGOSITY

Pregnancies complicated by TTTS are, with rare exception, monozygotic twins. Monozygotic twinning results from an early (within 14 days following fertilization) embryonic 'splitting' of a single zygote. The cause of this division is unknown, although some have viewed it as an anomalous embryonic event.[6] The timing of the division determines both the chorionicity and amnionicity.[7] Division prior to the differentiation of the chorion results in the development of a dichorionic–diamniotic twin gestation; this occurs in approximately 30% of monozygotic twins. Twinning after differentiation of the chorion but before the amnion results in a monochorionic–diamniotic twin gestation. This constitutes 60–70% of monozygotic twins, and is the placental type commonly seen in TTTS. A monochorionic–monoamniotic twin gestation ensues after the differentiation of the amnion in about 1% of monozygotic twins. TTTS typically occurs in 5–17% of monochorionic-diamniotic placentas, and although extremely rare, the syndrome has also been noted in dichorionic-diamniotic and monochorionic-monoamniotic placentas.

Although monozygotic twins typically have identical genetic make-up, phenotypic discordance is not uncommon.[8] Phenotypic discordance is presumed to occur if variable influences are exerted on the developing twins. Examples of placental factors that may facilitate discordance in monochorionic twins include abnormal vascular communications, unequal partitioning of the placental mass, or variable locations of the placental cord insertions. These factors are addressed in subsequent sections of this chapter.

Although rare, a handful of reported cases describe dizygotic monochorionic twin gestations.[9,10] This is hypothesized to occur from fusion of separately fertilized embryos such that the outer cells, which have committed to form the trophoblast, intermix to form a single placenta. Quintero et al reported a case of dizygotic monochorionic–diamniotic twins complicated by TTTS. The twins were discordant for gender. Microsatellite analysis of pericentromeric markers suggested dispermic fertilization of two separate ova. These findings suggest that chorionicity, not zygosity, may be responsible for placental vascular anastomoses.[9] However, our group has also noted one case of 'dichorionic' twins with TTTS. Fetoscopic surgery identified a single vascular communication. Pathological study of the fetal dividing membranes identified one area in which the chorion became progressively diminutive and then disappeared. We hypothesized that the chorionicity was a hybrid, with a region consistent with monochorionicity in a predominantly dichorionic placentation. Other groups have also reported cases of monochorionic twins with two completely separate placental disks connected by a thin bridge of placental tissue.[11] In an unpublished study of 600 MC placentas, Machin reports having seen eight cases of bipartite monochorionic placentas.[12] Recently, Lopriore et al described three bipartite placentas in a consecutive series of 109 monochorionic placentas (Figure 1).[13] Both studies imply that the incidence of bipartite monochorionic placentas (1 to 3%) is not as rare as previously suspected.

THE MONOCHORIONIC PLACENTA

The monochorionic twin placenta is usually shaped as a single disk (Figure 5.2). However, the chorionicity cannot be assigned by the number of placental masses (Figure 5.3). Dichorionic placentas that are in close proximity may abut one another and become fused into a single placental mass.[14] This occurs in approximately 50% of dichorionic placentas. As detailed above, a monochorionic placenta may rarely possess separate lobes that are connected together via a diminutive bridge of placental tissue. For these reasons, establishing chorionicity may pose as a diagnostic dilemma both prenatally via ultrasound and postnatally at time of gross placental evaluation. The prenatal sonographic markers of chorionicity are reviewed in later chapters of this book. Postnatal gross and histological markers of monochorionic vs dichorionic are detailed below.

Detailed documentation of the placental anatomy in twins is useful in that it may provide

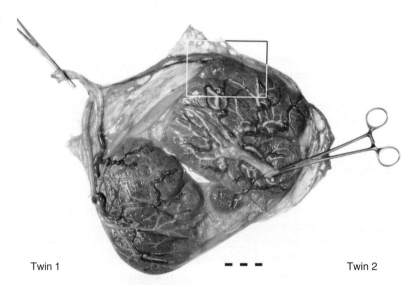

Twin 1   - - -   Twin 2

Figure 5.1 Bipartite monochorionic placenta after injection with colored dye. Arteries are injected with dark blue colored dye and veins with orange or yellow colored dye. (Reproduced with permission from[13].) (See also color plate section, page xvi.)

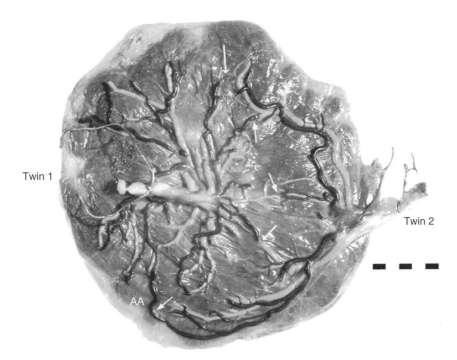

Figure 5.2 Placenta injection study with colored dye confirmed the presence of vascular communications confirming monochorionicity in this diamniotic twin placenta. This monochorionic twin gestation without twin-to-twin transfusion syndrome delivered after 38 weeks of gestation. Arteries are injected with dark-blue dye and veins with orange dye. The arrow at the bottom of the picture indicates an arterio-arterial anastomosis. Arterio-venous anastomoses from twin 2 to twin 1 are pointed out in the center of the picture, whereas an arterio-venous anastomosis from twin 1 to twin 2 is indicated at the top of the picture. (Not all anastomoses are labeled.) (Reproduced with permission from[15].) (See also color plate section, page xvii.)

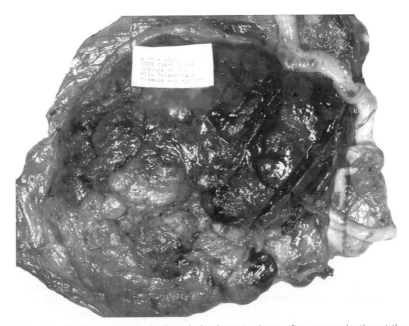

Figure 5.3 The chorionic side of a fused dichorionic-diamniotic placenta shows after exsanguination at the time of birth, which resulted in the pallor of Twin B's placenta. This allowed for a clear demarcation of the border between the fused placentas. (See also color plate section, page xvii.)

clinicopathological correlation to outcome. Evaluation of the monochorionic twin placenta, particularly if the pregnancy was complicated by TTTS, requires additional scrutiny. The first step is to establish chorionicity. Pathological ascertainment of chorionicity may be performed via several methods. Analysis of the 'dividing fetal membranes' by an experienced examiner is the surest method for assigning placental chorionicity. Dividing membranes are defined as the portion of the fetal membranes in which the two separate twin gestational sacs are in contact. All twins, except monochorionic–monoamniotics, have a dividing membrane. In the case of a monochorionic–diamniotic twin gestation, the dividing membrane is composed of only two abutting amnions, whereas the dividing membranes of dichorionic–diamniotic twins have intervening chorions between the two amnions (Figure 5.4). Thus, the dividing membranes of a monochorionic placenta are thin and have no blood vessel remnants within them. Because the amnion is composed of epithelium and connective tissue only, the dividing membrane is translucent. This is particularly useful during endoscopic fetal surgery for the treatment of TTTS, for the translucency of the membranes of monochorionic–diamniotic twins allows for visualization of the vascular anatomy on the opposite side of the dividing membrane. Lastly, manual separation of the dividing membranes of a monochorionic placenta to their insertion on the placental surface may be continued such that the amnion is stripped from the surface of the placenta.[16] This is in contrast to the fused dichorionic placenta. The dividing membrane of fused dichorionic placentas is thick, considerably more opaque, has remnants of villi and atrophied vessels in their four layers, and separation of the fetal membranes cannot be continued once the chorionic plate is reached, with further dissection resulting in placental disruption. The presence of vascular anastomoses is another placental finding seen nearly exclusively in monochorionic placentas.

The next step in the characterization of the monochorionic placenta is to identify the location of the dividing membrane on the surface of the placenta relative to the vascular equator. The vascular equator is defined as the region of the placenta where anastomotic vessels cross. It may be identified grossly by the relative avascular zone (aside from the anastomoses), measuring a few centimeters in width on the chorionic plate between the two placental cord insertions. The line of insertion of the dividing membrane into the placenta may not be in the region of the vascular equator. In fact, we have not uncommonly noted during fetoscopic laser surgery that the dividing membrane may run nearly perpendicular to the vascular equator (Figure 5.5). Because the

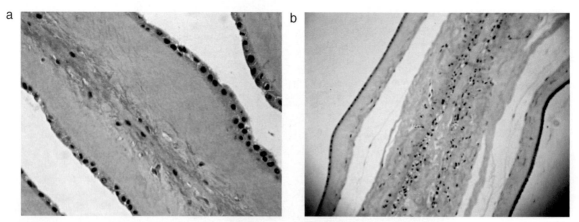

a   b

Figure 5.4 Histologic sections of the dividing membranes from a monochorionic diamniotic (a) and dichorionic diamniotic (b) twin gestations are shown. The monochorionic dividing membranes are composed of a layer of amnion and connective tissue only, in contrast to the dichorionic membranes which contain intervening chorions. (Reproduced courtesy of Pawini Khanna MD, Tampa General Hospital, Tampa, FL, USA.) (See also color plate section, page xviii.)

a 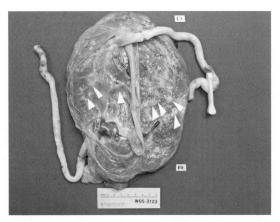 b

Figure 5.5 (a) Monochorionic-diamniotic placenta, status post laser therapy for TTTS, with the dividing membrane intersecting the vascular equator at a 45 degree angle to. Arrows point to lasered anastomoses. (b) Monochorionic diamniotic placenta, status post laser therapy for TTTS, with dividing membranes running perpendicular to the vascular equator. Arrows point to laser anastomoses. (See also color plate section, page xxviii.)

amniotic membranes may be moved freely over the chorionic surface in utero, one can envisage that the polyhydramnios noted in the recipient sac in TTTS may displace the dividing membrane insertion site towards the donor fetus (Figure 5.6). This may explain our observation that approximately two-thirds of all vascular anastomoses are located exclusively in the recipient's gestational sac.

The placental mass that supported each fetus may be qualitatively assigned by partitioning the placenta along the vascular equator. Umbilical cord description and position should be defined. Assignment of the umbilical cord to the appropriate fetus is obviously important. Accurate tagging and recording of the correct umbilical cord should be done at the time of delivery.

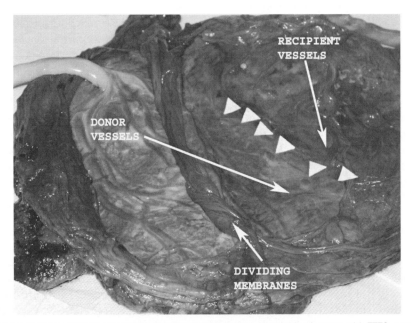

Figure 5.6 Dividing membranes pushed toward donor territory in this monochorionic placenta with TTTS, status post laser therapy. Small arrows point to laser photocoagulated areas and the vascular equator. (See also color plate section, page xviii.)

Also, the location of the placental cord insertion sites is recorded relative to the nearest placental margin and to each other, with a special note for marginal or velamentous cord insertions. Finally, the vascular anatomy should be concisely characterized. The methodology of placental vascular evaluation is described in the next section. Briefly, the origin and type of each vessel should be documented. All vascular anastomoses should be described relative to type, size, and location, and the overall vascular pattern should be assessed. A color photograph is most helpful in providing a visual record (Figure 5.2). Lastly, histological findings, particularly as they relate to TTTS, should be reported.

To better understand the role of the monochorionic placenta as it pertains to TTTS, the following placental factors will be reviewed in detail: (1) vascular anatomy; (2) partitioning of the placental mass; and (3) placental cord insertions.

VASCULAR COMMUNICATIONS

Dating back to Schatz, several observers have considered the vascular anastomoses of monochorionic placentas to be an important factor in the development of TTTS. Most authorities today agree that, to some extent, TTTS arises from unbalanced exchange of blood between twins through these vascular anastomoses. Indeed, several studies have shown that ablation of the vascular anastomoses 'cures' TTTS.[17,18] However, if virtually all monochorionic placentas have vascular communications, why does TTTS develop in only a minority of monochorionic pregnancies? Is there a vascular arrangement that preferentially results in TTTS or is associated with a worsened outcome? Regarding the corollary, is there a type of vascular communication that protects against TTTS? These are a few of many questions regarding the pathophysiology of TTTS that remain hotly debated. Only with further basic science and clinical research will we be able to fully answer these questions.

The developmental embryology regarding vascular anastomoses in the monochorionic twin placenta is currently not fully known. Placental pathological studies suggest that the vascular arrangement develops in the early embryonic period of development.[19] The vessels from the

yolk sac develop into the formed chorionic sac at about day 13 following fertilization. The primitive vascular precursors sprout along the inner surface of the primitive chorionic membrane. These vascular precursors begin to fill with blood when the fetal heart begins to pump. Whether the vessels become arteries or veins may be determined by directionality and pressure of blood flow. Some of the anastomoses may be kept open, and others atrophy. What influences, if any, dictate the number and type of anastomoses is unknown. One theory involves the unequal split of cells between the divided embryos.[20] This may result in differential timing of the fetal heartbeat, forcing the blood through the developing vascular channels. The unequal division of cell mass may not only affect vascular angioarchitecture but also placental mass allocation. Further clarification of the embryology of monochorionic twins as it pertains to the vascular communications will no doubt help in the understanding of the etiology of TTTS.

Although previously underestimated, it is now believed that virtually all monochorionic placentas have vascular anastomoses. The frequency of vascular anastomoses in twin gestations was well described in a report[17] that used comprehensive injection studies to evaluate the vascular anatomy of 278 twin placentas. After exclusion of 97 placentas that were noted to have completely separate placental masses and 19 placentas that were damaged, 162 fused placentas were successfully injected and studied. Ninety-six (59%) were assigned as dichorionic–diamniotic. Of the 56 monochorionic twin placentas studied, vascular communications were identified in 55 cases (98%). The single monochorionic placenta in which a vascular communication could not be found had an infarcted region in the area of the vascular equator; this area may have once contained an anastomosis in utero. Four cases, or 7% of the cases with a documented monochorionic placenta, were reported to be complicated by TTTS.

In the normal placenta, the chorionic surface vascular anatomy consists of branching vessels from the umbilical cord insertion site. The fetal arteries usually (but not always) course over veins, particularly those of large caliber (Figure 5.2). The fetal artery treks along the fetal surface of the placenta to the periphery, where it then dives into its designated cotyledon. The primary branches of the fetal vessels further subdivide into secondary and tertiary stems, from which the terminal villi arise. Thus, each primary villous stem arises into a separate cotyledon. The corresponding vein emerges from the same cotyledon within a few millimeters and courses back to the umbilical cord. Although the fetal artery and vein enter and depart the placental mass in close proximity to one another, the course of these vessels along the surface of the placenta may or may not be related to one another. Each cotyledon usually has only one artery and one vein. Three-vessel (or higher-order) cotyledons may be seen, particularly if one of the vessels serves as a vascular communication between monochorionic twins. The vascular equator divides the monochorionic placenta into two regions. This landmark is important not only because it is the region through which the anastomotic vessels traverse but also because it too helps define the relative placental parenchymal volume for each twin (Figures 5.2, 5.5, and 5.6).

The placental vascular anatomy may be delineated visually. This is the basis for the fetoscopically guided technique of selective laser photocoagulation of communicating vessels for the treatment of monochorionic twins complicated by TTTS[21] (Figure 5.7). As suggested above, it is the vascular equator, not the site of the dividing membrane insertion, which must be identified to allow for the separation of the two vascular circulations during fetal laser surgery. After delivery, injection studies using colored dye, milk, water, or air may further assist in identifying the vascular anatomy[19,22] as shown in Figure 5.7c. The umbilical cord may be trimmed to allow unobstructed access to the vessels, or the distal aspect of the cord may be clamped and individual vessels accessed via a fine needle to inject the media. The vascular patterns identified after delivery may not necessarily represent the anatomy that was present in utero. Spontaneous alterations of placental anatomy may occur from thrombosis of a vascular communication or infarction of a placental region that may have contained an anastomosis. These placental events may explain the reported cases of both the spontaneous resolution of TTTS as well as the sudden,

acute development of TTTS in previously documented 'normal' monochorionic pregnancies.[23] If a placental event developed remote from delivery, that placental region may be uninterpretable. It is important to note that post-delivery evaluation of placental communications cannot be performed accurately if a remote in utero demise of one twin occurred, or if the placenta was placed in a preservative such as formalin.

There are two types of vascular communications in a monochorionic placenta. The first type, artery-to-vein (AV) communications, are referred to as deep anastomoses, so-called because the communication takes place at the level of the fetal capillaries in the shared placental cotyledon. This is shown in Figure 5.8. AV anastomoses are unidirectional shunts. Directionality is always from high pressure artery to low pressure vein. Although the anastomoses are 'deep', at the level of terminal villi, identification of the origin of the primary arteries and veins on the surface of the chorionic plate allows for identification of all AV communications. In the case of TTTS, if the arterial component of the AV communication belongs to the donor, and the venous component to the recipient, the shunt would carry blood from the donor to the recipient fetus. We classify this type of AV anastomosis as an AV-DR, meaning from donor to recipient. In contrast, if the artery belongs to the recipient fetus and the vein to the donor, the direction of the shunt would be from recipient to donor, and is referred to as an AV-RD. Therefore, as long as the artery and vein can be identified, directionality may be assigned. Assignment of type of AV anastomoses may be performed both fetoscopically and by gross examination.

The second type of placental communication is referred to as a superficial anastomosis, so-called because the vessel directly links both fetal circulations without intervening villous tissue. Superficial anastomoses may be identified fetoscopically by noting the vessels running along the entire surface of the placenta in an often tortuous fashion from one umbilical cord to the other without interruption. There are two types of superficial anastomoses: the more common artery-to-artery (AA) anastomosis and the vein-to-vein (VV) anastomosis (Figure 5.8). Unlike an AV communication, the superficial anastomoses

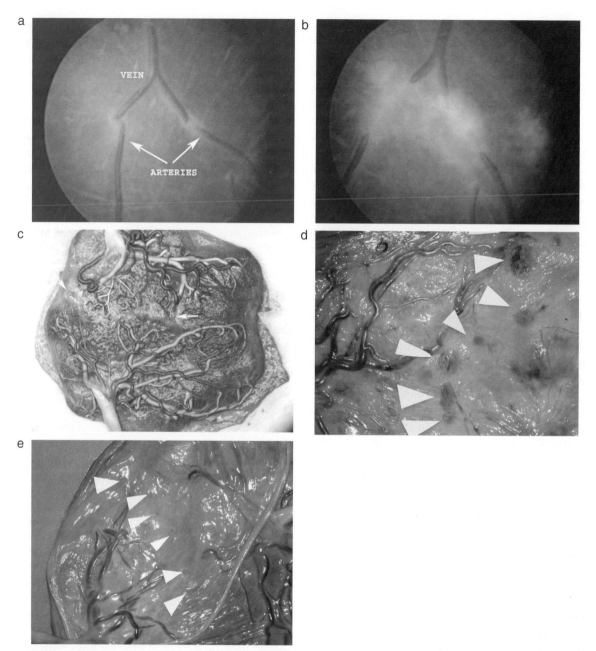

Figure 5.7 (a) Two artery-to-vein anastomoses, in a 'Y' shape, identified endoscopically in a pregnancy complicated by twin-twin transfusion syndrome. (b) The same vascular communication after laser ablation. (c)Functional dichorionization of a monochorionic-diamniotic placenta after laser therapy for TTTS. Arrows point to the lasered anastomoses. (d) and (e) Close up of monochorionic diamniotic placenta, status post laser therapy for TTTS. Arrows point to laser photocoagulated areas. (See also color plate section, page xx.)

may be unidirectional or bidirectional, depending on several factors. One factor may be the vascular relationships of the superficial anastomosis to surrounding AV anastomoses. For example, an AA anastomosis with a branching vessel that enters a donor cotyledon may serve as a 'functional' DR or RD, depending on where the arterial collision front, which we term the hemodynamic equator, resides within the AA vessel.[22] If the hemodynamic equator is on the

a 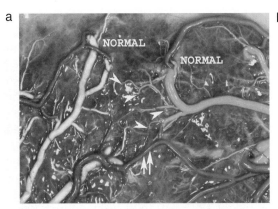 b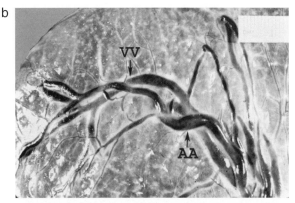

Figure 5.8 (a) This segment of placenta shows from bottom to top: 1) an artery to artery anastomosis (double arrows); 2) four artery to vein anastomoses designated by arrows; 3) two normally perfused cotyledons. (b) An artery to artery anastomosis (AA) courses toward the periphery with the AA crossing over its sister vein to vein anastomosis (VV) twice. (See also color plate section, page xxvi.)

donor side of the branching vessel, this system will serve as a functional RD. However, if the hemodynamic equator is on the recipient side of the branching vessel, the AA communication will serve as a functional DR. This relationship can only be ascertained in utero (Figure 5.9). Because the oxygenation content of the arterial systems of the donor vs recipient fetuses often varies, the color of the arterial blood from each twin may be discordant. This allows for fetoscopic identification of the hemodynamic equator. We have noted during endoscopic fetal surgery that the hemodynamic equator is not static: rather, it moves along the AA anastomosis. We have termed this phenomenon 'flashing'.[24] The reason for the movement of this collision front may have to do with the blood pressure that is mounted from the arterial systems of each fetus. Thus, it is possible that an AA that was once a functional DR may become a functional RD if the arterial blood pressure of the donor decreases and/or the recipient increases. Because hemodynamics may dictate directionality, assignment of type of AA anastomosis (functional DR vs functional RD) may only be possible in utero.

Monochorionic placentas may be classified as it pertains to TTTS via the type of vascular anastomoses identified.[25] Placenta type A is defined as having no anastomoses, type B as having AV anastomoses only, type C as having superficial anastomoses only, and type D as having AV and superficial anastomoses. Our group analyzed 131 monochorionic–diamniotic twin placentas

using this classification during a 4-year span; 105 placentas were from patients previously treated for TTTS by laser and 26 were monochorionic twins, with no TTTS, delivered at our institution. Forty-five cases were excluded because of placental fragmentation or fixation. Of the 105 monochorionic placentas with TTTS, 0 were type A, 85 (81%) were type B, 1 (1%) was type C, and 19 (18%) were type D. Of the 26 non-TTTS monochorionic placentas, 4 (15%) were type A, 0 were type B, 17 (65%) were type C, and 5 (19%) were type D. This study showed an association between the development of TTTS and type of monochorionic placenta. TTTS did not develop in type A (no anastomoses) and was unlikely to develop in type C (superficial only), whereas the syndrome occurred in all cases of type B (AV only) and most cases of type D (AV + superficial) placentas. This study suggests that AV communications play a central role in the development of TTTS.

In that AV communications appear to be an important factor in TTTS, what then is the role for superficial anastomoses? Some groups have reported that AA anastomoses are less common in TTTS and may be associated with improved perinatal outcomes.[26,27] However, we caution against the notion that AA communications are always protective. In the study by Bermudez et al,[26] the severity of disease was unrelated to the type of anastomosis. We have found that an AA anastomosis may or may not equilibrate the exchange of blood, depending on the nature

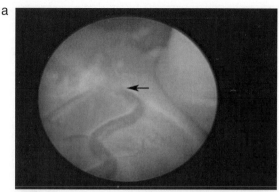

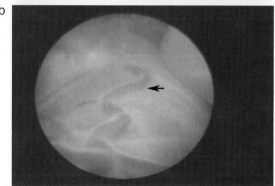

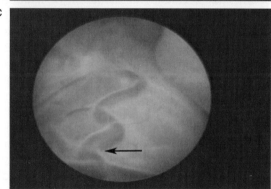

Figure 5.9 This time sequence endoscopic view of an artery to artery anastomosis shows the collision front (arrows) between presumably oxygenated and less well oxygenated fetal blood: (a) collision front at the top of the vessel, (b) collision front half-way down the vessel, and (c) collision front at bottom of vessel. (See also color plate section, page xxi.)

of the vascular anatomy and hemodynamics. In fact, severe TTTS with only superficial anastomoses has been reported by our group.[28] A factor that must be taken into account is whether the role of the AA in utero serves as a functional DR, RD, or both. Also, it must be remembered that the superficial vessel remains a conduit

through which acute transfusion may occur in the face of the fetal demise of one twin. In this setting, demise of one twin may result in demise or serious neurological harm of the co-twin from back bleeding. VV anastomoses were shown to be associated with decreased perinatal survival in one study.[26] Thus, superficial anastomoses do play an important role in TTTS, and should be targeted for ablation at the time of selective laser photocoagulation of communicating vessels.

The number of vascular anastomoses and the risk of TTTS have also been studied. Bajoria et al[27] initially demonstrated that the likelihood of TTTS was greater if fewer anastomoses were present. However, a co-author of that paper subsequently showed no relationship with TTTS and number of vascular communications.[26] The study by Bermudez et al showed that the number of anastomoses was not different in monochorionic–diamniotic placentas complicated by TTTS vs controls.[25]

Although rare, the 'circular vasculature', a unique vascular pattern that has important clinical manifestations, should be addressed. A circular vascular pattern is one in which all the major placental vessels have anastomotic communications. Thus, each individual fetus has a paucity of its own designated placental territory. Rather, most of the blood volume is being exchanged through the anastomoses from one fetus to the other. If selective laser photocoagulation of communicating vessels is performed in such a case, there may be a high likelihood of a double fetal demise. Depending on the clinical manifestation and the severity of the TTTS, one may elect to forego laser surgery for amnioreductions.

There are several limitations of the current studies that try to address the pathophysiology of TTTS in regards to the placental vascular anatomy. Most of these studies are conducted after delivery. As mentioned above, vascular changes may occur during the course of the pregnancy. Superficial anastomoses may not be interpretable in regards to directionality and this approach lends itself to a more qualitative assessment. A quantitative assessment of flow through the vascular communications can only be done in utero. What does the vascular caliber, the differential of the twins' blood pressures, blood viscosity, or other changes in intrauterine fetal hemodynamics have to do with the pathophysiology of TTTS? Our group has reported a pilot study that attempted to measure blood flow through all vascular communications in utero.[29] Recently, Lopriore et al developed a novel method to measure blood flow. They studied a unique case of TTTS syndrome treated with fetoscopic laser surgery. The ex-recipient subsequently became severely anemic and was treated with an intrauterine blood transfusion at 29 weeks' gestation. After birth, a placental injection study identified residual unidirectional AV anastomoses from the ex-recipient to the ex-donor without AV anastomoses in the opposite direction. Prospective measurements of decreasing hemoglobin levels between the intrauterine transfusion and birth allowed calculation of the net blood flow through the AV anastomoses. In this case the anastomotic blood flow at 29 weeks' gestation was 27.9 ml/24 h.[30]

While the net imbalance of blood flow between the fetuses is accepted as a central factor for the etiology of TTTS, the vascular communications may also serve as a conduit for the transfusion of other factors from one fetus to the other. Several studies have documented imbalances in hormone and protein levels, including atrial natriuretic peptide, renin, and antidiuretic hormone concentrations.[31–35] What is the role of the discordance in these and other factors in the pathophysiology and/or propagation of TTTS? Further refinement of in-utero techniques to measure fetal hemodynamics and proteins with correlation to placental anatomy may shed further light on this syndrome.

PARTITIONING OF PLACENTAL MASS

In addition to the vascular anatomy, it is important to consider the division of the placental mass of monochorionic placentas. Monochorionic twins may not share equal masses of villous tissue; one twin may have more placental tissue for development (Figure 5.10). This finding has several important implications regarding monochorionic twin gestations, particularly if they are complicated by TTTS. What is the role of the individual placental mass in the pathogenesis of TTTS? Is the relatively high rate of intrauterine growth restriction noted in TTTS due the unequal partitioning of the placental mass?

To help answer these questions, Quintero et al[36] studied the individual placental mass (IPM) of the donor and recipient twins after selective laser photocoagulation of communicating vessels and compared that to the IPMs of uncomplicated monochorionic twins. Because of fibrosis and degeneration of the placenta associated with fetal demise, all such cases were excluded from the analysis. Thus, placentas from 75 TTTS cases treated with laser surgery and 61 uncomplicated monochorionic twins

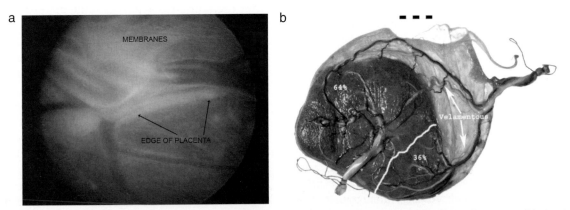

Figure 5.10 (a) Endoscopic view of a velamentous cord insertion with the vessels of the cord off the placenta, and instead embedded in the membranes. (b) Monochorionic placenta without TTTS. Twin 1 has a velamentous cord insertion and a placental share of 36%, whereas twin 2 has a paracentral cord insertion and a placental share of 64%. (Figure 5.10b reproduced with permission from[40]) (See also color plate section, page xix.)

were analyzed. The fresh placentas were cut along the vascular equator and individually weighed, thereby obtaining the IPM. The individual placental territory (IPT) for each fetus was calculated by dividing its IPM by the total placental mass and multiplying by 100. The donor fetuses were noted to weigh less than smaller control fetuses, whereas there was no significant difference in weight between the recipients and the larger controls. Corrected for gestational age, the IPT was not different between TTTS and control fetuses. This finding has two important ramifications: first, the partitioning of placental mass does not seem to be a primary cause for the development of TTTS; secondly, if placental territories were no different between the donors and smaller controls, why were the donor fetuses more growth restricted? This finding suggests that placental mass alone does not explain the growth restriction that may occur in the donor fetus. Other factors that are present in the TTTS cases but not the uncomplicated monochorionic cases may explain this, such as the imbalanced blood flow via the vascular communications or the poor nutrient exchange due to the histological changes noted in donor villus.

Another interesting finding of this study was that as little as 10–14% of the placental territory was able to sustain fetal life and result in perinatal survival. This finding demonstrates the ability of the fetus to adapt to chronic placental insufficiency. Why some donor fetuses with diminutive placental territory survive while others with more equable placental mass succumb is unknown. At this time, there is no accurate means of predicting placental territory prenatally.

PLACENTAL CORD INSERTION

The site of umbilical cord insertion into the placenta may be described as central, paracentral, marginal, or velamentous. Unlike a central or marginal umbilical cord insertion, which inserts onto the placental disk, the velamentous cord inserts into the fetal membranes (Figure 5.10). The bare umbilical vessels, unsupported by either umbilical cord or placental tissue, then traverse the fetal membranes between the amnion and chorion before insertion into the placenta.

Although relatively uncommon in singleton pregnancies, the velamentous cord insertion occurs at a significantly higher rate in multiple gestations. Kobak et al[37] reported the incidence of velamentous insertion of one cord as being nine times higher in twins than the 1–2% found in singleton placentas. In a more recent study of 447 twins,[38] the incidence of one velamentous cord insertion in dichorionic twin pregnancies was 6% and in the monochorionic twins it was 18%.

Abnormal cord insertions are of concern because of the increased risk of poor perinatal outcomes. Hanley[38] reported a 46% rate of birthweight discordance in monochorionic twins complicated by a velamentous cord. Machin[39] reviewed 60 consecutive monochorionic twin placentas and noted that the presence of a velamentous cord was associated with higher rates of growth discordance and mortality. Of interest, a velamentous cord appeared to be a risk factor for 'unequal placental parenchymal sharing'.

What is the role of a velamentous cord insertion in TTTS? A review of our experience in Tampa has led to several interesting insights. We established a referral system to retrieve the placentas of patients who were prenatally diagnosed and treated for TTTS at our institution. Patients and their referring physicians were asked to ship the fresh placentas after delivery for pathological evaluation. Two hundred and seventy-three complicated monochorionic twin placentas were received between July 1997 and December 2001, of which 249 were TTTS cases. After excluding cases in which the placenta was unsuitable for analysis due to tissue fragmentation or fixation, 168 TTTS cases were available for analysis. This was compared with 64 uncomplicated monochorionic twins delivered during the same time period. The incidence of velamentous cord insertion in the TTTS group was 34.5% (58/168). This was significantly higher than the uncomplicated monochorionic twins group, which had a velamentous cord insertion rate of 18.8% (12/64, $p = 0.02$). Within the groups, our review showed that a velamentous cord insertion was more frequently associated with the smaller fetus. In the TTTS cases, 25.6% (43/168) of the donor fetuses had velamentous insertions vs 10.7% (18/168, $p < 0.001$) of the recipients, whereas in the uncomplicated monochorionic twins group, the rate of velamentous insertion for the smaller fetus was 14.1% (9/64) vs 4.7% (3/64, $p = 0.06$) for the larger fetus. There were three cases in the TTTS group that had a velamentous cord insertion for both the donor and recipient twins. In a recent study of 76 consecutive TTTS placentas, Lopriore et al also found similar results and report that 24% (18/76) of the donors and 3% (2/63) of the recipients had a velamentous cord insertion.[40]

The excess frequency of velamentous cords in twin placentas complicated by TTTS has led several authors to theorize regarding its role in this syndrome. Fries et al[41] noted that one-third of monochorionic twin placentas had such abnormal cord insertions, of which 64% were involved with TTTS. They thus sought an etiological role for the abnormal insertion. Bruner et al[42] found a similarly high frequency of velamentous cord insertions of the donor twins, and Mari et al[43] also alluded to an etiological role in causing the imbalance that leads to the transfusion syndrome. These findings were confirmed by Machin.[39] He noted growth discrepancies more commonly in central/velamentous cord insertions of monochorionic twins. Furthermore, AV anastomoses were more common in this situation. These authors' findings do mirror our own, in that monochorionic twins complicated by TTTS have a higher rate of abnormal cord insertions vs uncomplicated monochorionic twins. However, whether the presence of a velamentous cord insertion serves simply as a risk factor for TTTS or is directly involved in the etiology of the syndrome remains in question. Moreover, several recent studies report a similar incidence of velamentous cord insertion in monochorionic placentas with and without TTTS.[42,43,44,45]

Does the presence of an abnormal cord insertion impact perinatal outcome in pregnancies complicated by TTTS? From the review of our patients in Tampa, this does not appear to be the case, at least in those that underwent previous laser therapy. A velamentous insertion was not associated with the severity of disease as assessed by the Quintero stage. The rate of velamentous cords divided by stage was as follows: stage I, 37.5% (12/32); stage II, 21.7% (10/46);

stage III, 40.0% (22/55); stage IV, 41.2% (14/34, $p = 0.18$). To evaluate the possible influence of a velamentous insertion on perinatal mortality, 23 cases from the TTTS group were excluded from the analysis because they underwent umbilical cord occlusion. Of the remaining 145 TTTS cases, the finding of a velamentous cord did not influence the number of total survivors. In the velamentous cord group, 47.8% (22/46) had two survivors, 30.4% (14/46) had one survivor, and 21.7% (10/46) had no survivors, vs the non-velamentous group, in which 56.6% (56/99) had two survivors, 28.3% (28/99) had one survivor, and 15.2% (15/99) had no survivors ($p = 0.52$). There were no differences in perinatal outcome if the abnormal cord insertion was present for the donor vs the recipient. Lastly, no differences were found in the birthweight and gestational age at delivery according to type of cord insertion.

The proximity of the umbilical cord insertions may influence the caliber of the vascular anastomoses. The closer the cord insertions (See chapter 9, Figure 9.11b), the higher the chance of large-caliber anastomoses. The vascular equator may be difficult to define because of the large overlapping vessels, which may have a complex pattern. When the cord insertions are several centimeters apart, the vascular equator is usually well demarcated, with smaller-caliber anastomoses. However, anastomoses caliber and type cannot be predicted solely on cord insertion proximity. An extreme example was illustrated by Wenner,[46] who was surprised to find no anastomoses in the placental vascular ramifications of a thoracopagus.

The cord distance may have important implications regarding perinatal outcome, particularly in those TTTS cases that undergo laser treatment. In a review of 226 patients that underwent laser therapy for TTTS at our institution, we noted that cord distance may be related to perinatal survival. The cord distance was significantly greater in those cases with at least one survivor (14.6 ± 0.90 cm) vs pregnancies with no survivors (11.75 ± 5.43 cm, $p = 0.036$). In this study, we were not able to identify a relationship between the cord distance and the number of communicating vessels.

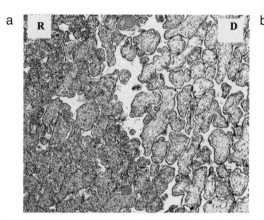 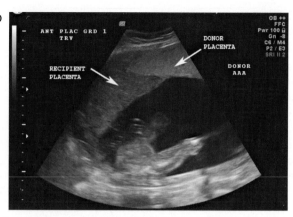

Figure 5.11 (a) In this figure the recipient is labeled 'R' and the donor is 'D'. The villi of the donor are generally slightly larger and much paler because of the paucity of fetal blood and some minor amount of edema, while those of the recipient are darker, more compact and their capillaries are congested. These figures are photographed from the meeting point of the respective villous districts and also demonstrate that there are no villous anastomoses but that the villi of donor and recipient merge irregularly. (b) The echogenic interface between donor and recipient portions of the monochorionic placenta has been observed with ultrasound, perhaps correlating to differences in oxygenation and blood flow as noted in (a). This case of Stage III TTTS with critically abnormal Dopplers in both twins shows the donor's portion as hyperechogenic and the recipient's as hypoechogenic.

PLACENTAL HISTOLOGICAL CHANGES ASSOCIATED WITH TWIN–TWIN TRANSFUSION SYNDROME

The portion of the placenta supporting the donor fetus is usually pale. This is in stark contrast to the recipient's placental portion, which is congested, giving an enlarged and hyperemic appearance. However, at the level of the villi, the donor has been described as having a significantly enlarged villous structure compared with that of the recipient,[47] and this has been attributed to fetal edema of the donor villi (Figure 5.11). This finding is unexpected in that fetal edema of the donor fetus is uncommon, particularly relative to the recipient twin. The enlarged villi of the donor fetus may in turn impinge on the intervillous space, thus affecting maternal perfusion.[48] This may explain the observations made by Matijevic et al, who studied blood flow in the spiral arteries of each twin's portion of the placenta using Doppler. They reported increased resistance on the side of the donor or growth-restricted twin compared with that of the recipient or appropriately grown twin.[49] Sala et al[50] reported that the recipient twin had thinned trophoblastic villous covering and that the villous vessels were markedly distended. In contrast,

the donor had thick trophoblast and frequently 'empty' villous capillaries. These observed histological differences between the donor and recipient twins may have an understated role in TTTS, particularly as it relates to the further propagation of the disease.

CONCLUSION

To better understand TTTS, the study of the placenta must continue. Friedrich Schatz and others were instrumental in making the first steps in our understanding of TTTS by methodical evaluation of the placenta after delivery. Yet, there is only so much that can be learned from a non-functioning organ – one that is neither linked to the maternal nor fetal circulations. As technology advances, it is our hope that the placenta may be studied more frequently in utero. Only after viewing the placenta 'in action' will we be able to take the next few steps in our understanding of TTTS.

REFERENCES

1. Schatz F. Zur Frage über die Quelle des Fruchtwassers und über Embryones papyracei. Arch Gynäkol 1875; 7: 336–8.

2. Schatz F. Eine besondere Art von einseitiger Polyhydramnie mit anderseitiger Oligohydramnie bei eineiigen Zwillingen. Arch Gynaekol 1882; 19:329–69.

3. Schatz F. Die Gefässverbindungen der Placentarkreisläufe eineiiger Zwillinge, ihre Entwicklung und ihre Folgen. Arch Gynaekol 1886; 27:1–72.

4. Schatz F. Acardii und ihre Verwandten. Berlin: Hirschwald, 1898.

5. Schatz F. Systematisches und alphabetisches Inhaltsverzeichnis von Friedrich Schatz: Placentakreisläufe eineiiger Zwillinge, ihre Entwicklung und ihre Folgen, in Band 19, 24, 27, 29, 30, 53, 55, 58, 60. Arch Gynakol 1900; 60:559–84.

6. Melnick M, Myrianthopoulos NC. The effects of chorion type on normal and abnormal developmental variation in monozygous twins. Am J Med Genet 1979; 4:147–56.

7. Benirschke K, Kaufmann P, Baergen RN. Pathology of the Human Placenta. New York: Springer-Verlag, 2006.

8. Boklage CE. Race, zygosity, and mortality among twins: interaction of myth and method. Acta Genet Med Gemellol (Roma) 1987; 36:27–88.

9. Quintero RA, Mueller OT, Martinez JM et al. Twin–twin transfusion syndrome in a dizygotic monochorionic-diamniotic twin pregnancy. J Matern Fetal Neonatal Med 2003; 14:279–81.

10. Souter VL, Kapur RP, Nyholt DR et al. A report of dizygous monochorionic twins. N Engl J Med 2003; 349:154–8.

11. Altshuler G, Hyde S. Placental pathology case book: A bidiscoid, monochorionic placenta. J Perinatol 1993; 13:492–93.

12. Machin GA. Why is it important to diagnose chorionicity and how do we do it? Best Pract Res Clin Obstet Gynaecol 2004; 18:515–30.

13. Lopriore E, Sueters M, Middeldorp JM et al. Twin pregnancies with two separate placental masses can still be monochorionic and have vascular anastomoses. Am J Obstet Gynecol 2006; 194:804–8.

14. Benirschke K. Placental membranes in twins. Obstet Gynecol Survey 1958; 13:88–91.

15. Lopriore E, Middeldorp JM, Sueters M, Vandenbussche F, Walther FJ. Twin-to-twin transfusion syndrome: from placental anastomoses to long-term neurodevelopmental outcome. Curr Pediatric Rev 2005; 1:191–203.

16. Bleisch VR. Diagnosis of monochorionic twin placentation. Am J Clin Pathol 1964; 42:277–84.

17. Quintero RA, Dickinson JE, Morales WJ et al. Stage-based treatment of twin–twin transfusion syndrome. Am J Obstet Gynecol 2003; 188:1333–40.

18. Senat MV, Deprest I, Boulvain M et al. Endoscopic laser surgery versus serial amnioreduction for severe twin-to-twin transfusion syndrome. N Engl J Med 2004; 351:136–44.

19. Benirschke K. The biology of the twinning process: how placentation influences outcome. Semin Perinatol 1995; 19:342–50.

20. Robertson E, Neer K. Placental injection studies in twin gestation. Am J Obstet Gynecol 1983:147:170–3.

21. Quintero R, Morales W, Mendoza G, et al. Selective photocoagulation of placental vessels in twin–twin transfusion syndrome: Evolution of a surgical technique. Obstet Gynecol Surv 1998; 53:S97–S103.

22. Sutherland JM, Coen RW. Placental vascular communications between twin fetuses. A simplified technique for demonstration. Am J Dis Child 1970; 120:332–3.

23. Nikkels PG, van Gemert MJ, Soilie-Szarynska KM et al. Rapid onset of severe twin–twin transfusion syndrome caused by placental venous thrombosis. Pediatr Dev Pathol 2002; 5:310–14.

24. Murakoshi T, Quintero RA, Bornick PW, Mien MH. In vivo endoscopic assessment of arterioarterial anastomoses: insight into their hemodynamic function. J Matern Fetal Neonatal Med 2003; 14:247–55.

25. Bermudez C, Becerra CH, Bornick PW et al. Placental type; and twin–twin transfusion syndrome. Am J Obstet Gynecol 2002; 187:489–94.

26. Denbow ML, Cox P, Taylor M, Hammal DM, Fisk NM. Placental angioarchitecture in monochorionic twin pregnancies: relationship to fetal growth, fetofetal transfusion syndrome, and pregnancy outcome. Am J Obstet Gynecol 2000; 182:417–26.

27. Bajoria R, Wigglesworth J, Fisk NM. Angioarchitecture of monochorionic placentas in relation to the twin–twin transfusion syndrome [see comments]. Am J Obstet Gynecol 1995; 172:856–63.

28. Bermudez C, Becerra C, Bornick PW et al. Twin–twin transfusion syndrome with only superficial placental anastomoses: endoscopic and pathological evidence. J Matern Fetal Neonatal Med 2002; 12:138–40.

29. Nakata M, Martinez JM, Diaz C, Chmait R, Quintero RA. Intra-amniotic Doppler measurement of blood flow in placental vascular anastomoses in twin–twin transfusion syndrome. Ultrasound Obstet Gynecol 2004; 24:102–3.

30. Lopriore E, Middeldorp JM, Oepkes D et al. Residual anastomoses after fetoscopic laser surgery in twin-to-twin transfusion syndrome: frequency, associated risks and outcome. Placenta 2006.

31. Nageotte M, Hurwitz S, Kaupke C, Vaziri N, Pandian M. Atriopeptin in the twin transfusion syndrome. Obstet Gynecol 1989; 73:867–70.

32. Berry SM, Puder KS, Bottoms SF et al. Comparison of intrauterine hematologic and biochemical values between twin pairs with and without stuck twin syndrome. Am J Obstet Gynecol 1995; 172:1403–10.

33. Bajoria R, Hancock M, Ward S, D'Souza SW, Sooranna SR. Discordant amino acid profiles in monochorionic twins

with twin–twin transfusion syndrome. Pediatr Res 2000; 48:821–8.

34. Bajoria R, Ward S, Chatterjee R. Natriuretic peptides in the pathogenesis of cardiac dysfunction in the recipient fetus of twin–twin transfusion syndrome. Am J Obstet Gynecol 2002; 186:121–7.

35. Bajoria R, Ward S, Chatterjee R. Brain natriuretic peptide and endothelin-l in the pathogenesis of polyhydramnios-oligohydramnios in monochorionic twins. Am J Obstet Gynecol 2003; 189:189–94.

36. Quintero RA, Martinez JM, Lopez J et al. Individual placental territories after selective laser photo-coagulation of communicating vessels in twin–twin transfusion syndrome. Am J Obstet Gynecol 2005; 192:1112–18.

37. Koback AJ, Cohen MR. Velamentous insertion of cord with spontaneous rupture of vasa previa in twin pregnancy. Am J Obstet Gynecol 1939; 38:l063–66.

38. Hanley ML, Ananth CV, Shen-Schwarz S et al. Placental cord insertion and birth weight discordancy in twin gestations. Obstet Gynecol 2002; 99:477–82.

39. Machin GA. Velamentous cord insertion in monochorionic twin gestation. An added risk factor. J Reprod Med 1997; 42:785–9.

40. Lopriore E, Sueters M, Middeldorp JM et al. Velamentous cord insertion and unequal placental territories in monochorionic twins with and without twin-to-twin transfusion syndrome. Am J Obstet Gynecol 2007; 196:159 e1–5.

41. Fries MH, Goldstein RB, Kilpatrick SJ et al. The role of velamentous cord insertion in the etiology of twin–twin transfusion syndrome. Obstet Gynecol 1993; 81:569–74.

42. Bruner J, Anderson T, Rosemond R. Twin-to-twin transfusion syndrome: The real problem is poor placentation. Am J Obstet Gynecol 1995; 172:311.

43. Mari G, Uerpairojkit B, Abuhamad A, Martinez E, Copel J. Velamentous insertion of the cord in polyhydramnios-oligohydramnios twins. Am J Obstet Gynecol 1995; 172:291.

44. Bajoria R. Vascular anatomy of monochorionic placenta in relation to discordant growth and amniotic fluid volume. Hum Reprod 1998; 13:2933–40.

45. De Paepe ME, DeKoninck P, Friedman RM. Vascular distribution patterns in monochorionic twin placentas. Placenta 2005; 26:471–5.

46. Wenner R. Les examens vasculaires des placentas gemellaires et le diagnostic des jumeaux homozygotes. Bull Soc R Belge Gynecol Obstet 1956; 26:773–83.

47. Aherne W, Strong SJ, Corney G. The structure of the placenta in the twin transfusion syndrome. Biol Neonat 1968; 12:121–35.

48. Abraham JM. Intrauterine feto-fetal transfusion syndrome: clinical observations and speculations on pathogenesis. Clin Pediatr 1967; 6:405–10.

49. Matijevic R, Ward S, Bajoria R. Non-invasive method of evaluation of trophoblast invasion of spiral arteries in monochorionic twins with discordant birthweight. Placenta 2002; 23:93–9.

50. Sala MA, Matheus M. Placental characteristics in twin transfusion syndrome. Arch Gynecol Obstet 1989; 246: 51–6.

6

Mathematical modeling of twin–twin transfusion syndrome

Martin JC van Gemert, Jeroen PHM van den Wijngaard, Asli Umur, and Michael G Ross

Introduction • **Anastomoses** • **Proposed twin–twin transfusion syndrome etiology and pathophysiology** • **Twin–twin transfusion syndrome modeling** • **Results** • **Discussion** • **Summary of model assumptions and predictions**

INTRODUCTION

Twin–twin transfusion syndrome (TTTS) is a unique complication of monochorionic twin pregnancies, diagnosed by discordant amniotic fluid volume (oligo/anhydramnios–polyhydramnios sequence). Often, but not always, serious cardiovascular sequelae develop, resulting in the assessment of TTTS as having a widely variable and unpredictable clinical presentation. TTTS is a consequence of placental anastomoses, which can be arteriovenous from donor to recipient (AVDR), arteriovenous from recipient to donor (AVRD), arterioarterial (AA), and venovenous (VV). These anastomoses allow a net fetofetal transfusion to develop from one twin (the donor) to the other (the recipient). While about 96% of all monochorionic placentas have anastomoses, only 5–10% of them develop TTTS (see Chapter 3). TTTS severity has been classified.[1] Stage I includes the oligo–polyhydramnios sequence without further complications. Stage II also includes lack of donor bladder filling. Stage III includes critically abnormal arterial or umbilical venous flow and/or ductus venosus patterns in either twin. Stage IV includes hydrops, and stage V intrauterine fetal demise in either or both twins. Although ultrasonography can study the fetal and placental anatomy, and Doppler sonography the blood flow of major fetal, umbilical, and placental vessels, other parameters contributing to TTTS presentation and sequelae cannot be studied directly (i.e. the fluid flows responsible for the amniotic fluid discordance, cardiovascular parameters including fetal blood pressures, and the net fetofetal transfusion). Because an animal model of TTTS is not available, understanding the complex pathophysiology of TTTS to its full extent is problematic. As an alternative, mathematical models of monochorionic twin pregnancies have been developed with the hope that they can aid in identifying and understanding the sequence of events that leads to the various TTTS manifestations and the potential efficacy of therapies.

The first TTTS model was developed by the British medical physicist Dr David G Talbert.[2,3] It consists of two identical pulsating fetoplacental units, comparable to 28 weeks of gestation, which are abruptly connected by AVDR, AVRD, AA anastomoses. The subsequent progression of the two fetoplacental circulations and their amniotic fluid volumes towards a new steady state is then computed. This model identified for the first time a sequence of events that related AVDR transfusion with onset of the TTTS stages I and II.

Our group has markedly expanded upon this initial model, developing three consecutive generations of TTTS mathematical models, using nonpulsating circulations, but including fetoplacental and anastomotic growth and varying placental sharing and amnionicity.[4–6] Table 6.1 summarizes the parameters used in the three models in the form of first-order differential equations. The purpose of this chapter is to present our modeling of

Table 6.1 Parameters used in the three models in the form of first-order differential (growth) equations for each of the twins

| Compartment | Parameters included as differential equations | | |
	1st model	2nd model	3rd model
Blood	Volume	Volume, colloids, osmoles	Arterial volume, venous volume, colloids, osmoles, RAS
Amniotic fluid		Volume, osmoles	Volume, osmoles
Interstitial fluid			Volume, colloids
Intracellular fluid			Volume

The net fetofetal transfusion from donor to recipient transfuses all parameters mentioned in the blood compartment.
RAS, renin–angiotensin system.

TTTS pathophysiology in a tutorial way. We have not included simulations of TTTS therapies and refer to our publications for details.[7–10]

ANASTOMOSES

An AVDR anastomosis connects the umbilical artery of the donor with the umbilical vein of the recipient. The AV connections occur at the capillary level within a cotyledon that receives its blood from a donor chorionic artery and drains it by a recipient chorionic vein. AVRD anastomoses, from recipient to donor, often exist next to primary AVDRs, where the AVRDs are defined as having the smaller diameter (higher resistance) compared to the primary AVDR with the largest diameter. Further, AA or VV anastomoses directly connect chorionic arteries or veins of the two twins. In our models, the AVDR, AVRD, AA, and VV anastomoses are represented by tubes, which directly connect with the two umbilical circulations, without branches to the normal placental chorionic vessels. This is a simplification, because it is known that most if not all anastomoses have branches to the normal placental circulation of the fetuses.

Placental anastomoses cause a fetofetal transfusion of blood and its constituents between combinations of arterial and venous blood compartments of the twins. The amount of transfusion results from the driving pressure gradient divided by the anastomotic resistance to blood flow (Ohm's law). Obviously, AVDR transfusion is the principal flow here and the combined AVRD, AA, and VV transfusions return part of the AVDR flow back to the donor, driven by gradients between recipient and donor vascular pressures. The resulting net fetofetal transfusion is from donor to recipient and is defined as:

$$\text{NetFetofetalTransf} = \text{AVDR-flow} - (\text{AVRD-flow} + \text{AA-flow} + \text{VV-flow}) \quad (1)$$

When TTTS develops in the model, recipient arterial and venous pressures exceed those of the donor, so the resulting directions of blood flow through AA and VV anastomoses are from recipient to donor, explaining their negative sign in eqn (1). However, we acknowledge that clinical cases have been described where flow through an AA was found to be from donor to recipient.[11] We hypothesize that this unusual phenomenon may occur when the AA connects a short donor chorionic arterial segment with a long, high resistance, recipient segment. Then, due to the hydrostatic pressure loss in the recipient, the driving AA pressure gradient is from donor to recipient. However, because fetofetal transfusion reduces the donor's arterial pressure and increases the recipient's pressure, we also hypothesize that this can only occur temporarily. In our model, AA anstomoses connect directly with the umbilical arteries of both twins, so we cannot simulate this phenomenon. Furthermore, TTTS in the absence of an AVDR is another remarkable presentation.[12] We confirm this observation, as it also occurred in two of our TTTS cases (unpublished).

Again, our model cannot simulate this intriguing TTTS presentation.

We use Poiseuille's law of laminar blood flow to define the vascular resistance (Resist) of the anastomoses, which depends on blood viscosity, length, and radius of the tube:

$$\text{Resist} = \frac{8}{\pi} \text{Viscosity} \frac{\text{Length}}{\text{Radius}^4} \qquad (2)$$

Note that the radius is included to the 4th power, implying radius has an exceedingly strong influence on resistance, e.g. a radius increase by a factor of 2 decreases the resistance by a factor of 2^4 (= 16), at constant viscosity and length.

Although a joint cotyledon (AVDR and AVRD anastomoses) is anatomically not a tube, their resistances nevertheless are equivalent in our model, because of their assumed identical growth behavior.[4] Briefly, anastomoses increase their length and radius linearly (see section on 'Proposed TTTS etiology and pathophysiology'). As eqn (2) includes length divided by radius to the 4th power, the anastomotic resistances decrease proportional to gestational age to the 3rd power. In a cotyledon, the radius of the capillaries does not vary with gestational age. Instead, the number of capillaries grows commensurate with the placental volume, assumed proportional to gestational age to the 3rd power.[4] Thus, approximating the vascular resistance of a cotyledon by the parallel circuit of identical capillary resistances, overall cotyledonic resistance is inversely proportional to the number of capillaries, and, hence, inversely proportional to the 3rd power of gestation, identical to AVDR and AVRD resistances.

In previous work,[13] we used a fractal geometry model for the vascular tree to simulate how AVDR and AVRD resistances relate to the diameter of their feeding and draining vessels. In this model, the cotyledon has a 20–24 times higher resistance than the feeding artery plus draining vein. Thus, the tube used in our models to represent AVDR or AVRD resistances also has a 20–24 times higher resistance than the feeding artery plus draining vein, implying the AVDR and AVRD anastomotic tube radii in the model cannot represent their actual radii, which are about $\sqrt[4]{20} \approx 2.1$ to $\sqrt[4]{24} \approx 2.2$ times larger than the radii used in the model. Furthermore, because the fetal arterial pressure is much higher than the venous pressure, pressure deviations from normal likely produce much larger intertwin arterial than venous pressure gradients. This implies that an AA has a much greater efficacy than a VV of identical dimensions to reduce the net fetofetal transfusion compared with the AVDR alone. We estimated that a VV anastomosis of identical length requires an 8 times smaller resistance (eqn A5 of previous work[4]), or a 1.7 times larger diameter than an AA for equal reduction of the AVDR transfusion. However, in cases of a hydropic recipient twin, the simulated recipient venous pressure is significantly enlarged, implying a VV is more effective in reducing the AVDR flow than without a hydropic twin (see 'Results' section).[6]

Several unidirectional AV anastomoses are equivalent to a circuit of parallel AV tube resistances and, hence, equivalent to one overall AV tube resistance using the law of parallel resistances, i.e. $(R_{AVoverall})^{-1} = (R_{AV1})^{-1} + (R_{AV2})^{-1} + (R_{AV3})^{-1} + \ldots$. This holds for AVRD, AA, and VV resistances too. So, multiple AVDR, AVRD, AA, and VV anastomoses are equivalent to a set of overall single AVDR, AVRD, AA, and VV resistances. We recall that in real monochorionic twin placentas, the anastomotic pattern is not exactly a set of tubes connecting the umbilical cords. Nevertheless, we found that multiple placental anastomoses of certain types are approximately equivalent to a set of overall single anastomotic resistances of the same types.

PROPOSED TWIN–TWIN TRANSFUSION SYNDROME ETIOLOGY AND PATHOPHYSIOLOGY

The etiology of TTTS was proposed to be a consequence of the normal development of the placental anastomoses as compared to the natural growth of the fetuses. Here, because little is known about growth of anastomoses, we assumed that normal anastomotic development is that length and diameter of the anastomoses increase proportional to gestational age. We hypothesized that anastomoses develop similarly as chorionic and umbilical vessels and available data of serial measurements show that the diameter of AA anastomoses,[14] umbilical veins,[15] as well as the length of umbilical veins and chorionic vessels – the latter considered proportional to the diameter of singleton placentas[16] – all grow approximately proportional to gestational age (Figure 6.1). Implication is that anastomotic resistances decrease significantly during gestation, i.e. according to eqn (2) as inversely proportional to gestational age to the 3rd power. Furthermore, the donor's arterial minus recipient's venous pressure, the driving pressure gradient of AVDR transfusion, increases approximately linearly with gestational age, based on fetal lamb experiments.[4] Consequently, AVDR transfusion is proportional to gestational age to the 4th power. This assumption has been confirmed by published placental blood flow measurements,[17] supposing it is proportional to cotyledonic blood flow (Figure 6.2). In contrast, natural growth of fetuses (and their blood volumes) is approximately proportional to gestational age to the 2nd power,[4] which is a slower increasing function than AVDR flow. Thus:

$$AV\text{-}FetofetalTransf \propto (Gestational\ Age)^4 \quad (3)$$

$$NaturalBloodVolGrowth \propto (Gestational\ Age)^2 \quad (4)$$

where symbol $\propto$ denotes 'proportional to'.

These different growth rates cause donor twins to effectively lose blood volume through the AVDR and recipients to effectively gain this blood volume. Because of this mechanism, the natural fetal growth of each twin loses the competition with this continuous exogenous change in its blood volume. Obviously, if only unidirectional AVDR anastomoses are present, the well-known deleterious effects of TTTS develop with increasing severity without the possibility of recovery. On the other hand, if other anastomoses (AVRD, AA, VV) are also present, part of the AVDR transfusion will be returned back to the donor, eqn (1). Under these circumstances, TTTS either will not develop, or it will have a reduced severity compared to TTTS caused by the single AVDR. Consequently, whether TTTS develops or not, and TTTS severity, is determined by the capacity (length and diameter) of AVDR anastomoses compared to the combined capacity of AVRD, AA, and VV anastomoses (recipient to donor). This mechanism explains why some but not all monochorionic twin placentas with anastomoses develop TTTS.

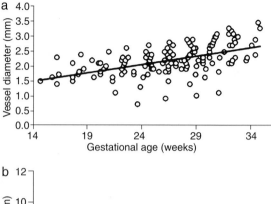

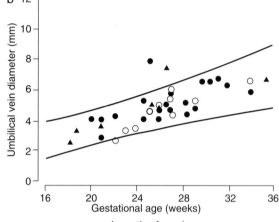

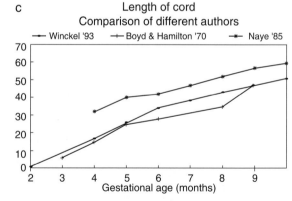

Figure 6.1 (a) Serial ultrasonographic measurements of the AA diameter in 19 non-TTTS and 2 TTTS monochorionic twin placentas. (Reprinted from Denbow et al,[14] with permission from the authors and from Elsevier.) (b) Umbilical vein diameter before the first intravascular transfusion in 36 red cell alloimmunized pregnancies. Lines indicate reference ranges (95% tolerance interval) in normal pregnancies. ○, moderate anemia (hematocrit deficit ≤20%), ●, severe anemia (hematocrit deficit >20%). ▲, hydropic fetuses. (From Oepkes,[15] with permission.) (c) Length of umbilical cord as determined in three studies (when exact numbers were not given, the approximate number was entered). (From Benirschke and Kaufmann,[16] page 333, with permission).

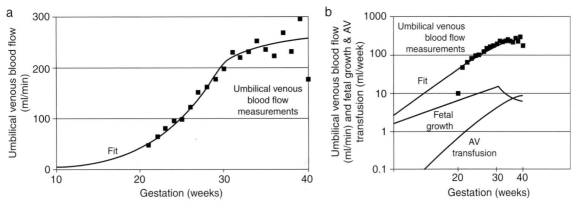

Figure 6.2 (a) Normal placental perfusion, represented by an average of 209 umbilical venous blood flows (■),[17] is approximately proportional to gestational age to the 4th power until 30 weeks (FIT). (b) Umbilical venous blood flow is as in (a). Natural fetal growth is proportional to gestational age to the 2nd power until 30 weeks. AV transfusion: simulated behavior of a clinical case, using our first model of 1 AVDR anastomosis and unequal placental sharing,[4] where the donor has 65% and the recipient 35% of the placenta.[7] Note the logarithmic scale, used for better comparison of the three curves.

Thus far, quantifying unidirectional AV fetofetal transfusion throughout gestation has been impossible, although assessment of individual AV anastomotic flow at one gestational age was published very recently. First, Quintero's group used intra-amniotic ultrasound,[18] and, secondly, our group related AVDR flow with decreasing hemoglobin concentrations between the moment of an intrauterine blood transfusion and birth.[19]

TWIN–TWIN TRANSFUSION SYNDROME MODELING

First-generation hemodynamic model

The blood volumes of the twins are the primary model parameters because the anastomoses transport blood volume from one twin to the other. Our model relates overall growth of the blood volumes of donor and recipient twins to a linear combination of their natural growth, i.e. the anticipated normal physiological growth of their blood volume, and the net fetofetal transfusion from donor to recipient, eqn (1). Here, the NetFetofetalTransf is assumed to directly affect fetal growth of both twins. This is an approximation that neglects possible control mechanisms that try to maintain normal growth. The following

two growth equations of the fetal blood volumes constitute our first-generation model:

$$\text{OverallBloodVolGrowth} = \text{NaturalBloodVolGrowth} \pm \text{NetFetofetalTransf} \quad (5)$$

The plus sign denotes the equation for the recipient and the minus sign for the donor. NaturalBloodVolGrowth was taken proportional to the fetal arterial minus venous pressure gradient.

Through Poiseuille's law, eqn (2), the anastomotic resistances at 40 weeks can be calculated, and because we used that the length and radii increase linearly with gestation, their resistances at any gestational age t (weeks), denoted as XY-Resist(t), XY = AVDR, AVRD, AA, or VV, relate to the resistances at $t = 40$ weeks as

$$\text{XY-Resist}(t) = \text{XY-Resist}(t = 40)\frac{(40-4)^3}{(t-4)^3} \quad (6)$$

We assumed that placental anastomoses become functional at 4 weeks – hence the term $(t–4)$. Growth eqns (5) translate mathematically as first-order differential equations. They can be solved numerically, combined with eqns (1), (2) and (6), assessing blood pressures from pressure–volume curves, and using as initial condition that blood volumes of both twins are zero at $t = 0$, the moment of embryonic splitting. The numerical solution, from 0 to 40 weeks, is by a standard forward finite-difference method using a time step of about 1 minute, and using type and size of anastomoses and degree of placental sharing as input parameters.

Second-generation hemodynamic and amniotic fluid dynamics model

In our second model,[5] we added amniotic fluid dynamics to our first model. We had to adapt the mechanism of fetal blood volumetric growth. We included that the growing fetus and amniotic cavity acquire fluid and nutrients from the maternal circulation to maintain the volume of the total body fluid as well as the amniotic fluid. Fluid and nutrients are provided by the transplacental fluid flow from the maternal to the fetoplacental circulation, implying

$$\text{TransPlacentFlow} = \\ \text{TotalBodyFluidGrowth+AmnioticFluidGrowth} \quad (7)$$

Because the primary model parameters are the blood volume of the twins, we had to relate blood volume with total body fluid volume. We assumed the fetal blood is a constant fraction of 10% of the total body fluid:

$$\text{BloodVolume} = 0.1*\text{TotalBodyFluid} \quad (8)$$

Then, eqns (5) become

$$\text{OverallBloodVolGrowth} = 0.1* \\ \text{TotalBodyFluidGrowth} \pm \text{NetFetoFetalTransf} \quad (9)$$

The growth of anastomoses, placenta and fetuses, the blood volume vs blood pressure curves, the relation for net fetofetal transfusion, and the model input parameters, were all taken identical as in the first model. In eqn (9), TotalBodyFluidGrowth directly follows from eqn (7) as the difference between TransPlacentFlow and AmnioticFluidGrowth. Growth of the amniotic fluid volume is the sum of urine production and lung fluid secretion minus the sum of swallowing and intramembranous flow, the flow from amniotic cavity to the fetal blood across the total surface of the placenta, umbilical cord, and fetal skin.

The additional parameters included in the second model for each twin are those that control the various fluid flows included in the model. First, the transplacental fluid flow was described by the Starling equation, proportional to the difference between the maternofetal hydrostatic and colloid osmotic pressure (COP) gradients:

$$\text{TransPlacentFlow} \propto (\text{MatFetPressGrad} - \\ \text{MatFetCOPGrad}) \quad (10)$$

Although the Starling equation is an accepted choice here, for example,[2] we acknowledge that transplacental fluid transfer is a complex and still incompletely understood mechanism. Recently, new pathways have been identified which are known to be capable of somehow regulating this fluid transfer.[20] The maternal blood COP is assumed to be unaffected by fetofetal transfusion. The first new model parameter then is the fetal blood COP. Secondly, we assumed that swallowing (i.e. thirst mediated) is controlled by the fetal blood osmolality, which therefore is the second new parameter. We assumed that swallowing becomes equal to fetal lung fluid secretion once the fetal blood osmolality has decreased by 4% or more of its normal value.[5] So, fetal blood osmolality is the third new parameter. Thirdly, the intramembranous flow is also taken as a Starling equation, proportional to the difference between the hydrostatic and osmotic pressure gradients between amniotic fluid and fetal capillaries. The osmotic pressure gradient relates to the osmolalities of amniotic fluid and fetal blood. Hence, the amniotic fluid osmolality is the fourth new model parameter. So, our second model comprises 10 growth (differential) equations, 5 for each twin, of (1) fetal blood volume, (2) amniotic fluid volume, (3) fetal blood osmolality, (4) amniotic fluid osmolality, and (5) fetal blood COP (see Table 6.1). Furthermore, urine production was controlled by a pressure–diuresis curve, where urination ceases once the pressure decreased to half or less of the normal value, and otherwise increases proportional to the normalized arterial pressure squared. Lung secretion was included as a function of gestation without a control mechanism.

The net fetofetal transfusion along the anastomoses links three of the five equations of each twin, not only transfusing blood volume but also blood colloids and osmoles. The equations are solved numerically as before.

Third-generation model of a hydropic recipient

In our third model,[6] we simulated a sequence of events that leads to the onset and development of hydrops in the recipient twin. Three essential elements had to be added to our second model.[5] The first is vasoconstrictive peptides, described as the renin–angiotensin system (RAS) mediators that reduce urine production.[21,22] The second is the limited capacity of the fetal heart to increase its cardiac output beyond normal values following abnormally increased blood pressures,[23,24] leading to a state of high-output cardiac failure. The obvious third element is an interstitial fluid compartment. Table 6.1 summarizes the 10 parameters included in this model for each twin, comprising 20 first-order differential equations.

As before, growth of the fetal total body fluid volume (fetal blood, but here also intracellular and interstitial fluids) and growth of the fetal amniotic fluid volume are caused by the transplacental fluid flow across the placenta, eqn (7), where

$$\text{TotalBodyFluid} = \text{BloodVol} + \text{IntracelVol} + \text{InterstVol} \qquad (11)$$

Normal fetal urine production, affecting amniotic fluid volumetric growth, is modified here by three mechanisms:

- the pressure–diuresis curve used in our second model (see end of section on 'second-generation hemodynamic and amniotic fluid dynamics model')
- the influence of the blood COP (i.e. filtration of fetal blood across the glomerular capillary membrane)
- the influence of the blood concentration of RAS mediators, which reduce urine production.

As before in eqns (5) and (9), overall growth of the two fetal blood volumes is a linear combination of natural (i.e. anticipated normal) blood volumetric growth, and the net fetofetal transfusion. However, the blood volume is no longer fixed to 10% of the total body fluid volume as in eqn (8), but follows from eqn (11) as the difference between total body fluid and intracellular plus interstitial fluid volumes. Natural total blood volumetric growth follows from the difference between transplacental flow and growth of the

amniotic, intracellular, and interstitial fluids, eqns (7) and (11). Growth of the interstitial fluid volume is governed by Starling forces, comparable to eqn (10), which determine magnitude and direction of the transvascular flow from the fetal circulation to the interstitial compartment, proportional to the difference between the vascular-interstitial hydrostatic and colloid osmotic pressure gradients:

$$\text{TransVascularFlow} \propto (\text{VascInterstPressGrad} - \text{VascInterstCOPGrad}) \qquad (12)$$

Growth of the fetal intracellular space was modeled proportional to the actual value and to growth of the fetal blood volume.

The fetal heart has been demonstrated to operate near the maximal cardiac output plateau in the Frank–Starling curve.[23,24] Therefore, fetal cardiac reserve is limited as compared to adult physiology. We expressed cardiac output to depend upon changes in preload and afterload. Increased preload increases the cardiac output by the Frank–Starling effect until 1.1 times the normal venous pressure, after which it increases only slightly when venous pressure is elevated.

We calculated the (arterial) cardiac output and venous return separately, to allow an excess blood volume, ExcVenVol, to accumulate in the venous part of the circulation following forward heart failure of the recipient. The equations describing arterial and venous blood volumetric growth then follow as a linear combination of (a) the excess blood volume that is removed from the arterial circulation and added to the venous volume, RemExcVenVol, and (b) volumetric growth of arterial and venous blood volumes, expressed as blood volumetric growth (arterial plus venous), multiplied by the ratio of arterial or venous blood volume to total blood volume, expressed as V_{bArt}/V_b or V_{bVen}/V_b. Thus, eqns (5) and (9) become

$$\text{OverallArtVolGrowth} = -\text{RemExcVenVol} + (\text{NaturalBloodVolGrowth} \pm I_{net}) \cdot \frac{V_{bArt}}{V_b} \qquad (13)$$

$$\text{OverallVenVolGrowth} = +\text{RemExcVenVol} + (\text{NaturalBloodVolGrowth} \pm I_{net}) \cdot \frac{V_{bVen}}{V_b} \qquad (14)$$

Symbol I_{net} denotes the net fetofetal transfusion, eqn (1). The recipient equations are indicated by the plus sign, the donor equations by the minus sign.

Model input parameters and the solution of the differential equations remained as previously, albeit using a time step of 0.6 s, required to prevent the numerical solution includes an oscillatory component.

RESULTS

From the viewpoint of pathophysiological mechanisms, our model is clear and simple (Figure 6.3). First, stages I and II TTTS develop if the net fetofetal transfusion increases at a rate in excess of the rate of increasing growth of each twin. Then, a stuck donor twin and markedly increased colloids in the recipient follow, albeit that recipient hypertension and urine production are not yet excessive. In our model, the strongly increased colloids cause an excess transplacental fluid flow from the maternal to the recipient circulation, a consequence of using Starling's

eqn (10), which mainly exits through the bladder, causing polyhydramnios. TTTS severity remains limited to stages I or II if the net fetofetal transfusion stabilizes compared with fetal growth, due to the compensating anastomoses that return part of the AVDR transfusion back to the donor. Secondly, TTTS stage IV may develop (Figure 6.4) if the net fetofetal transfusion continues to increase stronger than the rate of increasing fetal growth of each twin. Then, a sequence of events develops that leads to a severely hypotensive donor twin that produces excessive RAS mediators, which are transfused to the recipient by the AVDR anastomosis. The RAS mediators mitigate the recipient's polyuria, which causes overfilling, and hence increased arterial and venous pressures (Figure 6.4b), resulting in recipient forward cardiac failure. Subsequently, both the hydrostatic and colloid osmotic pressure gradients between fetal blood and interstitial fluid increase; however, the lymph flow returning from the interstitium into the vascular compartment (not discussed here) is reduced due to the increased venous pressure.[6] The overall effect is

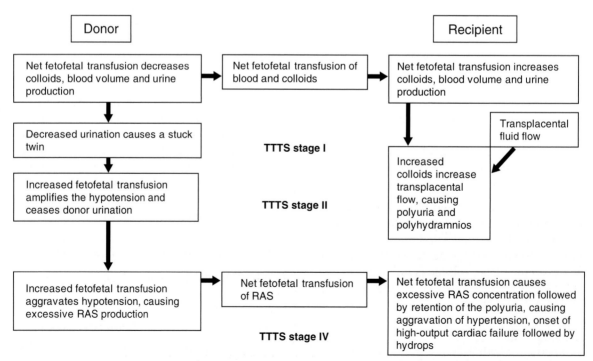

Figure 6.3 Mechanisms responsible for the development of TTTS stages I, II, and IV.[6]

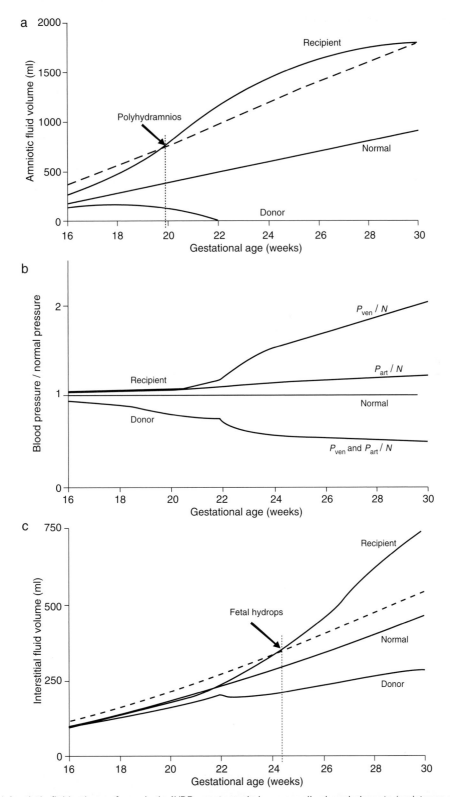

Figure 6.4 (a) Amniotic fluid volumes for a single AVDR anastomosis in an equally shared placenta (resistance at 40 weeks is 0.28 mmHg/ml/24 h). Recipient polyhydramnios develops at 19.9 weeks, a stuck donor at 22 weeks. The dashed line gives twice the normal amniotic fluid volume, our definition of polyhydramnios.[5,6] (b) Arterial (P_{art}) and venous (P_{ven}) blood pressures divided by their normal values, indicated by N. (c) Interstitial fluid volumes. Beyond 24.4 weeks, recipient interstitial fluid has increased more than 1.18 times normal, our definition of hydrops.[6] The dashed line indicates 1.18 times normal interstitial fluid volumes.

that the excess transplacental flow now mainly exits into the interstitium rather than the bladder, and onset of hydrops occurs (Figure 6.5). Interestingly, therefore, increased exit of excess transplacental flow into the interstitial space to cause hydrops necessarily implies a reduced exit into the amniotic cavity, reducing the severity of, or even resolving, the polyhydramnios (see Figure 6.5). (This phenomenon has been described clinically by Trespidi et al in their Figure 1.[25]) Despite the simplicity of these mechanisms, we acknowledge the increased complexity of this model compared to the previous models,[4,5] and refer to our publication for details.[6]

Our model predicts that recipient blood volumes remain close to their normal values but donor twins become growth retarded, probably a consequence of relating overall blood volumetric growth directly with the net fetofetal transfusion, eqns (13) and (14). It is important to note that growth discordance may actually not occur in at least 20% of TTTS cases, pointing to a limitation of the model. Furthermore, the model predicts that the amniotic fluid osmolality changes little during pregnancy, even in a severe TTTS case (Table 3 of Umur et al[5]), in excellent agreement with clinical observations.[26]

Single and unidirectional AVDR anastomoses, as well as an AVDR inadequately compensated by oppositely directed anastomoses, produce a hydropic recipient twin (see Figure 6.4). In our model, a hydropic recipient will not spontaneously recover. This is because the donor twin cannot spontaneously recover from its severe hypotension (see Figure 6.4b), so the excess RAS in the recipient, transfused from the donor, sustains, implying the recipient cardiovascular status cannot spontaneously improve either, so hydrops persists (see Figure 6.4c). However, we acknowledge that this may not actually hold, particularly if there is decompensation or demise of the donor, or thrombosis of the AVDR.[27]

Simulations of the compensatory capacity of AVRD and AA anastomoses to prevent hydrops in the recipient show that AA is the best in preventing a hydropic recipient twin. However, VV is the best in delaying onset of hydrops following onset of TTTS, owing to the strongly increased venous pressure that always precedes onset of hydrops (see Figure 6.4b).

The fetofetal transfusion along an AVDR anastomosis was found to be as large as 11 ml/24 h at 22 weeks, at onset of a stuck donor with 32 ml blood volume (Figure 6.6). This large AV

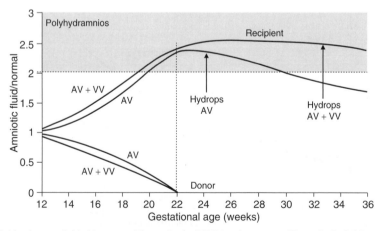

Figure 6.5 Amniotic fluid volumes divided by normal for a single AVDR (resistance at 40 weeks is 0.28 mmHg/ml/24 h) and an AVDR inadequately compensated by a VV (AVDR and VV resistances are 0.16 and 0.02 mmHg/ml/24 h, respectively). Both anastomotic patterns were selected to produce a stuck donor twin at 22 weeks. The gray area indicates at least an amniotic fluid volume of twice the normal value, our definition of polyhydramnios.[5,6] Hydrops is defined as an 18% or more increased interstitial fluid volume.

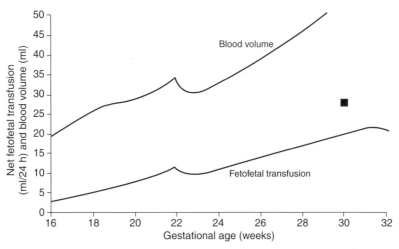

Figure 6.6 The AVDR transfusion and the donor blood volume of Figure 6.4. The measurement at 30 weeks refers to five patent AVDR anastomoses as a consequence of incomplete TTTS laser therapy.[19]

transfusion is possible due to compensation of the corresponding loss of donor fluid by the (maternofetal) transplacental fluid flow, as well as possible transfusion from the interstitial into the vascular compartment. Interestingly, if an AVRD anastomosis is also present, compensating part of the donor's loss of red blood cells by the AVDR, the net fetofetal transfusion (donor to recipient) even increases to 14.7 ml/24 h at 22 weeks at 34 ml donor blood volume. In other words, our third model simulates a net fetofetal transfusion that can develop without the donor's short-term demise, predicting a turnover of donor blood volume every 3 days! Interestingly, AVDR transfusions produced by our model are in unexpected agreement with the experimental value of 27.9 ml/24 hours (see Figure 6.6) that we found recently in five unidirectional AVDRs. These anastomoses remained patent following incomplete TTTS laser therapy, and the new donor required an intrauterine blood transfusion 48 hours before emergency delivery at 30 weeks of gestation.[19]

DISCUSSION

The development of realistic TTTS mathematical models is challenging. The complexity of fetal physiology may at first make modeling seem a hopeless enterprise: not only is there a paucity of information available on normal fetoplacental cardiovascular function and amniotic fluid homeostasis but also the influence of TTTS on such developments is poorly understood. Therefore, simplified and sometimes empirical descriptions of fetoplacental and amniotic fluid development are unavoidable. In view of the complexity of TTTS pathophysiology, a sequence of models of increasing sophistication, with model testing at each state of development, represents the optimal practical approach. As a result, we believe that our modeling has provided important principles and trends to illustrate realistic clinical scenarios.

In the time period between the first and final draft of this chapter we finalized the description of pulsating arterial flow propagation along the fetal arterial tree.[28] We combined this model with our TTTS model,[6] extended with the dynamics of blood hematocrit and arterial wall collagen–elastin concentrations (stiffness) and thickness, and described stage III TTTS in our fourth-generation model.[29] Furthermore, very recently, Wee et al[30] reported that diameter of draining veins of AV anastomoses increase linearly with gestational age, showing our assumption of AV anastomotic development also to be true.

In conclusion, mathematical modeling of TTTS pathophysiology has contributed significantly to understanding the sequence of events that govern the numerous TTTS clinical presentations as well as the efficacy of therapeutic strategies (not shown in this chapter).

SUMMARY OF MODEL ASSUMPTIONS AND PREDICTIONS

- TTTS etiology is that anastomoses develop linearly in length and diameter, proportional to normal placental volumetric development, vs normal growth of the twins.
- TTTS pathophysiology is explained by AVDR fetofetal transfusion, which increases at a rate in excess of the rate of increasing fetal blood volumetric growth of each twin.
- Net fetofetal transfusion can be as high as 33% of the donor blood volume per 24 hours.
- TTTS is caused by one or more (unidirectional) AVDR anastomoses.
- AVDR flow in our model is in agreement with measured AVDR flow, about tens of ml per 24 hours.
- The hemodynamic competition between the AVDR capacity (length and diameter) vs the combined capacity of all compensating anastomoses (AVRD, AA, VV) determines whether or not TTTS develops, and TTTS severity. This explains why some but not all monochorionic placentas with anastomoses develop TTTS.
- The probability that an AVRD adequately reduces the flow of the primary AVDR is much smaller than the probability that an AA of equal diameter of the feeding and draining vessels reduces the AVDR flow adequately. This refers to onset of TTTS as well as to onset of a hydropic recipient twin.
- A VV anastomosis produces the largest interval between onset of a stuck donor and onset of recipient hydrops.
- TTTS severity is only weakly correlated with an earlier gestational age at TTTS onset (not discussed in this chapter).
- A hydropic recipient will not recover spontaneously.
- A recipient twin that develops hydrops simultaneously reduces its polyhydramnios.

REFERENCES

1. Quintero RA, Morales WJ, Allen MH et al. Staging of twin–twin transfusion syndrome. J Perinatol 1999; 19:550–5.
2. Talbert DG, Bajoria R, Sepulveda W, Bower S, Fisk NM. Hydrostatic and osmotic pressure gradients produce manifestations of fetofetal transfusion syndrome in a computerized model of monochorial twin pregnancy. Am J Obstet Gynecol 1996; 174:598–608.
3. Tan TYT, Denbow ML, Cox PM, Talbert D, Fisk NM. Occlusion of arterio-arterial anastomosis manifesting as acute twin–twin transfusion syndrome. Placenta 2004; 25:238–42.
4. van Gemert MJC, Sterenborg HJCM. Haemodynamic model of twin–twin transfusion syndrome in monochorionic twin pregnancies. Placenta 1998; 19:195–208.
5. Umur A, van Gemert MJC, Ross MG. Amniotic fluid and hemodynamic model in monochorionic twin pregnancies and twin–twin transfusion syndrome. Am J Physiol Regul Integr Comp Physiol 2001; 280: R1499–509.
6. van den Wijngaard JPHM, Umur A, Krediet RT, Ross MG, van Gemert MJC. Modeling a hydropic recipient twin in twin–twin transfusion syndrome. Am J Physiol Regul Integr Comp Physiol 2005; 288:R799–814.
7. van Gemert MJC, Umur A, Tijssen JGP, Ross MG. Twin–twin transfusion syndrome: etiology, severity and rational management. Curr Opin Obstet Gynecol 2001; 13:193–206.
8. Umur A, van Gemert MJC, Ross MG. Fetal urine and amniotic fluid in monochorionic twins with twin–twin transfusion syndrome: simulations of therapy. Am J Obstet Gynecol 2001; 185:996–1003.
9. van den Wijngaard JPHM, Umur A, Ross MG, van Gemert MJC. Modelling the influence of amnionicity on the severity of twin–twin transfusion syndrome in monochorionic twin pregnancies. Phys Med Biol 2004; 49:N57–64.
10. van den Wijngaard JPHM, Ross MG, van den Sloot JAP, Ville Y, van Gemert MJC. Simulation of therapy in a model of a nonhydropic and hydropic recipient in twin–twin transfusion syndrome. Am J Obstet Gynecol 2005; 193:1972–80.
11. Murakoshi T, Quintero RA, Bornick PW, Allen MH. In vivo endoscopic assessment of arteriovenous anastomoses: insights into their hemodynamic function. J Matern Fetal Neonatal Med 2003; 14:247–55.
12. Bermúdez C, Becerra C, Bornick PW et al. Twin–twin transfusion syndrome with only superficial placental anastomoses: endoscopic and pathological evidence. J Matern Fetal Neonatal Med 2002; 12:138–40.
13. Umur A, van Gemert MJC, Nikkels PGJ, Ross MG. Monochorionic twins and twin–twin transfusion syndrome: the protective role of arterioarterial anastomoses. Placenta 2002; 23:201–9.

14. Denbow ML, Taylor M, Cox P, Fisk NM. Derivation of rate of arterio-arterial anastomotic transfusion between monochorionic twin fetuses by Doppler waveform analysis. Placenta 2004; 25:664–70.

15. Oepkes D. Ultrasonograpy and Doppler in the management of red cell alloimmunized pregnancies. PhD thesis, Leiden, The Netherlands, 1993.

16. Benirschke K, Kaufmann P. Pathology of the human placenta. New York: Springer Verlag, 3rd edn, 1995.

17. Gerson AG, Wallace DM, Stiller RJ et al. Doppler evaluation of umbilical venous and arterial blood flow in the second and third trimester of normal pregnancies. Am J Obstet Gynecol 1987; 70:622–6.

18. Nakata M, Martinez JM, Diaz C, Chmait R, Quintero RA. Intra-amniotic Doppler measurement of blood flow in placental vascular anastomoses in twin–twin transfusion syndrome. Ultrasound Obstet Gynecol 2004; 24: 102–3.

19. Lopriore E, van den Wijngaard JPHM, Middeldorp JM et al. Assessment of feto-fetal transfusion flow through placental arterio-venous anastomoses in a unique case of twin-to-twin transfusion syndrome. Placenta 2006; May 4 [Epub ahead of print].

20. Beall MH, van den Wijngaard JPHM, van Gemert MJC, Ross MG. Water flux and amniotic fluid volume: understanding fetal water flow. In Guignard JP, Baumgart S, eds. Understanding fetal water flow in Questions and Controversies in Neonatology series: Renal/Fluids and Electrolytes volume.

21. Mahieu-Caputo D, Dommergues M, Delezoide AL et al. Twin-to-twin transfusion syndrome. Role of the fetal renin–angiotensin system. Am J Pathol 2000; 156: 629–36.

22. Faber JJ, Anderson DF. Angiotensin mediated interaction of fetal kidney and placenta in the control of fetal arterial pressure and its role in hydrops fetalis. Placenta 1997; 18:313–26.

23. Gilbert RD. Control of fetal cardiac output during changes in blood volume. Am J Physiol 1980; 238:H80–6.

24. Thornburg KL, Morton MJ. Filling and arterial pressures as determinants of left ventricular stroke volume in fetal lambs. Am J Physiol 1986, 251:H961–8.

25. Trespidi L, Boschetto C, Caravelli E et al. Serial amniocenteses in the management of twin–twin transfusion syndrome: When is it valuable? Fetal Diagn Ther 1997; 12:15–20.

26. Huber A, Diehl W, Zikulnig L et al. Amniotic fluid and maternal blood characteristics in severe mid-trimester twin–twin transfusion syndrome. Fetal Diagn Ther 2004; 19:504–9.

27. Nikkels PGJ, van Gemert MJC, Sollie-Szarynska KM et al. Rapid onset of severe twin–twin transfusion syndrome caused by placental venous thrombosis. Pediatr Dev Pathol 2002; 5:310–14.

28. van der Wijngaard JPHM, Westerhof BE, Faber DJ, et al. Abnormal arterial flow velocities by a transmission line model of the feto-placental circulation. Am J Physiol 2006; 291:R1222–33.

29. van der Wijngaard JPHM, Westerhof BE, Ross MG, van Gemert MJC. Mathematical model of twin–twin transfusion syndrome with pulsatile circulations. Am J Physiol Regul Integr Comp Physiol 2007 (in press).

30. Wee LY, Sullivan M, Humphries K, Fisk NM. Longitudinal blood flow in shared (arteriovenous anastomoses) and non-shared cotyledons in monochorionic placentae. Placenta. 2007 (in press).

7

Ultrasound assessment in twin–twin transfusion syndrome

Rubén A Quintero

Introduction • Step one: diagnosis of twin–twin transfusion syndrome • Step two: staging of twin–twin transfusion syndrome • Step three: cervical length assessment • Step four: preoperative mapping • Other aspects of the ultrasound assessment • Conclusion

INTRODUCTION

The ultrasound assessment of patients with twin–twin transfusion syndrome (TTTS) can be particularly challenging. The presence of oligohydramnios in the sac of the donor twin frequently impairs adequate visualization of the fetal anatomy, fetal gender, and occasionally, adequate Doppler interrogation of the different vessels of this fetus. Polyhydramnios is typically associated with a frequently moving recipient twin, which makes the Doppler assessment of this fetus particularly difficult. Polyhydramnios may also result in significant maternal discomfort with back pain or light-headedness in the recumbent position, hindering further the completion of the ultrasound examination. Lastly, the examination is typically done under an atmosphere of psychological tension from maternal anxiety, given the grave prognosis in most cases. Despite these limitations, a thorough and complete ultrasound examination is necessary to correctly diagnose and assess the status of patients with TTTS.

The ultrasound assessment of patients with TTTS can be systematized to be performed in several steps or levels, including diagnosis, staging, cervical length, and preoperative mapping. Each of these steps will be discussed below.

STEP ONE: DIAGNOSIS OF TWIN–TWIN TRANSFUSION SYNDROME

TTTS is a complication of monochorionic multiple pregnancies defined sonographically as the combined presence of polyhydramnios in one sac and oligohydramnios in the other sac in a monochorionic–diamniotic twin gestation. Polyhydramnios is defined as a maximum vertical pocket (MVP) ≥ 8 cm, and oligohydramnios as an MVP ≥2 cm (poly8-oligo2). Monochorionicity is established by the presence of a single placenta, absence of a twin-peak sign, thin dividing membrane, and same gender.

Variations in the definition

Although the condition affects mostly twin pregnancies, TTTS can also occur in triplet or higher-order multiple gestations provided at least two fetuses are monochorionic. In monoamniotic twins, the lack of a dividing membrane precludes the presence of oligohydramnios, but the syndrome can be suspected by the presence of polyhydramnios and differences in bladder filling or Doppler studies of the two fetuses. In monochorionic triplet pregnancies, two or all three fetuses may be involved.

Definitions no longer used

Until a few years ago, TTTS was only diagnosed postnatally if an intertwin hemoglobin difference >5 g/dl[1] and a birth weight difference >20%[2] existed between the twins. However, in a classic study by Danskin and Neilson[3] in 178 twin pairs, only four pairs had a hemoglobin difference >5 g/dl and a weight difference >20% but none of these pregnancies showed evidence of polyhydramnios or oligohydramnios. Similarly, percutaneous umbilical blood sampling in six TTTS patients failed to show hemoglobin differences >5 g/dl except in one pregnancy.[4] A difference of only 1.7 g/dl was found in 4 patients by Saunders and collaborators.[5] Because of these findings, the previous neonatal criteria based on birthweight discordance and hemoglobin differences are no longer used.

Ultrasound diagnosis of twin–twin transfusion syndrome

Over the years, the sonographic definition of TTTS has been particularly marred by lack of standardization. Unfortunately, such lack of standardization has resulted in the inclusion of patients without TTTS in treatment series, or even worse, to unnecessary termination of pregnancy in patients without TTTS. Hence, the need to establish a standard sonographic approach to TTTS cannot be overemphasized.

The original ultrasound reports on the diagnosis of TTTS were based on biometric discrepancies (>10 mm of either the biparietal diameter or the transverse diameter of the trunk between the twins) in addition to polyhydramnios of the larger twin.[6] Furthermore, Brennan et al suggested that the presence of same sex, disparity in size or in the number of vessels in the umbilical cords, single placenta with different echogenicity of the cotyledons supplying the two cords, and evidence of hydrops in either twin or congestive heart failure in the recipient twin be added to the criteria.[7] Doppler studies were also used in an attempt to define the syndrome. With the introduction of the sonographic staging system,[8] it is now easy to understand the conflicting findings of the original reports that used Doppler to define the disease, and the actual role

that Doppler assessment plays in the assessment of patients with TTTS.[9–13]

Current ultrasound definition of twin–twin transfusion syndrome

Several important achievements have been made in the last decade in defining TTTS. First, for the reasons mentioned above, the condition requires a sonographic diagnosis. This is important as it establishes ultrasound as the sole reliable diagnostic tool for the condition. As a corollary, the diagnosis of TTTS in patients with monochorionic twin pregnancies with an adverse pregnancy outcome or with significant size discordance between the twins but without prenatal sonographic diagnosis of TTTS lacks definite proof of the condition and may only rely on circumstantial evidence. Secondly, there has been a gradual acceptance of the sonographic criteria by which TTTS is defined: namely, the presence of polyhydramnios, defined as a maximum vertical pocket of ≥8 cm in one sac, and oligohydramnios, defined as a vertical pocket of ≤2 cm in the other sac. Finally, some sonographic parameters are no longer part of the definition – namely, abnormal Doppler studies or growth discordance – as will be explained below.

Definition of polyhydramnios and oligohydramnios

Polyhydramnios and oligohydramnios are defined as sonographic estimates of amniotic fluid volumes above and below the 95th percentile for gestational age, respectively.

Ultrasound assessment of amniotic fluid volume has been either subjective, or semiquantitative using the maximum vertical pocket (MVP), amniotic fluid index (AFI), or the 2-dimensional pocket (2D). The MVP is defined as the largest vertical pocket of amniotic fluid without the presence of umbilical cord or other fetal parts. The AFI is the sum of the 4 MVPs taken in each quadrant with the transducer aligned in the sagittal plane. The 2D diameter is the product of the MVP times the maximum transverse diameter in any particular quadrant. Both the MVP and the AFI have been shown to behave similarly in singletons, dichorionic twins, and

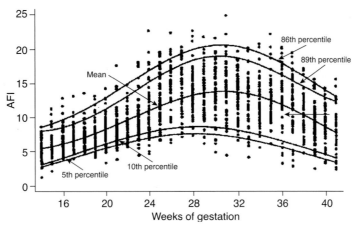

Figure 7.1 Regression of amniotic fluid index (AFI) on gestational age. Amniotic fluid index = 1.39 − (0.158 Gestational age) + (0.01 Gestational age^2) − (0.0003 Gestational age^3) + 0.000002 Gestational age^4. R^2 = 0.96. (Reproduced with permission from[16].)

monochorionic twins, whereas the 2D pocket is smaller in twins than in singletons.[14] The decision to use the MVP instead of the AFI in terms of the sonographic definition of TTTS is based on several grounds. First, the AFI is known to increase, with gestational age until approximately 33 weeks[15,16] (Figure 7.1), whereas the MVP remains relatively stable throughout the second trimester (Figure 7.2). Secondly, the AFI is impractical in twins, because of the varying location of the dividing membrane. Lastly, the uterine fundus may not have surpassed the umbilicus in some patients, which hinders the designation of the four quadrants for the AFI.

Some disagreement has existed as to which MVP cut-off values should be used in the definition of oligohydramnios and polyhydramnios. Most authors agree on ≤2 cm for the definition of oligohydramnios, and ≥8 cm for the definition of polyhydramnios. Oligohydramnios defined as ≤2 cm corresponds to the 5th percentile in MVP estimates, and changes little throughout gestation.[16–19] The 95th percentile corresponds to an MVP of approximately 8 cm.[14] Because of the known inaccuracy of amniotic fluid volume estimates, regardless of the sonographic technique used, the 2 and 8 cm cut-offs should be viewed as the minimum criteria to diagnose TTTS.

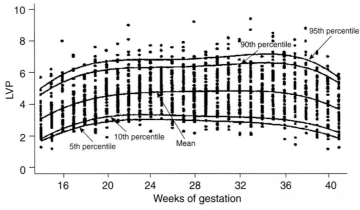

Figure 7.2 Regression of single deepest pocket (lowest vertical pocket, LVP) on gestational age. Single deepest pocket = 2.12 + (0.398 Gestational age) + (0.02 Gestational age^2) + (0.0005 Gestational age^3) + (0.00005 Gestational age^4). R^2 = 0.92. (Reproduced with permission from[16].)

The importance of adhering to a standard definition of TTTS cannot be overemphasized because of the grave implications of treating non-TTTS patients or not treating bona fide TTTS patients. Non-descriptive terms such as poly/oli, or twin-polyhydramnios-oligohydramnios-sequence (TOPS), used in the past, are slowly being abandoned. While there has been universal acceptance of an MVP of ≤2 cm as part of the definition of TTTS, some authors have argued that using <1 cm is a more stringent criterion. We have looked at this question in our own patient population. If one agrees that stage III and stage IV TTTS patients represent the extremes of the

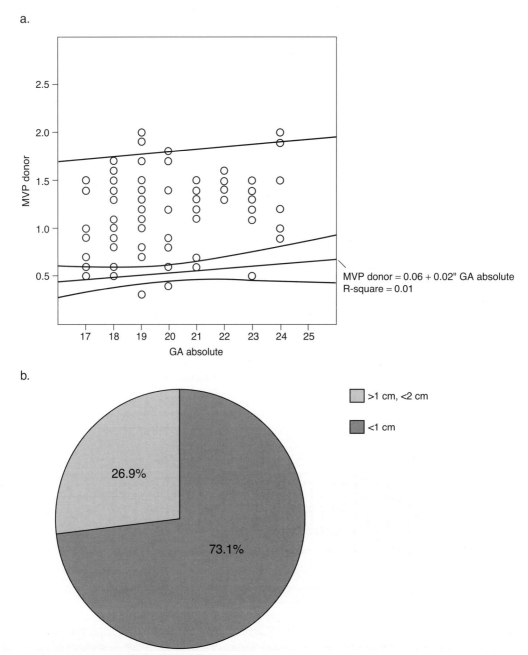

a.

MVP donor = 0.06 + 0.02" GA absolute
R-square = 0.01

b.

26.9%

73.1%

>1 cm, <2 cm

<1 cm

Figure 7.3 (a) Maximum vertical pocket (MVP) of donor by gestational age (GA). (b) Percent of patients with MVP of donor between 1–2 cm versus <2 cm.

spectrum in terms of disease severity, the use of a 1 cm cut-off would declassify 27% of patients as having TTTS (Figures 7.3a,b).

Some authors have suggested using ≥10 cm for the definition of polyhydramnios particularly after 20 weeks. Such decision would declassify 38% stage III and 8.3% of stage IV TTTS patients. Using a cut off of 20 weeks, 22% of patients would be under diagnosed using an MVP of >10 cm. Although the MVP rises slightly with

gestational age before 16 weeks of gestation, the use of an MVP <8 cm is unwarranted, as it is likely to result in significant overlap with the normal population (Figures 7.4a,b).

Sonographic pitfalls: the cocoon sign

Because of the presence of oligohydramnios, the donor twin is usually stuck against the walls of the uterus: thus, the name 'stuck twin.' However, in

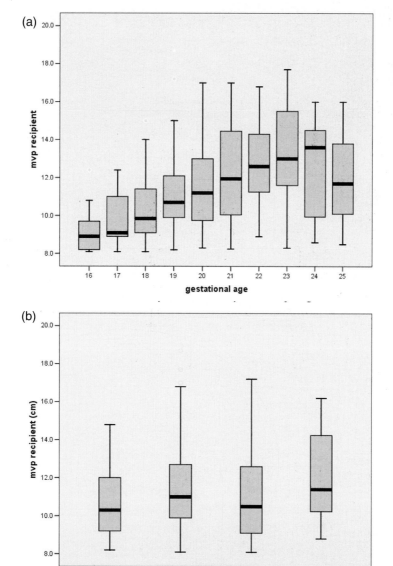

Figure 7.4 (a) Maximum vertical pocket (MVP) of recipient by gestational age (GA). Using an MVP of > 10 cm at 20 weeks would under diagnose 22% of TTTS patients. (b) MVP of recipient by Stage. A cut-off of > 10 cm a 20 weeks would declassify 22% of Stage III−IV patients (13 out of 59 patients).

approximately 15% of TTTS patients, the donor twin is enveloped by the dividing membrane, such that it is connected to the uterine wall by a stalk of these membranes (Figure 7.5a–c). As a result, the donor twin, despite having anhydramnios, may not be stuck to the uterine wall. We have called this potential sonographic pitfall 'the cocoon sign', as the term implies.[20] Thus, a non-stuck donor twin may not necessarily be better off than a stuck one. The importance of the recognition of the cocoon sign lies in the ability to correctly diagnose anhydramnios of the donor twin and not measure fluid of the recipient twin mistakenly as belonging to the donor twin, by placing the calipers from the edge of the enveloping membrane to the uterine wall. Because the donor is

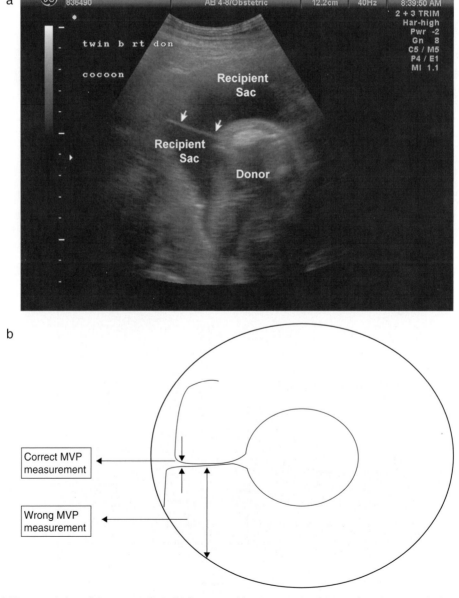

Figure 7.5 (a) Ultrasound view of the cocoon sign. (b) Correct and incorrect measurement of maximum vertical pocket (MVP) in the presence of the cocoon sign. (See also color plate section, page xxii.)

c

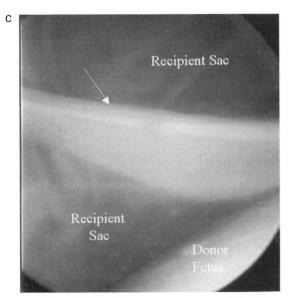

Figure 7.5 Cont'd (c) Endoscopic view of the cocoon sign. (Reproduced with permission from[20].) (See also color plate section, page xxi.)

allowed to move, albeit enveloped by the membranes, the sonologist may erroneously conclude that the fetus does have ample amniotic fluid.

STEP TWO: STAGING OF TWIN–TWIN TRANSFUSION SYNDROME

Our current understanding of the heterogenous presentation of TTTS explains the seemingly conflicting reports of pioneer investigators regarding the role of Doppler in TTTS.[9–13] Indeed, we now know that only a subgroup of TTTS patients present with abnormal Doppler findings. Thus, Doppler studies are more important in terms of assessing disease severity rather than in defining the syndrome. TTTS is known to be a heterogeneous condition with different presentations. Variations of the syndrome include visualization or lack thereof of the bladder of the donor twin, and the presence or absence of abnormal Doppler studies or hydrops. TTTS may also present with demise of one or both twins. The heterogeneity may result as a direct consequence of determinant factors (e.g. abnormal Doppler studies due to placental insufficiency, or severe hemodynamic decompensation or superficial anastomoses), or more often, the expression of dynamic changes occurring over time, which eventually may result in demise of one or both twins. In 1999,[8] we proposed a sonographic staging system to account for all of the different presentations. Inherent in the staging system is the notion that the higher the stage, the worse the prognosis. For all stages, patients meet the basic criteria of polyhydramnios (MVP ≥8 cm), and oligohydramnios (MVP ≤2 cm). The staging system is as follows.

Stage I

The bladder of the donor is visible (Figure 7.6).

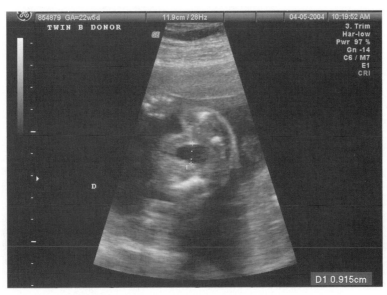

Figure 7.6 The bladder of the donor is visible.

Stage II

The bladder of the donor is not visible (Figure 7.7). The typical ultrasound examination of patients with TTTS lasts approximately 60 minutes. Non-visualization of the bladder of the donor therefore is defined as lack of visualization of the bladder of the donor twin in 60 minutes of ultrasound examination.

Stage III

Critically abnormal Doppler studies. These include:

- absent or reverse end-diastolic velocity in the umbilical artery (UA-AREDV) (Figure 7.8a–c).
- Reverse flow in the atrial contraction waveform of the ductus venosus (RFDV) (Figure 7.9).
- Pulsatile umbilical venous flow (PUVF) (Figure 7.10a,b).

There is no controversy regarding the definition of UA-AREDV. However, it is important to note that AREDV may be artificially created by setting the wall-motion filter (WFM) too high. The standard setting of the WMF is 100 mHz.

Occasionally, patients may show intermittent UA-AREDV. In these cases, the patient is staged as having positive diastolic flow. Similarly, if UA-AREDV is noted closer to the fetus, but diastolic flow is detected closer to the placental insertion of the umbilical cord, diastolic flow is considered to be present.

Doppler interrogation of the ductus venosus can be particularly challenging in the assessment of patients with TTTS. Care must be taken not to confuse the waveform of the ductus venosus with that of the hepatic veins or the inferior vena cava (Figure 7.11a–e: DV, hepatic vein, IVC). Similarly, the WMF should be set at 100 MHz. For the purposes of the staging system, flow in the ductus venosus must be reversed during the atrial contraction waveform to be called critically abnormal, and not merely absent (see Figure 7.10).

Pulsatile umbilical venous flow is considered to be present whenever Doppler interrogation of the umbilical vein shows a non-linear pattern (Figure 7.10a). The waveform is obtained at the level of the umbilical cord, not in the intra-abdominal portion of the umbilical vein. It is important to note that PUVF represents a different pathophysiological phenomenon from RFDV,

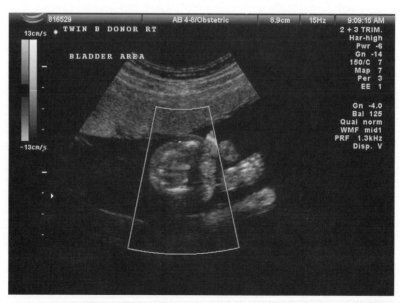

Figure 7.7 The bladder of the donor is not visible.

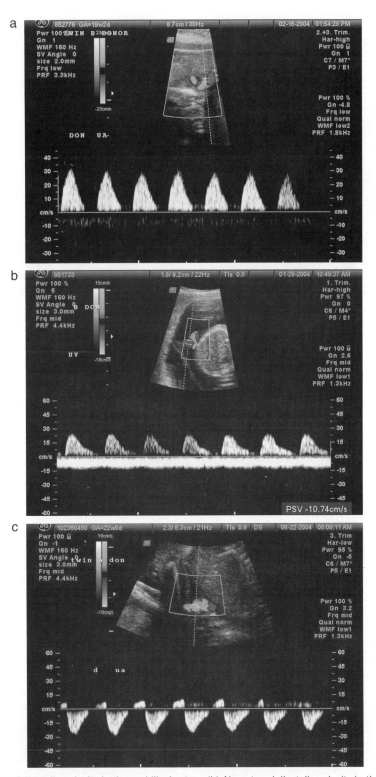

Figure 7.8 (a) Absent end-diastolic velocity in the umbilical artery. (b) Absent end-diastolic velocity in the umbilical artery and linear flow in the umbilical vein in the same view. (c) Reverse end-diastolic velocity in the umbilical artery. (See also color plate section, page xiii.)

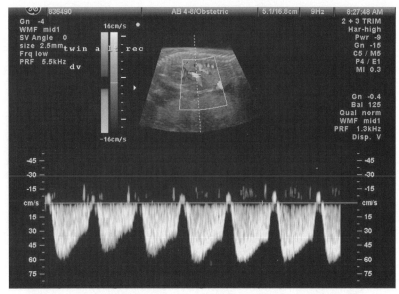

Figure 7.9 Reverse flow in the atrial contraction waveform of the ductus venosus. (See also color plate section, page xiv.)

as the latter occurs during diastole, whereas the former flow is typically a systolic abnormality. As such, RFDV and PUVF may coexist or occur independently in any given fetus.

Stage IV: Hydrops

Stage IV is defined by the presence of ascites, pericardial or pleural effusion, and scalp or skin edema (Figure 7.12a–c). Most if not all of these ultrasound findings are subjective. However, for the purposes of follow-up, the degree of third spacing may be monitored. Thus, the scalp may be measured at the level of the biparietal diameter as the distance from the skin to the parietal bone; pleural effusion may be measured as the transverse distance from the tip of the lung to the inner chest wall at the level of the base of the lung; pericardial effusion may be measured at the level of the four-chamber view as the distance between the right atrium and the pericardium in diastole; ascites may be measured at the abdominal circumference level as the distance between the anterior edge of the liver and the inner abdominal wall. Skin edema may also be measured at the level of the abdominal circumference.

Stage V: Intrauterine fetal demise of one or both twins (Figure 7.13)

Sub-staging

Classic vs atypical presentation

In the classic form, the bladder of the donor twin may not be visible in stages III and IV. When the bladder of the donor is visible in any of these two stages, it represents an atypical presentation. The importance of substaging may be useful in terms of explaining the pathophysiological mechanisms responsible for the different presentation as well as potentially useful in terms of prognosis.

Donor vs recipient

Stage III can be further described, depending on which of the two fetuses is affected. For example, if the patient is stage III because the donor twin has UA-AREDV, the patient can be classified as having stage III-donor. Similarly, if the fetus with the Doppler abnormality is the recipient twin, the patient can be classified as having stage III-recipient. Both fetuses may show critically abnormal Doppler findings, in which case the patient is rightfully classified as having stage III-donor-recipient. Although stage IV is typically

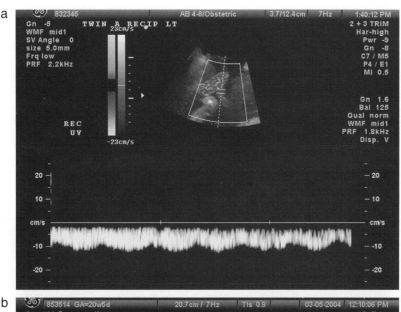

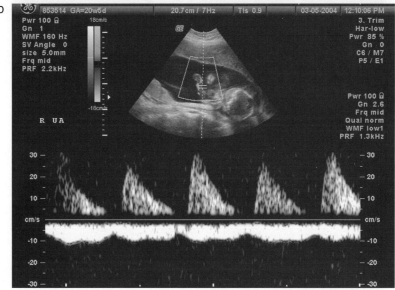

Figure 7.10 (a) Pulsatile umbilical venous flow. (b) Pulsatile umbilical venous flow in the umbilical vein and absent end-diastolic velocity in the umbilical artery in the same view. (See also color plate section, page xxv.)

associated with hydrops of the recipient twin, isolated hydrops of the donor may also occur. Some evidence is surfacing to explain the different substaging manifestations, but the actual mechanisms responsible for their production are still unclear. Substaging in terms of donor or recipient may facilitate communication between investigators in terms of individual prognosis for each twin. Neither tricuspid valve regurgitation nor Doppler studies of the middle cerebral artery (peak systolic velocity or other indices) have been shown to have prognostic value in the assessment of patients with TTTS. Therefore, neither of these two parameters is included in the staging system.

STEP THREE: CERVICAL LENGTH ASSESSMENT

The third aspect of the ultrasound evaluation of patients with TTTS involves an adequate assessment of the cervical length. Because of the early gestational age at which patients would typically present, transabdominal assessment of the cervical length is usually adequate. However, we prefer to document the cervical length via transvaginal ultrasound unless there are specific contraindications for doing so.

Assessment of the cervical length is particularly important because, in addition to fetal demise, miscarriage or premature labor is the second mechanism responsible for pregnancy loss in TTTS.

A short cervical length may be secondary to uterine contractions or from 'cervical incompetence' as a mechanical result of the overdistention of the uterus (Figure 7.14). Although our data shows a statistically significant inverse correlation between cervical length and the degree of polyhydramnios as measured by the MVP, the association is not strong ($R = -0.139$). Nonetheless, it does suggest that a short cervical length may indeed be partly explained by a mechanical phenomenon. Therefore, we recommend that patients

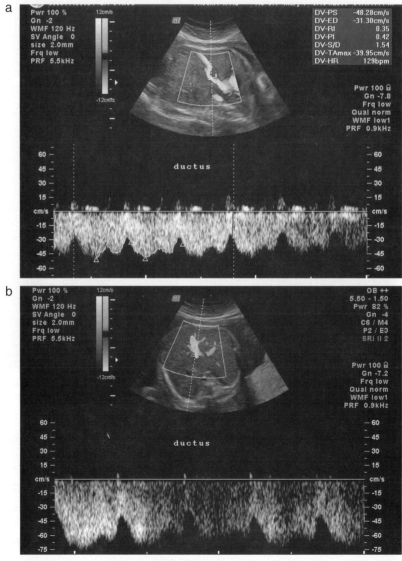

Figure 7.11 (a) Normal ductus venosus waveform, sagittal. (b) Normal ductus venosus waveform, transverse. (See also color plate section, page xxvi.)

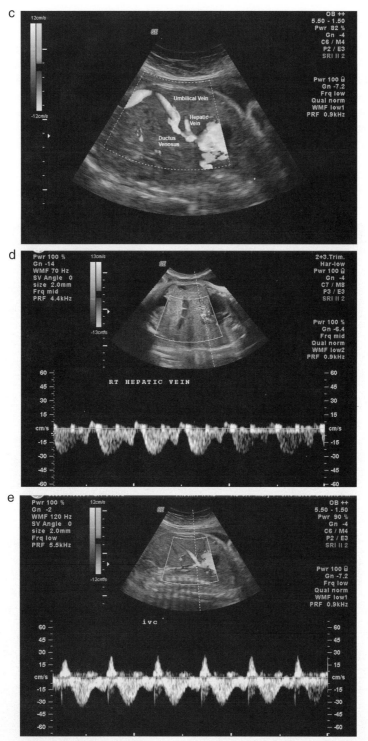

Figure 7.11 Cont'd (c) Normal ductus venosus, high resolution. (d) View of hepatic vein waveform. (e) View of inferior vena cava waveform. (See also color plate section, page xxvii.)

with a cervical length <2.5 cm undergo a cervical cerclage prior to referral. If a cervical length <2.5 cm is found incidentally during the evaluation, we may choose to place a cerclage at the time of the laser surgery or the following day, to allow potential benefit of the concomitant amnioreduction. Because of this management algorithm, our data show no difference in outcome relative to a cervical length less or greater than 2.5 cm.

STEP FOUR: PREOPERATIVE MAPPING

The last aspect of the ultrasound evaluation of patients with TTTS consists of an attempt to predict the location of the dividing membrane and thus the vascular equator and direction of the vascular anastomoses. We call this step preoperative mapping. Preoperative mapping may help in choosing the point of entry into

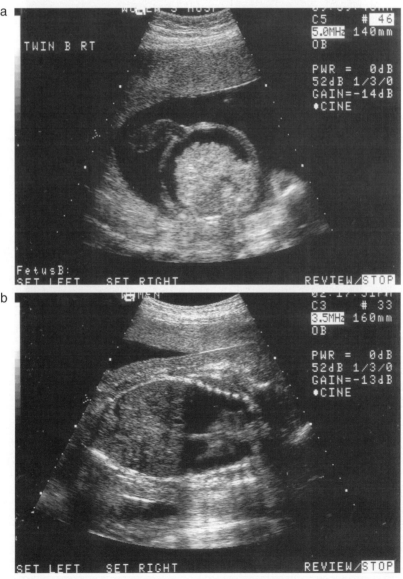

Figure 7.12 (a) Ascites. (b) Pericardial/pleural effusions. (Reproduced with permission from[21].)

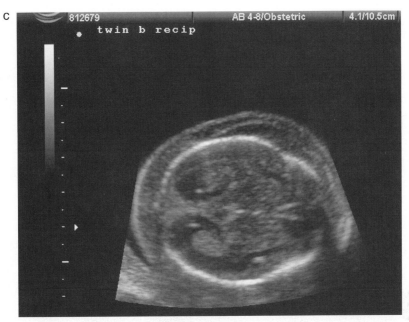

Figure 7.12 Cont'd (c) Scalp edema. Degree of edema may be followed by measuring the distance from the parietal to the skin.

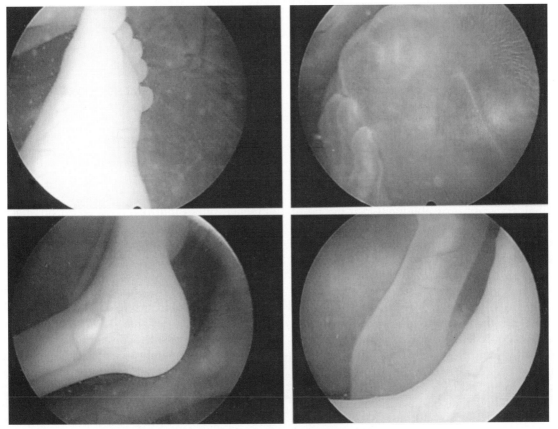

Figure 7.13 Stage V, defined as intrauterine fetal demise of one or both twins. Feto–fetal results in a plethoric twin that has died and been transfused by the pale twin. (Reproduced with permission from[22].) (See also color plate section, page xix.)

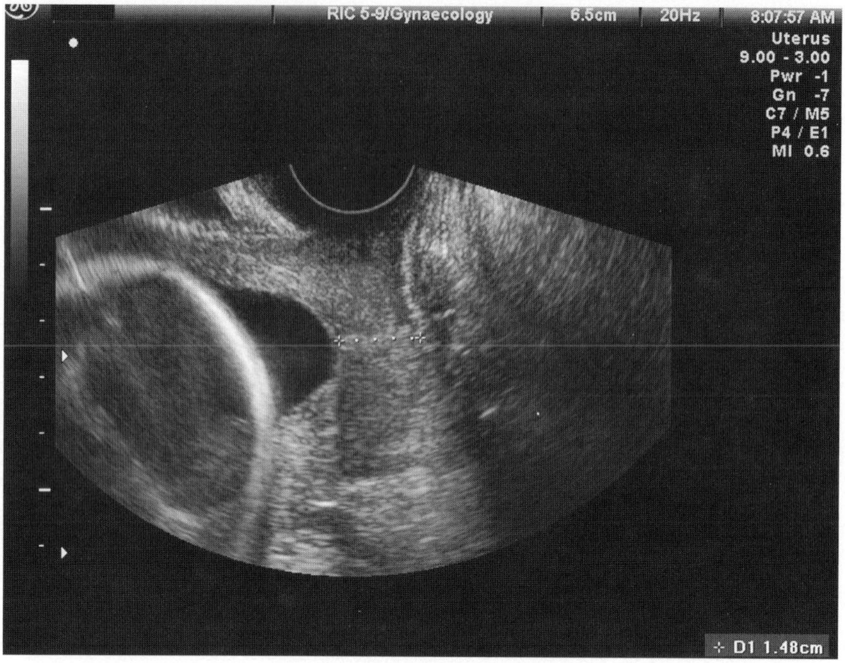

Figure 7.14 Incompetent cervix.

the uterus, particularly in patients with a posterior placenta.

Mapping is most accurate when the donor twin is stuck, and most difficult in stage I or if a cocoon sign is present. In cases where the donor is stuck, preoperative mapping uses the lie of the donor as a guide to the location of the dividing membrane. Indeed, in most cases, the dividing membrane follows the lie of the donor, i.e. longitudinal, transverse, or oblique. Once the lie of the donor is determined, the placental insertion of the umbilical cords is then assessed. If the donor twin is between the insertions of the umbilical cords, one might anticipate that there will be anastomoses in the sac of the donor twin and that they will be obscured by this fetus. If, on the other hand, the donor twin is not between the two cords, this fetus should typically not interfere with identification of the anastomoses (Figures 7.15a–c). Preoperative mapping is particularly important to avoid unintentional injury to the dividing membrane (unintentional septostomy), which may result in further tearing of the dividing membrane, cord entanglement, and fetal demise.

OTHER ASPECTS OF THE ULTRASOUND ASSESSMENT

Estimated fetal weight and fetal weight discordance

The legacy of neonatal criteria for the diagnosis of TTTS still lingers. A 20% discordance in birthweight was to establish the diagnosis of TTTS. Prenatal ultrasound diagnosis based on specific amniotic fluid discordances, as opposed to postnatal criteria, has eliminated birthweight discordance as a criterion. Figure 7.16 shows the frequency distribution of EFW discordance as determined by ultrasound. As can be seen, the spectrum ranges from 0 to 65%, approximately. Restriction of the definition of TTTS to only those fetuses with at least 20% discordance would disqualify approximately 31% of all TTTS patients. The reasons for the wide range of EFW discordances are not entirely clear. Intrauterine growth retardation (IUGR) may exist independently of TTTS, as a completely separate entity. We now know that growth restriction may occur as a result from lack of individual

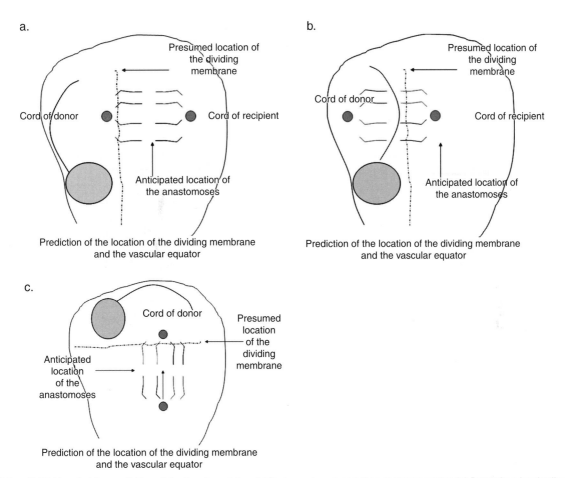

Figure 7.15 Mapping for prediction of the location of the dividing membrane and the vascular equator. (a) Donor in a longitudinal lie. (b) Donor in a longitudinal lie. Donor interfering. Anastomoses within the sac of the donor. (c) Donor in a transverse lie.

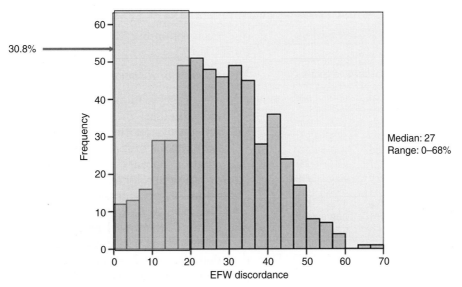

Figure 7.16 Estimated fetal weight (EFW) discordance, $N = 513$ (7/97–1/04).

placental territory, from the placental vascular anastomoses themselves, or from both. The contribution of either of these factors, either independently or in conjunction, cannot be predicted prenatally.

Although EFW discordance may provide information about the disparity in growth, a more useful parameter to establish is the actual percentile growth for each fetus, particularly if it is below the 10th percentile. Table 7.1 shows the cut-off values used in our laboratory to diagnose IUGR (estimated fetal weight <10th percentile). TTTS patients in whom one or both twins are classified as having IUGR should then be labeled as having both diagnoses, i.e. TTTS and IUGR. This approach may facilitate the communication between investigators and the counseling of patients for treatment. Our data show that approximately 50% of TTTS patients have IUGR of one of the fetuses.

Ultrasound assessment of deep communications and/or superficial anastomoses

There are a few reports on the use of ultrasound to assess deep communications or superficial anastomoses.[24] Most studies have been performed on patients without TTTS and anterior placentas, as color Doppler insonation of the placental parenchyma is easier in these patients.

Deep vascular communications

The presumed diagnosis of deep placental vascular communications involves color Doppler identification of an arterial vessel coming in one direction, and a venous drainage of the same cotyledon going in an opposite direction (Figure 7.17). While such approach may indeed identify deep vascular communications, it is by no means reliable. In-vivo endoscopic assessment of placental vascular anastomoses shows that the course of the vessels on the placental surface is unpredictable. As a result, the participating artery and vein, while seemingly in opposite directions, may actually belong to the same fetus. This notion is precisely why prior statements regarding the endoscopic ability to identify placental vascular anastomoses based on the angle of incidence between the artery and vein were disqualified. In extreme cases, non-shared cotyledons may show one of the vessels curving on the surface of the placenta making a complete 'U-turn' (Figure 7.18). Sonographically, this would appear as an artery and a vein traveling in opposite directions, suggesting the presence of an AV anastomosis, when, in reality, this is a normally and individually perfused cotyledon. Because of the poor sensitivity of ultrasound in delineating the path of placental vessels, the diagnosis of deep vascular communications is, in our opinion, suspect.

Superficial vascular anastomoses

The identification of superficial anastomoses, in particular, of AA anastomoses, has been previously reported.[25] As with AV communications, this is best attempted in patients with an anterior placenta. AA anastomoses can be suspected with color Doppler by noting the direction of blood flow towards the transducer from both ends of the vessel. Pulsed Doppler interrogation of the vessel may reveal a characteristic additive waveform resulting from the summation of the two heart beats within the same vessel. The identification of VV anastomoses has not been described.

Table 7.1 Diagnosis of IUGR present in one twin (fetal weight at or below the 10th percentile for gestational age)

Menstrual week	In utero fetal weight standards at ultrasound percentiles (g)				
	3rd	10th	50th	90th	97th
16	110	121	146	171	183
17	136	150	181	212	226
18	167	185	223	261	279
19	205	227	273	319	341
20	248	275	331	387	414
21	299	331	399	467	499
22	359	398	478	559	598
23	426	471	568	665	710
24	503	556	670	784	838
25	589	652	785	918	981
26	685	758	913	1068	1141

Adapted from Hadlock et al.[23]

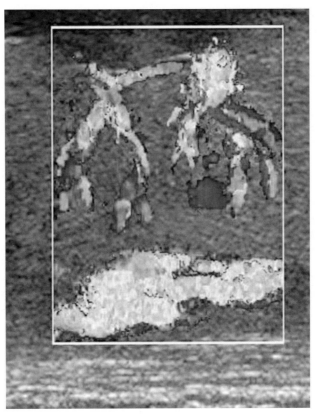

Figure 7.17 Color Doppler identification of an arterial vessel coming in one direction, and a venous drainage of the same cotyledon going in the opposite direction. (See also color plate section, page xxiv.)

The sensitivity for the identification of AA anastomoses has been reported to be as high

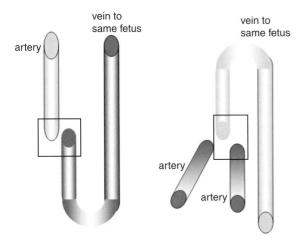

Figure 7.18 Possible pitfalls using morphological criteria to assess deep AV anastomoses. The boxes show an artery and vein running in opposite directions. (See also color plate section, page xxi.)

as 85%.[25] However, this figure represents the cumulative sensitivity over several ultrasound examinations in the same patient up to the third trimester. In our experience, identification of AA anastomoses is both insensitive and extremely time-consuming, even in patients in which a 50% incidence of AA anastomoses can be predicted (e.g. atypical stage III donor). We have not found any difference in the prognosis of patients treated with laser relative to the presence or absence of AA anastomoses. Thus, the quest for the sonographic identification of AA anastomoses may be of limited diagnostic interest.

CONCLUSION

Systematic ultrasound assessment of patients with TTTS allows establishing an adequate diagnosis and prognostic factors. Careful attention to sonographic details is necessary to avoid common pitfalls. Preoperative mapping is important in the planning of any invasive procedure, particularly in the case of laser therapy.

REFERENCES

1. Rausen A, Seki M, Strauss L. Twin transfusion syndrome. J Pediatr 1965; 66:613–28.

2. Tan K, Tan R, Tan A. The twin transfusion syndrome. Clin Pediatr 1979; 18:111–14.

3. Danskin FH, Neilson JP. Twin-to-twin transfusion syndrome: What are appropriate diagnostic criteria? Am J Obstet Gynecol 1989; 161:365–9.

4. Fisk NM, Borrell A, Hubinont C et al. Fetofetal transfusion syndrome: do the neonatal criteria apply in utero? Arch Dis Child 1990; 65:657–61.

5. Saunders N, Snijders R, Nicolaides K. Twin–twin transfusion syndrome during the 2nd trimester is associated with small intertwin hemoglobin differences. Fetal Diagn Ther 1991; 6:34–6.

6. Wittman B, Baldwin V, Nichol B. Antenatal diagnosis of twin transfusion syndrome by ultrasound. Obstet Gynecol 1981; 58:123–7.

7. Brennan JN, Diwan RV, Rosen MG, Bellon EM. Fetofetal transfusion syndrome: prenatal ultrasonographic diagnosis. Radiology 1982; 143:535–6.

8. Quintero R, Morales W, Allen M et al. Staging of twin–twin transfusion syndrome. J Perinatol 1999; 19:550–555.

9. Farmakides G, Schulman H, Saldana LR et al. Surveillance of twin pregnancy with umbilical arterial velocimetry. Am J Obstet Gynecol 1985; 153:789–92.

10. Giles WB, Trudinger BJ, Cook CM, Connelly AJ. Doppler umbilical artery studies in the twin–twin transfusion syndrome. Obstet Gynecol 1990; 76:1097–9.

11. Ishimatsu J, Yoshimura O, Manabe A et al. Ultrasonography and Doppler studies in twin-to-twin transfusion syndrome. Asia Oceania J Obstet Gynaecol 1992; 18: 325–31.

12. Pretorius DH, Manchester D, Barkin S et al. Doppler ultrasound of twin transfusion syndrome. J Ultrasound Med 1988; 7(3):117–24.

13. Yamada A, Kasugai M, Ohno Y et al. Antenatal diagnosis of twin–twin transfusion syndrome by Doppler ultrasound. Obstet Gynecol 1991; 78:1058–61.

14. Chau AC, Kjos SL, Kovacs BW. Ultrasonographic measurement of amniotic fluid volume in normal diamniotic twin pregnancies. Am J Obstet Gynecol 1996; 174:1003–7.

15. Moore TR, Cayle JE. The amniotic fluid index in normal human pregnancy. Am J Obstet Gynecol 1990; 162: 1168–73.

16. Magann EF, Sanderson M, Martin JN, Chauhan S. The amniotic fluid index, single deepest pocket, and two-diameter pocket in normal human pregnancy. Am J Obstet Gynecol 2000; 182:1581–8.

17. Gramellini D, Chiaie D, Piantelli G et al. Sonographic assessment of amniotic fluid volume between 11 and 24 weeks of gestation: construction of reference intervals related to gestational age. Ultrasound Obstet Gynecol 2001; 17:410–15.

18. Magann EF, Chauhan SP, Bofill JA, Martin JN Jr. Comparability of the amniotic fluid index and single deepest pocket measurements in clinical practice. Aust N Z J Obstet Gynaecol 2003; 43:75–7.

19. Magann EF, Doherty DA, Chauhan SP et al. How well do the amniotic fluid index and single deepest pocket indices (below the 3rd and 5th and above the 95th and 97th percentiles) predict oligohydramnios and hydramnios? Am J Obstet Gynecol 2004; 190:164–9.

20. Quintero RA, Chmait RH. The cocoon sign: a potential sonographic pitfall in the diagnosis of twin–twin transfusion syndrome. Ultrasound Obstet Gynecol 2004; 23: 38–41.

21. Quintero R. Selective laser photocoagulation of communicating vessels in twin–twin transfusion syndrome. In: Quintero R, ed. Diagnostic and Operative fetoscopy. New York: The Parthenon Publishing Group, 2002: 43–54.

22. Quintero RA, Martinez JM, Bermudez C, Lopez J, Becerra C. Fetoscopic demonstration of perimortem feto-fetal hemorrhage in twin–twin transfusion syndrome. Ultrasound Obstet Gynecol 2002; 20:638–9.

23. Hadlock FP, Harrist RB, Martinez-Poyer J. In utero analysis of fetal growth: a sonographic weight standard. Radiology 1991; 181:129–33.

24. Taylor MJ, Farquharson D, Cox PM, Fisk NM. Identification of arterio-venous anastomoses in vivo in monochorionic twin pregnancies: preliminary report. Ultrasound Obstet Gynecol 2000; 16:218–22.

25. Taylor MJ, Denbow ML, Tanawattanacharoen S et al. Doppler detection of arterio-arterial anastomoses in monochorionic twins: feasibility and clinical application. Hum Reprod 2000; 15:1632–6.

8

Amnioreduction therapy for twin–twin transfusion syndrome

Jan E Dickinson

Introduction • Amnioreduction: physiological rationale • Amnioreduction: technique • Complications • Efficacy of amnioreduction as a therapy in twin–twin transfusion syndrome • Conclusion

INTRODUCTION

Twin–twin transfusion syndrome (TTTS) is one of the most challenging complications of the monochorionic twinning process. Characterized by high perinatal mortality and morbidity rates, TTTS has stimulated intense research interest globally over the past two decades. The advent of obstetric ultrasound has enabled the accurate prenatal identification of TTTS and this detection capability has facilitated potential therapeutic interventions. Additionally, the treatment modalities have been refined as knowledge of the pathophysiology of TTTS has improved. It is evident that TTTS is a complex condition and, as yet, there is no intervention which consistently produces optimal perinatal outcomes.

Several therapeutic interventions have been used to improve maternal and perinatal outcomes in TTTS, including medical therapies such as digoxin[1] and prostaglandin synthase inhibitors,[2] intrauterine transfusion therapies,[3] specific surgical interventions (selective fetal delivery,[4] selective feticide[5,6]), amnioreduction,[7–9] septostomy,[10,11] placental laser ablation,[12–14] and delivery if the gestation is in the third trimester. Only two therapeutic interventions for TTTS have withstood the test of time and medical scrutiny: amnioreduction and placental laser ablation. Although both of these therapies have been demonstrated to improve the perinatal survival rates of severe TTTS, neither is without procedural complications

nor is successful in all cases.[15] It has taken two decades for a randomized controlled trial of therapies for TTTS to be completed and published.[16] Further randomized studies on management strategies are clearly required and are awaited with interest by healthcare providers and parents affected by this most fascinating complication of twinning.

AMNIOREDUCTION: PHYSIOLOGICAL RATIONALE

Amnioreduction, the percutaneous removal of large volumes of amniotic fluid from the sac of the recipient fetus in TTTS, was the first widely employed intervention to significantly alter the dismal perinatal prognosis of this condition. Indeed, this technically simple procedure remains a central component of the therapeutic armamentarium of TTTS, either alone or as an adjunct to placental laser ablation techniques.

The hallmark diagnostic feature of TTTS is the oligohydramnios/polyhydramnios sequence.[17,18] The donor fetus is characterized by a restrictive oligohydramnios (maximum vertical pocket [MVP] ≤ 2 cm) secondary to hypovolemia, whereas the recipient fetus displays hypervolemic polyuric polyhydramnios (MVP ≥ 8 cm), creating a unique sonographic portrait (Figure 8.1). The polyhydramnios of the recipient fetus may reach extreme levels, with secondary maternal respiratory compromise. Preterm labor or preterm membrane rupture may occur secondary to the

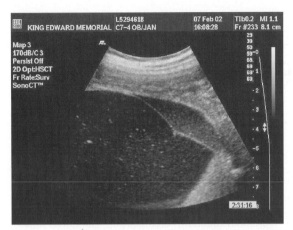

Figure 8.1 Sonographic appearance of polyhydramnios/ oligohydramnios sequence demonstrating markedly discordant amniotic fluid volumes.

excessive amniotic fluid volume, frequently at very preterm gestations.

Amniotic fluid pressure follows a weakly sigmoid-shaped regression curve, plateauing in the midtrimester, and increasing as gestation advances in both normal singleton and twin gestations.[19] Polyhydramnios is associated with an elevation of intrauterine pressure above the gestation mean, although not always exceeding the upper limit of normal.[20] Furthermore, amniotic pressure is positively correlated with the MVP of fluid. In cases where polyhydramnios is associated with an elevated amniotic fluid pressure, drainage of amniotic fluid results in normalization of amniotic fluid pressure.[20] Garry et al[21] observed an elevated intra-amniotic pressure in all cases of TTTS; this decreased to the normal range following amnioreduction and restoration of normal amniotic fluid volume.

As amniotic fluid pressure increases, fetal pO_2 decreases, an effect independent of gestation.[20] There is a significant association between elevated amniotic fluid pressure and abnormal fetal blood gas status.[22] Raised amniotic pressure has been associated with an impairment in uteroplacental perfusion in both animal and human studies.[23–25] Following therapeutic amnioreduction in 8 pregnancies with polyhydramnios, Bower et al[25] observed a 74% median increase of uterine artery volume flow. It is postulated that elevated amniotic fluid pressure compresses the placenta and intervillous space.[21] These findings were reiterated

by Guzman et al,[26] who observed significantly improved uterine artery impedance indices and increased flow velocities using Doppler studies prior to and following amnioreduction in severe polyhydramnios.

Based on the physiological observations outlined above, it has been postulated that the elevated amniotic pressure secondary to the recipient polyhydramnios in TTTS may impair placental perfusion to the donor, contributing to further hypovolemia and oliguria. Decreasing the amniotic fluid pressure with amnioreduction may relieve this abnormality of uteroplacental perfusion, thus providing a potential mechanism for the efficacy of this procedure in TTTS.

Preterm labor or preterm membrane rupture is also a consequence of polyhydramnios and increased amniotic pressure. Perinatal outcomes for TTTS are greatly influenced by gestation at delivery.[27,28] Amnioreduction, by reducing the amniotic pressure, may prolong gestation and improve perinatal outcomes in this indirect manner.[29]

AMNIOREDUCTION: TECHNIQUE

Amnioreduction is a technically simple procedure, although appropriate patient selection, patient positioning, and drainage mechanisms are important to minimize procedure-related complications. The procedure may be accomplished without sophisticated technology, although there has been a recent trend in the use of vacuum-assisted devices to withdraw the amniotic fluid rather than manual techniques.[30] There is wide variation in the amnioreduction technique in terms of needle gauge used, the volume and rate of amniotic fluid withdrawn, and the completion MVP or amniotic fluid index (AFI). Interestingly, despite these procedural differences, the reported success rates of this technique are remarkably similar.[27,28]

Patient sedation with a benzodiazepine is helpful for maternal comfort and to reduce excessive fetal movement of the recipient fetus during the procedure. Positioning of the woman is critical to the successful completion of the procedure (Figure 8.2). Lateral tilt will reduce the potential for aortocaval compression and supporting pillows behind the spine and between the knees will aid maternal comfort.

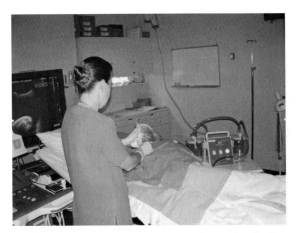

Figure 8.2 Patient positioning and set-up for amnioreduction.

There is a linear relationship between the volume of amniotic fluid removed and the alteration in AFI, with a decrease in the AFI of approximately 1 cm/100 ml fluid removed.[31,32] This alteration in AFI appears to be independent of gestation and preprocedure AFI, and can provide a preprocedure approximation of the volume to be drained. Other units use single measures of amniotic fluid as a guide, typically reducing the amniotic fluid volume until an MVP of 5–6 cm is obtained.

COMPLICATIONS

Amnioreduction has been associated with four main procedure-associated complications: preterm labor and/or amniorrhexis, fetal demise, infectious complications, and placental abruption. It is difficult to dissociate the primary condition being treated from the first two adverse outcomes, as polyhydramnios has a clear association with preterm birth and intrauterine fetal demise. Inadvertent septostomy has been reported following amnioreduction with umbilical cord entanglement.[27]

The needle insertion site is selected so as to avoid transplacental needle passage or disruption of the dividing membrane. In addition, the needle insertion site should not be too cephalad due to the marked alteration in uterine morphology that follows decompression and the acute angulation which may occur secondarily to this phenomenon. Our practice is to use an 18-gauge spinal needle, although a variety of needle gauges have been reported, inserted under continuous ultrasound guidance following infiltration of local anesthetic to the skin and deeper tissues. Amniotic fluid is drained either by a manual system or a vacuum bottle system (Figure 8.3a,b) until the volume of the recipient sac is normal.

The reported complication rates from large volume amnioreduction are quite variable. In single-center series the complication rate has ranged from 1.5% (3/200 procedures)[33] to 4.6% (8/174).[34] Multiple-center series have been associated with a tendency to increased complication rates, varying from 3.2% (9/281)[27] to 6% (46/760).[28]

a
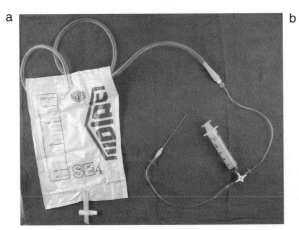

b
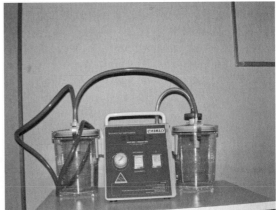

Figure 8.3 Two drainage systems in use for amnioreduction: (a) three-way tap and syringe closed system; (b) electronic vacuum aspiration system.

EFFICACY OF AMNIOREDUCTION AS A THERAPY IN TWIN–TWIN TRANSFUSION SYNDROME

Amnioreduction has been employed as a primary or adjunctive therapy in TTTS for two decades. As discussed previously, this technique does not alter the underlying pathophysiology of unbalanced vascular anastomoses in monochorionic–diamniotic twin placentation, but appears to prolong gestation by reducing intra-amniotic pressure and improving uteroplacental perfusion.

The available data on the efficacy of amnioreduction are based on two randomized controlled trials,[16,35] one cohort comparative study,[36] and many observational series of varying size and methodological quality.[3,7–9,11,27,28,34,37–48] The initial data on outcomes for TTTS were derived from non-controlled institutional observational studies. As the experience of any single institution is numerically small, there is marked heterogeneity within these series and inter-study comparisons are almost impossible to make. In general, these data focus on perinatal survival with scant attention paid to neonatal morbidity or long-term developmental outcomes. These small institutional observational studies have, however, demonstrated that amnioreduction offers a benefit compared to non-interventional strategies and have prompted the conduct of larger studies. There have been two large observational series of TTTS treated with amnioreduction strategies published.[27,28] The demography and outcomes of the pregnancies in these two registries was very similar, suggesting a fixed survival rate for amnioreduction strategies in TTTS (Table 8.1). The median gestation at diagnosis in each registry was 21 weeks and the median gestation at delivery 29 weeks, again emphasizing the very preterm delivery that characterizes amnioreduction as a therapy. Overall perinatal survival rates for TTTS treated with amnioreduction in two large observational studies has been approximately 60%.[27,28]

Two comparative cohort studies have been published comparing outcomes in non-randomized geographically separate populations treated with amnioreduction or placental laser techniques.[36,47] Although perinatal survival rates were comparable in both series between the techniques (Table 8.2), there was a significant increase in the gestation at delivery in pregnancies managed with placental laser ablation. This increase in gestation at delivery was reflected with an increased birthweight and lower incidence of abnormal neonatal brain scans in survivors.

There have been two randomized controlled clinical trials completed comparing amnioreduction with other techniques in TTTS.[16,35] A third randomized controlled trial comparing amnioreduction with placental laser ablation, sponsored by the NIH, was commenced in the USA but abandonded secondary to recruitment difficulties. The first published randomized controlled trial of antepartum interventions in TTTS was that of Senat et al[16] in 2004. This trial compared the perinatal outcomes of 142 pregnancies complicated with severe TTTS prior to 26 weeks' gestation in which cases were randomly allocated to amnioreduction or placental laser ablation. Most cases were stage II (43.7%) or III (47.2%) disease at randomization. Placental laser ablation was associated with a significant increase in at least one survivor at 6 months of age compared with serial amnioreduction (76% (55/72) vs 51% (36/70), $p = 0.002$). Dual survival at 6 months of age occurred in 36% of cases treated with placental laser and 26% of cases treated with serial amnioreduction. In 24% of placental laser cases and 49% of amnioreduction cases there were no survivors. There was a significantly lower incidence of neurological complications at 6 months

Study	Cases	Years	Gestation at diagnosis (weeks)	Gestation at delivery (weeks)	Perinatal survival (%)	Dual survivors (%)
Dickinson[27]	112	1995–98	21.5	29	62.5	48.4
Mari[28]	223	1990–98	21.5	29	60	52.7

Table 8.1 Twin–twin transfusion registries

Table 8.2 Comparative cohort series of amnioreduction and placental laser ablation therapies

Parameter	Technique	Hecher[47] (n = 116)	Quintero[36] (n = 173)
Gestation at diagnosis (weeks)	Amnioreduction	20.4	21.6
	Laser	20.7 (p = 0.438)	20.7 (p = 0.003)
Gestation at delivery (weeks)	Amnioreduction	30.7*	29
	Laser	33.7* (p = 0.018)	32 (p = 0.005)
Perinatal survival	Amnioreduction	51%	58.3%
	Laser	61% (p = 0.239)	65.8% (p = 0.26)
Dual perinatal survival	Amnioreduction	42%	48.7%
	Laser	42% (p = 1.0)	44.3% (p = 0.764)

* Includes only those pregnancies with liveborn babies.

of age in those infants treated with placental laser (48% vs 69%, placental laser vs amnioreduction, respectively, p = 0.003). Similarly, periventricular leukomalacia was observed less frequently in those surviving infants treated antenatally with placental laser (6% vs 14%, placental laser vs amnioreduction, respectively, p = 0.02).

When the data for cases randomized to amnioreduction in the Senat trial are scrutinized, there is one outstanding observation evident: how dismally amnioreduction performed as an intervention for TTTS. The outcomes for pregnancies randomized to amnioreduction are amongst the worst ever published. The performance of amnioreduction is even more concerning when scrutiny of the data demonstrates only one case in each treatment arm with stage IV disease. The reason for the amnioreduction outcome data is unclear and is most likely secondary to multiple phenomena such as pregnancy termination and individual research center management variations.

The second completed clinical trial compared amnioreduction with microseptostomy as primary therapeutic interventions for TTTS.[35] The study was concluded at the planned interim analysis after 73 women were enrolled. The survival of any fetus occurred in 78% of the pregnancies in the amnioreduction group vs 80% of pregnancies in the septostomy group (RR = 0.94, 95% CI 0.55, 1.61; p = 0.82). It is interesting to compare the difference in the perinatal outcomes of this clinical trial with those from the Senat trial amnioreduction arm outlined above. The birthweight of the donor fetus was greater in the

septostomy group as compared to the amnioreduction group (1291 ± 731 vs 996 ± 408 g; p = 0.02) despite a similar gestational age at delivery. Women undergoing septostomy were more likely to require a single procedure for treatment than the amnioreduction group (64% vs 46%, p = 0.04). However, these outcome data demonstrate a high incidence of very preterm delivery in both treatments arms, presumably as neither treatment option addresses the underlying placental pathology.

CONCLUSION

Amnioreduction was the first therapy to alter the universally dismal prognosis for severe TTTS. There is an increasing body of scientific evidence to support the use of placental laser ablation of the vascular anastomoses as a definitive therapy; however amnioreduction will remain as an adjunct to placental laser and possibly as a primary therapy for early-stage disease. It is clear that therapeutic options for TTTS will continue to evolve as medical knowledge of the pathophysiology increases.

REFERENCES

1. De Lia J, Emery MG, Sheafor SA, Jennison TA. Twin transfusion syndrome: successful in utero treatment with digoxin. Int J Gynaecol Obstet 1985; 23:197–201.
2. Jones JM, Sbarra AJ, Dilillo L, Cetrulo CL, D'Alton ME. Indomethacin in severe twin–twin transfusion syndrome. Am J Perinatol 1993; 10:24–6.

3. Weiner CP, Ludomirski A. Diagnosis, pathophysiology, and treatment of chronic twin-to-twin transfusion syndrome. Fetal Diagn Ther 1994; 9:283–90.

4. Urig MA, Simpson GF, Elliott JP, Clewell WH. Twin–twin transfusion syndrome: the surgical removal of one twin as a treatment option. Fetal Ther 1988; 3:185–8.

5. Deprest JA, Audibert F, Van Schoubroeck D, Hecher K, Mahieu-Caputo D. Bipolar coagulation of the umbilical cord in complicated monochorionic twin pregnancy. Am J Obstet Gynecol 2000; 182:340–5.

6. Taylor MJO, Shalev E, Tanawattanacharoen S et al. Ultrasound-guided umbilical cord occlusion using bipolar diathermy for Stage III/IV twin–twin transfusion syndrome. Prenat Diagn 2002; 22:70–6.

7. Mahony BS, Petty CN, Nyberg DA et al. The "stuck twin" phenomenon: ultrasonographic findings, pregnancy outcome, and management with serial amniocenteses. Am J Obstet Gynecol 1990; 163:1513–22.

8. Elliott JP, Urig MA, Clewell WH. Aggressive therapeutic amniocentesis for treatment of twin–twin transfusion syndrome. Obstet Gynecol 1991; 77:537–40.

9. Saunders NJ, Snijders RJM, Nicolaides KH. Therapeutic amniocentesis in twin–twin transfusion syndrome appearing in the second trimester of pregnancy. Am J Obstet Gynecol 1992; 166:820–4.

10. Saade GR, Belfort MA, Berry DL et al. Amniotic septostomy for the treatment of twin oligohydramnios–polyhydramnios sequence. Fetal Diagn Ther 1998; 13:86–93.

11. Hubinont C, Bernard P, Pirot N, Biard J-M, Donnez J. Twin-to-twin transfusion syndrome: treatment by amniodrainage and septostomy. Eur J Obstet Gynaecol Reprod Biol 2000; 92:141–4.

12. De Lia JE, Cruikshank DP, Keye WR Jr. Fetoscopic neodymium:YAG laser occlusion of placental vessels in severe twin–twin transfusion syndrome. Obstet Gynecol 1990; 75:1046–53.

13. Ville Y, Hyett J, Hecher K, Nicolaides K. Preliminary experience with endoscopic laser surgery for severe twin–twin transfusion syndrome. N Engl J Med 1995; 332:224–7.

14. Quintero RA, Comas C, Bornick PW, Allen MH, Kruger M. Selective versus non-selective laser photocoagulation of placental vessels in twin-to-twin transfusion syndrome. Ultrasound Obstet Gynecol 2000; 16:230–6.

15. Fisk NM, Galea P. Twin–twin transfusion – as good as it gets? N Engl J Med 2004; 351:182–4.

16. Senat MV, Deprest J, Boulvain M et al. Endoscopic laser surgery versus serial amnioreduction for severe twin-to-twin transfusion syndrome. N Engl J Med 2004; 351:136–44.

17. van Gemert MJ, Umur A, Tijssen JG, Ross MG. Twin–twin transfusion syndrome: etiology, severity and rational management. Curr Opin Obstet Gynecol 2001; 13:193–206.

18. Jain V, Fisk NM. The twin–twin transfusion syndrome. Clin Obstet Gynecol 2004; 47:181–202.

19. Fisk NM, Ronderos-Dumit D, Tannirandorn Y, et al. Normal amniotic pressure throughout gestation. Br J Obstet Gynaecol 1992; 99:18–22.

20. Fisk NM, Tannirandorn Y, Nicolini U, Talbert DG, Rodeck CH. Amniotic pressure in disorders of amniotic fluid volume. Obstet Gynecol 1990; 76:210–14.

21. Garry D, Lysikiewicz A, Mays J, Canterino J, Tejani N. Intra-amniotic pressure reduction in twin–twin transfusion syndrome. J Perinatol 1998; 18:284–6.

22. Fisk NM, Vaughan J, Talbert D. Impaired fetal blood gas status in polyhydramnios and its relation to raised amniotic pressure. Fetal Diagn Ther 1994; 9:7–13.

23. Greiss FC Jr. A clinical concept of uterine blood flow during pregnancy. Obstet Gynecol 1967; 30:595–604.

24. Skillman CA, Plessinger MA, Woods JR, Clark KE. Effect of graded reductions in uteroplacental blood flow on the fetal lamb. Am J Physiol 1985; 249:H1098–105.

25. Bower SJ, Flack NJ, Sepulveda W, Talbert DG, Fisk NM. Uterine artery blood flow response to correction of amniotic fluid volume. Am J Obstet Gynecol 1995; 173: 502–7.

26. Guzman ER, Vintzileos A, Benito C et al. Effects of therapeutic amniocentesis on uterine and umbilical artery velocimetry in cases of severe symptomatic polyhydramnios. J Mat Fetal Med 1996; 5:299–304.

27. Dickinson JE, Evans SF. Obstetric and perinatal outcomes from the Australian and New Zealand twin–twin transfusion syndrome registry. Am J Obstet Gynecol 2000; 182:706–12.

28. Mari G, Roberts A, Detti L et al. Perinatal morbidity and mortality rates in severe twin–twin transfusion syndrome: results of the international amnioreduction registry. Am J Obstet Gynecol 2001; 185:708–15.

29. De Lia J, Fisk N, Hecher K et al. Twin-to-twin transfusion syndrome – debates on the etiology, natural history and management. Ultrasound Obstet Gynecol 2000; 16:210–13.

30. Dolinger MB, Donnenfeld AE. Therapeutic amniocentesis using a vacuum bottle aspiration system. Obstet Gynecol 1998; 91:143–4.

31. Denbow ML, Sepulveda W, Ridout D, Fisk NM. Relationship between change in amniotic fluid index and volume of fluid removed at amnioreduction. Obstet Gynecol 1997; 90:529–32.

32. Abdel-Fattah SA, Carroll SG, Kyle PM, Soothill PW. Amnioreduction: How much to drain? Fetal Diagn Ther 1999; 14:279–82.

33. Elliott JP, Sawyer AT, Radin TG, String RE. Large-volume therapeutic amniocentesis in the treatment of hydramnios. Obstet Gynecol 1994; 84:1025–7.

34. Duncombe GJ, Dickinson JE, Evans SF. Perinatal characteristics and outcomes of pregnancies complicated by twin–twin transfusion syndrome. Obstet Gynecol 2003; 101:1190–6.

35. Moise KJ, Dorman K, Lamvu G et al. A randomized trial of amnioreduction versus septostomy in the treatment of twin–twin transfusion syndrome. Am J Obstet Gynecol 2005; 193:701–7.

36. Quintero RA, Dickinson JE, Morales WJ et al. Stage-based treatment of twin–twin transfusion syndrome. Am J Obstet Gynecol 2003; 188(5):1333–40.

37. Bebbington MW, Wittmann BK. Fetal transfusion syndrome: antenatal factors predicting outcome. Am J Obstet Gynecol 1989; 160:913–15.

38. Urig MA, Clewell WH, Elliott JP. Twin–twin transfusion syndrome. Am J Obstet Gynecol 1990; 163:1522–6.

39. Rådestad A, Thomassen PA. Acute polyhydramnios in twin pregnancy. A retrospective study with special reference to therapeutic amniocentesis. Acta Obstet Gynecol Scand 1990; 69:297–300.

40. Gonsoulin W, Moise KJ, Kirshon B et al. Outcome of twin–twin transfusion syndrome diagnosed before 28 weeks of gestation. Obstet Gynecol 1990; 75:214–16.

41. Pinette MG, Pan Y, Pinette SG, Stubblefield PG. Treatment of twin–twin transfusion syndrome. Obstet Gynecol 1993; 82:841–6.

42. Bruner JP, Rosemond RL. Twin-to-twin transfusion syndrome: a subset of the twin oligohydramnios–polyhydramnios sequence. Am J Obstet Gynecol 1993; 169:925–30.

43. Cincotta R, Oldham J, Sampson A. Antepartum and postpartum complications of twin–twin transfusion syndrome. Aust NZ J Obstet Gynaecol 1996; 36:303–8.

44. Trespidi L, Boschetto C, Caravelli E et al. Serial amniocenteses in the management of twin–twin transfusion syndrome: when is it valuable? Fetal Diagn Ther 1997; 12:15–20.

45. Dennis LG, Winkler CL. Twin-to-twin transfusion syndrome: aggressive therapeutic amniocentesis. Am J Obstet Gynecol 1997; 177:342–349.

46. Kilby MD, Howe DT, McHugo JM, Whittle MJ. Bladder visualization as a prognostic sign in oligohydramnios–polyhydramnios sequence in twin pregnancies treated using therapeutic amniocentesis. Br J Obstet Gynaecol 1997; 104:939–42.

47. Hecher K, Plath H, Bregenzer T, Hansmann M, Hackeloer BJ. Endoscopic laser surgery versus serial amniocentesis in the treatment of severe twin–twin transfusion syndrome. Am J Obstet Gynecol 1999; 180: 717–24.

48. Johnsen SL, Albrechtsen S, Pirhonen J. Twin–twin transfusion syndrome treated with serial amniocenteses. Acta Obstet Gynecol Scand 2004; 83:326–9.

9

Laser treatment for twin–twin transfusion syndrome

Rubén A Quintero

History • Technical aspects • Special technical considerations • Conclusion

HISTORY

The fundamental principle behind the laser treatment of twin–twin transfusion syndrome (TTTS) consists of interrupting the vascular anastomoses that allow blood exchange between the fetuses and thus eliminating the intertwin transfusion process. The surgical technique assumes that all placental vascular anastomoses can be identified and obliterated. Neodynium:YAG laser photocoagulation of placental vascular anastomoses was first proposed by De Lia in the late 1980s.[1] The approach involved performing a limited laparotomy, placement of a purse string in the myometrium, and introduction of a trocar and endoscope to perform fetoscopy. Unfortunately, a description of the actual technique to identify the placental vascular anastomoses was never provided. Instead, vessels that appeared 'suspicious' for being anastomoses were targeted.[2] Thus, a reproducible surgical technique to obliterate all placental vascular anastomoses was lacking. In 1995, Ville et al reported their preliminary experience with laser treatment for TTTS. In their technique, all vessels crossing the dividing membrane were targeted.[3] The technique assumed that all vessels crossing the dividing membrane were placental anastomoses, which is indeed the case in many patients. However, many non-anastomotic vessels could cross the dividing membrane and thus be potentially targeted. Under normal circumstances, the anatomical location of

the dividing membrane on the surface of placenta bears little relationship to the location of the vascular equator. In the case of TTTS, the dividing membrane could potentially be displaced even more towards the sac of the donor twin, thus exposing more normal vessels of this fetus. Photocoagulation of all vessels crossing the membrane, while effectively interrupting the vascular communications between the two fetuses, could also increase the likelihood of injury or death of the donor twin (typically) or the recipient twin by targeting vessels not involved in the syndrome but critical to the survival of the fetuses.

In 1998, I developed a surgical technique based on precise endoscopic identification of the vascular anastomoses between the fetuses. I dubbed this technique 'selective laser photocoagulation of communicating vessels, or SLPCV', in contradistinction to the previous non-selective technique.[4] Briefly, deep arteriovenous (AV) communications are identified on the surface of the placenta by noting that the terminal end of the artery from one of the fetuses does not have a corresponding returning vein to the same fetus. Instead, the returning vein travels to the other twin. A systematic analysis at the vascular equator of the placenta discloses deep AV communications from donor to recipient. A deep AV communication from donor to recipient is identified if the artery originates in the donor twin (AVDRs), or from recipient to donor, if the artery originates in the recipient twin (AVRDs), regardless of the location of the dividing membrane. Superficial arterioarterial or venovenous communications (AA, VV) are easily identified as vessels that do not have a terminal end in the placenta, but rather continue their course from one umbilical cord to the other. Patients treated with SLPCV compared favorably with those treated with the non-selective technique.[5] While some centers may still use a non-selective approach to photocoagulate all vascular anastomoses, SLPCV has essentially become the standard technique in most institutions.

TECHNICAL ASPECTS

Successful surgical treatment of TTTS is intimately dependent on the surgical technique as well as the proper technology and instrumentation. The following sections will address the technical aspects involved.

The working environment: fluid or gas

Ideally, surgery within the amniotic cavity would be performed under a gas environment, as in standard laparoscopy. Indeed, visualization within gas is superior to that within fluid, both in terms of light transmission as well as in the angle of view which is reduced by 30% in water. Working within gas would also be advantageous should bleeding in the amniotic cavity occur. Work within gas would also allow the use of electrosurgery, CO_2 laser and other standard surgical techniques. Carbon dioxide is the most widely used gas in laparoscopy because it does not support combustion and dissolves readily in the patient's blood. However, the use of CO_2 in the pregnant ewe results in fetal acidosis after 30 minutes.[6] Presumably, fetuses are unable to clear the CO_2 into the maternal circulation fast enough to avoid lowering of their pH. It is not known whether a similar complication would occur in humans given the differences in placentation. Pelletier et al tested Xenon and CO_2 in sheep, and did not show development of fetal acidosis with the former.[7] In our lab, nitrous oxide did not result in fetal acidosis (unpublished). However, nitrous oxide allows combustion, which is obviously not desirable. Therefore, only CO_2 is a viable candidate for gas medium during fetoscopy.

Unfortunately, gas within the amniotic cavity interferes with ultrasound imaging. This limitation could be overcome if adequate endoscopic visualization allowed dispensing the use of ultrasound for a short period of time. However, gas instillation may limit adequate monitoring of the fetus and of the procedure. Furthermore, gas may dissect the membranes from the uterine wall, resulting in collapse of the amniotic cavity. Lastly, evacuation of the gas from the amniotic cavity may be difficult, and small bubbles may persist at the level of the anterior uterine wall, hampering ultrasound visualization with ultrasound.

Despite the above, we have found a very limited application of working within a gas environment in TTTS, specifically, in patients with an anterior placenta and turbid amniotic fluid from prior or intraoperative bleeding. In these cases, a small bubble of air can be used to identify vascular anastomoses otherwise not visible through the turbid fluid. The bubble can be placed beneath the anastomoses with lateral tilting of the operating table. The endoscope is then placed in the gas/water interface and the vessels lasered within the gas bubble (Figure 9.1). This small surgical tip may allow completion of an otherwise very difficult surgery.

Amniotic fluid exchange

The amniotic cavity may be turbid, particularly with advancing gestational age. Visualization may be further hindered by bloody discoloration from previous procedures such as amniocenteses or cordocenteses, from intraoperative intraamniotic bleeding, or from excessive vernix. Light transmission in these settings can be significantly compromised. To overcome this problem, we have developed techniques to exchange the amniotic fluid with Ringer's lactate or 0.9 saline solution. One technique uses a custom-designed suction–irrigation probe or 'trumpet' (Figure 9.2) that is inserted through the trocar under ultrasound guidance and directed to a pocket of amniotic fluid. Fluid is retrieved in amounts of 300–500 ml at a time, and substituted with physiological solution. The quality of the remaining fluid can be assessed through the clear suction tubing. Amniotic fluid exchange can also be performed

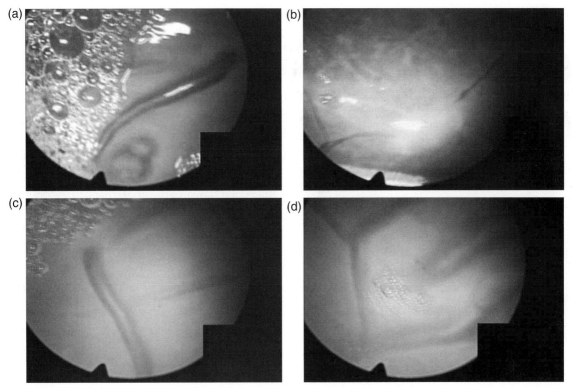

Figure 9.1 Vessels (a) and a lasered anastomosis (b) are clearly visualized within an air bubble. Anastomoses are difficult if not impossible to visualize through discolored amniotic fluid with debris from previous procedures (c and d). (See also color plate section, page xxviii.)

simultaneously by infusion of fluid through the trumpet and suctioning through the shaft of the trocar via a side-port. A third technique uses infusion of fluid through the operating channel of the endoscope and suctioning through the trocar

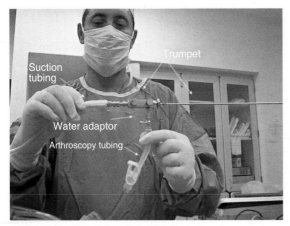

Figure 9.2 Irrigation trumpet. (See also color plate section, page xiii.)

(Figure 9.3a,b). Once the fluid has become clear, the endoscopic procedure can continue. These amniotic fluid exchange systems can clear the amniotic fluid at a maximum rate of 2250 ml/min without altering the total amniotic fluid volume. Despite the speed, up to 45 minutes may be required to clear a bloody discolored amniotic fluid cavity from previous invasive procedures, or from intraoperative bleeding.

Precise knowledge of the amount of fluid infused or drained can be obtained with the use of special infusion pumps. We currently use the arthroscopic pump made by Davol (Davol, Cranston, RI) (Figure 9.4a,b). This pump has a digital display of the fluid balance, which the surgeon can readily see. The calculation of the balance is based on the weight of the fluid on the stand of the pump. Inaccurate estimates may occur due to fluid leakage through the trocar. Fluid infusion is also based on the sonographic appearance of the amniotic cavity, which

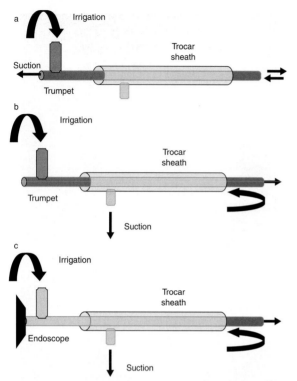

Figure 9.3 (a) Infusion and suction done through the trumpet. (b) Infusion through the trumpet; suction via a side-port of the trocar. (c) Infusion through the operating channel of the operating endoscope and suction via a side-port of the trocar.

provides an overall sense of the amount of fluid present.

Endoscopes

Although some endoscopes were specifically designed for fetoscopy in the 1970s, all endoscopes currently used are either custom-made or adaptations from other surgical specialties. Familiarity with technological aspects of the endoscopes is important in order to understand their capabilities and limitations. The endoscope has two fundamental systems: a light bundle that carries light to the tip of the endoscope, and the optic pathway which carries back the image under observation. The light bundle can be located at the periphery of the scope, but several other arrangements are also possible. Transmission of the image from the object to the eyepiece can be performed in three basic ways: fiberoptics, solid rod lens, or multiple lens.

Fiberoptics

Fiberoptic endoscopes use the internal reflection properties of certain materials, such as glass, to propagate light along a fiber. This property is based on the angle of incidence of light on the glass. By adjusting the angle, the light ray can be made to bounce within the fiber until it emerges at the other end. The endoscope is made using a tightly packed bundle of such fibers (collimation). Some of the fibers are used to transmit the light from the light source, while the rest are optical fibers that transmit the image back to the operator. Fiberoptic endoscopes are typically flexible, and are commonly used in the gastrointestinal and pulmonary tract, as well as in cardiovascular surgery. The larger the number of fibers, the clearer the image is. Advances in the collimation process allow more fibers to be packed together, with less intervening collimation material, therefore providing an improved image without increasing the outer diameter of the instrument.

Flexible endoscopes can be particularly useful in the treatment of patients with anterior placentas.[9] The endoscope must be both flexible and steerable, and have a working channel. It is important for the surgeon to know the angle of flexion of the endoscope (with and without a laser fiber) within the operating channel, to understand the capabilities of the instrument (Figure 9.5). Although visualization is not nearly as good as with rigid endoscopes, flexible endoscopes may play an important role in selected patients with anterior placentas.

Self-focusing rod lens

This technology also uses the reflective properties of glass or other materials to transmit light along a fiber of such material. However, in contrast to the fiberoptic endoscope in which the rays emerge at different points of the end surface of the fiber, the solid rod lens has the ability to focus the incident rays on a plane to provide an image. Solid rod lenses, to our knowledge, are not available with a diameter of less than 1.5 mm.

Multilens endoscopes

Ringleb and von Rohr in 1908 first developed endoscopes that included multiple lenses within

a

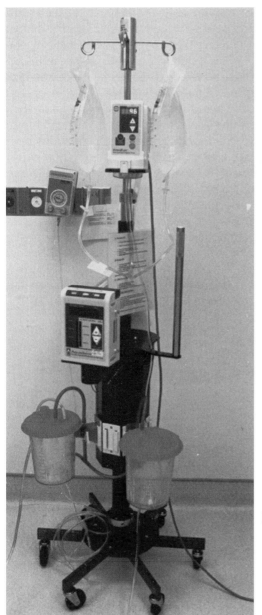

Figure 9.4 (a) Davol pump to infuse fluid with Aquasens to measure net balance of fluid. (b) From left to right, irrigation canisters showing dark, bloody fluid originally found upon entry into amniotic cavity from prior therapeutic amniocenteses and the less bloody fluid after amnioexchange. (Figure 9.4(a) has been reproduced with permission from[8].)

b

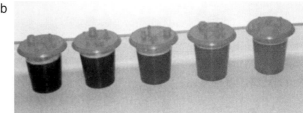

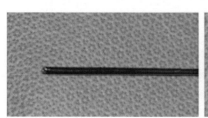 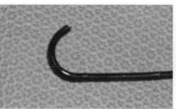 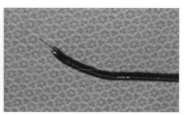

Figure 9.5 Left to right: tip of flexible endoscope straight, flexed without fiber, and flexed with fiber.

the shaft of the endoscope. The advantage of this system over the single lens optics of prior endoscopes was an improvement in the brightness, higher magnification, and an erect image. The space between the lenses was air. The lenses were spaced throughout the shaft of the endoscope according to their focal length. In 1959, the English physicist Hopkins designed an endoscope that replaced the air spaces with glass rods, and the lenses were replaced by annular spacers. The optical effect of the glass rod is to shorten the length of the optical path, which results in a higher angle of aperture and brighter relay-lens systems (Figure 9.6a). The lenses could be eliminated altogether by making glass rods with optical surfaces (Panoview endoscope). These endoscopes provide the best image available, and should be preferentially used.

In addition to their different optical properties, endoscopes also vary in their length, diameter, and whether they are purely diagnostic or operative. After testing different diameter endoscopes, we have settled on diagnostic and operative endoscopes 3.3 mm in diameter. Because operating endoscopes must sacrifice optical space for the operating or irrigation channel, they will typically have less resolution than diagnostic endoscopes of similar caliber. Therefore, we often combine diagnostic and operating endoscopes during surgery. The length of the endoscope is also critical. Because patients with TTTS may have different degrees of polyhydramnios, and because access to the amniotic cavity may be hindered by placental location, the ideal endoscope should span the entire length of the uterine cavity. Figure 9.6b shows our current set of diagnostic and operating endoscopes.

a
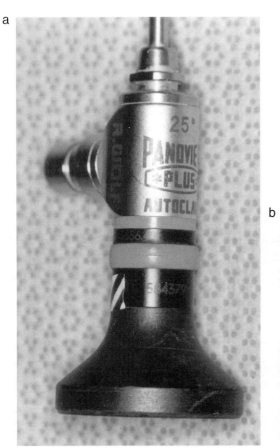

b
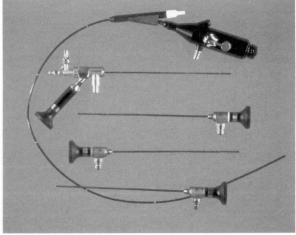

Figure 9.6 (a) Hopkins endoscope. (b) Fetal diagnostic and operating endoscopes. (Reproduced with permission from[8].)

Laser source

The physical characteristics of the Nd:YAG laser make it particularly suitable for use within the amniotic cavity and for coagulation of blood vessels. The CO_2 laser (wavelength 10 600 nm), which is the most commonly used laser in gynecology, is highly absorbed by water.[10] Thus, it cannot be used within the amniotic fluid. In contrast, the Nd:YAG laser (wavelength 1064 nm) can transmit energy through clear fluid. The laser is a solid crystal of yttrium–aluminum–garnet (YAG) that contains a dopant of the rare earth element of neodymium (Nd), which actually makes the light. When applied through a bare fiber, the Nd:YAG causes deep tissue coagulation. Protein coagulation of 1–2 mm can be achieved with a power of 20 watts for 1–3 seconds. The pure color aspect of the laser is only marginally important, because it is heat that determines the surgical effect. However, color specificity of lasers facilitates its effect on target tissue (hemoglobin-containing tissue) while sparing adjacent normal tissues. Most of the desired effect can be achieved with 15–30 watts, but occasionally a power as high as 40 watts may be necessary, particularly with larger blood vessels. The greater the blood flow through a vessel, the more it acts as a heat sink, and the greater the difficulty in achieving hemostasis.[11] Diode lasers (wavelength 980 nm) have also been recently used in TTTS and can also deliver energy within a fluid environment. They are typically less costly and less bulky, but may be limited in terms of the amount of energy they can provide (Figure 9.7a,b).

The Nd:YAG laser energy is delivered into the amniotic cavity by means of quartz fibers 400–600 μm in diameter. The fibers allow the beam to diverge 10–15° once emitted from the tip of the naked fiber, so the beam is no longer collimated. Thus, the smallest spot occurs at the tip and continuously enlarges as the fiber tip is moved away from the target. The fiber tip is typically placed within 1 cm of the target vessels for maximum safe effect.[10] Most laser fibers are end-firing. However, side-firing laser fibers, such as those used in urology, can be particularly useful in the treatment of patients with anterior placentas. Side-firing laser fibers are of a larger diameter such that they cannot be used through the operating channel of the current endoscope. Instead, they must be inserted in the amniotic cavity through an accessory port (Figure 9.8a,b).

Endoscopic monitoring of the coagulation effect is based on the known visual properties of proteins under different temperature conditions:

- at 60–65° C, blanching of the vessel occurs, which is indicative of adequate coagulation
- at 65–90° C, the tissue turns white-gray, indicative of protein denaturation
- at 90–100° C, puckering of the tissue occurs, consistent with drying of the tissue,
- finally, at 100° C, vaporization and carbonization of the tissue occurs.[9]

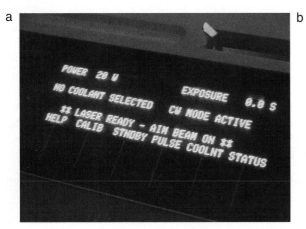
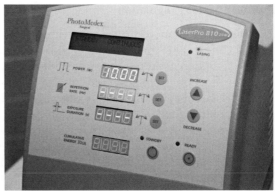

Figure 9.7 (a) Nd:YAG laser panel. (b) Diode laser.

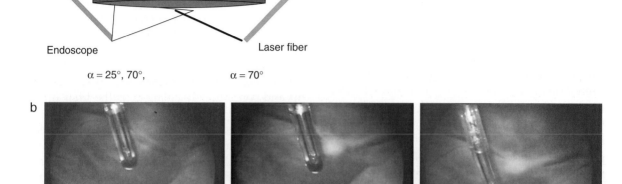

Figure 9.8 (a) Schematic drawing of angled endoscope, side-firing laser fiber, and anterior placenta. (b) Endoscopic view of side-firing laser fiber. (See also color plate section, page xxv.)

Accessory instruments

Accessory ports (2 mm) and blunt probes can be particularly useful under specific circumstances. Accessory ports may be required to pass side-firing laser fibers or blunt probes to complete surgery in some patients with anterior placentas. Blunt probes may be used to displace the donor twin to allow visualization of vascular anastomoses that may be blocked by this fetus. Although not often used, these accessory instruments may be critical in the completion of surgery in certain patients.

Pressure/volume regulation

The typical amniotic fluid pressure in patients with TTTS is 10–15 mmHg.[12] It is also known that the amniotic fluid pressure rises linearly by 1 mmHg/L of physiological fluid infused.[13] This is inconsequential in TTTS, as patients where exchange of the amniotic fluid is necessary due to bloody or vernix discoloration of the fluid rarely receive 1000 ml without being exchanged. More commonly, an even exchange of amniotic fluid can be performed through the trocar and trumpet as described above. Therefore, it is not necessary to monitor amniotic fluid pressure during surgery for TTTS.

Length of instruments

Adequate length of the trocar, endoscopes, and working instruments is paramount. In addition, the relationship between trocar length and endoscope length may vary between product companies. In one system, the endoscope and trocar are flushed at the tip, with a locking mechanism at the back end to prevent loss of fluid (hysteroscopic model). This system requires that the trocar and endoscope complex be moved back and forth within the amniotic cavity to reach the different vessels. In the endoscopes designed by Quintero (laparoscopic model), trocar length is always smaller than endoscope length. Fluid loss is prevented by a checkflow valve within the lumen of the trocar. The greater length of the endoscope allows surgery to be performed with decreased friction of the trocar against the membranes, as the trocar does not need to be advanced or retrieved within the amniotic cavity during the procedure. Endoscope length is critical for the adequate completion of the surgery. Ideally, the endoscope should span the entire amniotic cavity to reach all anastomoses, regardless of the point of entry into the amniotic cavity. Since fundal height can be as large as 40 cm in patients with TTTS, we have designed our endoscopes to reach that length. The trocar sleeve is approximately 4 cm shorter than the endoscope to allow freedom of the scope, but not much smaller, as it may be needed for assistance during surgery (see below).

Basic operating room setup

The operating room setup is the basic operative fetoscopy arrangement originally described by us.[14] Basically, the setup involves the use of ultrasound imaging, endoscopic imaging, and a laser equipment. In the United States, the ultrasound machine is placed to the right of the patient, as most sonographers are accustomed to scanning with their right hand, facing the patient. An endoscopic tower is also placed on the right side of the patient, more distally, to allow viewing of the surgery across the patient from the left side. An additional monitor is placed on the left side of the patient (slave monitor). Additional slave monitors may be used to allow viewing of the procedure from any angle of the operating room, as well as a dedicated monitor for the patient. The laser machine is placed on the left side of the patient. The patient is typically placed in decubitus. Occasionally, the dorsolithotomy position is used for patients with difficult access to an anterior placenta.

Ultrasound machine

A high-resolution ultrasound machine is used during laser surgery. A 2D 3.5 MHz transducer is preferred, as it provides adequate image quality and weighs less than the 3D counterparts. Draping of the ultrasound transducer is done first with a CIVCO cover (CIVCO Medical Instruments, Kalona, IO), followed by a standard laparoscopy camera drape (Advanced Medical Designs, Marietta, GA). The sonographer is gowned and gloved and has contact with the transducer with her right hand on the patient. The left hand of the sonographer is placed on the controls of the machine and never reaches the operating field. Sterile covers for the keyboard of the ultrasound machine have proven cumbersome and unnecessary.

Endoscopy

Endoscopic viewing is provided by a three-chip digital endoscopic camera, a 300 Watt Xenon light source, and a high-resolution monitor with Super VHS and DVD connection. The camera and light cord can be sterilized and brought across the operating field. Non-sterile cameras can be draped with a special sterile laparoscopy sheath and coupler. We normally use two cameras, one for the diagnostic endoscope and one for the operating endoscope. This arrangement cuts down on the operating time and helps maintain sterility.

Videomixing

The combination of endoscopy and ultrasound is best done with the help of a videomixer. This machine allows two or more imaging inputs, and can display them on a monitor separately or in combination (picture-in-picture). The mixer is placed within the endoscopic tower in one of the available shelves.

Laser machine

The laser machine is placed on the left side of the patient, next to the left endoscopy tower. The machine is operated by a laser-certified nurse. The laser fiber is passed from the operating field to the laser machine and is prevented from unwinding by attaching it to the light cord and camera cable with plastic clips. The laser fiber can be fed through the operating endoscope prior to entering the amniotic cavity to save on operating time. Activation of the laser energy is done via a pedal placed at the foot of the operator. The delivery is normally set to continuous mode, where the laser energy is transmitted via the fiber as long as the pedal is pressed. The machine is typically set at 15–20 watts, which may be increased up to 40 watts, depending on vessel size.

Patient positioning, prepping, and draping

Chapter 15 discusses in detail the operating room preparation of the patient. The patient is placed in the decubitus position. A left or right lateral tilt may be required if the patient develops hypotension from caval compression. The dorsolithotomy position is chosen in selected cases to avoid an anterior placenta and if no access from the right or the left side of the patient is available. A Foley catheter is placed in the bladder. The patient is then fully prepped and draped as for any major surgery.

Anesthesia

Chapter 18 discusses in detail our experience with general and local anesthesia. Most centers today use local anesthesia in the form of 1% lidocaine without epinephrine. A 10 ml syringe with a 21-gauge $1^1/_2$ inch needle is used. The skin is infiltrated to create a wheal. The needle is then inserted under ultrasound guidance to infiltrate the tissues to the level of the uterine serosa.

Trocar entry

In standard laparoscopy, the trocar insertion sites have been extensively worked out to avoid injury to the superficial epigastric vessels. In contrast, the site of entry into the amniotic cavity of the recipient twin will vary from patient to patient. The site of entry is chosen after careful preoperative mapping (Chapter 7) to avoid injury to the dividing membrane or the placenta. Injury to the superficial epigastric vessels is avoided by placing the trocar either at the midline or 8 cm lateral from the midline.[15] Power angio Doppler insonation of the myometrium under the proposed site of entry may disclose important vessels that need to be avoided (Figure 9.9).

A minimal skin incision is made at the chosen site using a No. 11 scalpel blade. It is important not to advance the scalpel blade too deep, as injury to the myometrium could occur, particularly in very thin patients.

The insertion of the trocar is done under ultrasound guidance. The resistance of the rectus sheath can be felt. Once the fascia is overcome, the trocar is advanced up to the level of the myometrium, without entering the amniotic cavity yet. Again, care is taken not to injure any obvious myometrial vessels that may be apparent on power angio imaging. The amniotic cavity of the recipient twin is then entered in a swift fashion, to avoid dragging of the membrane. If the patient has not had genetic testing, the first few milliliters of fluid are discarded and an amniotic sample of 20–30 ml is obtained for karyotypic analysis. If a genetic amniocentesis or a therapeutic amniocentesis has been previously performed, a sample of amniotic fluid is sent for microbiological analysis.

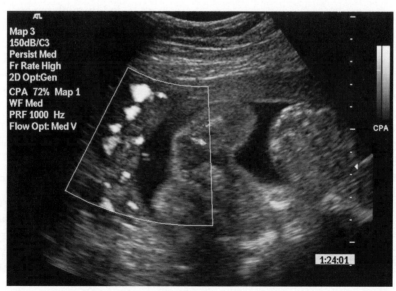

Figure 9.9 Ultrasound power angio image of the myometrium with vessels. Reproduced courtesy of Fung Yee Chan MD, Mater Mother's Hospital, Brisbane, Australia.

Selective laser photocoagulation of communicating vessels

There are three steps in performing selective laser photocoagulation of communicating vessels (SLPCV). The first step is a diagnostic one, which consists of the identification of all of the anastomoses, differentiating them from individually perfused areas of the placenta (diagnostic fetoscopy step). The second step consists in the actual lasering of the anastomoses. The third step involves reviewing all of the lasered anastomoses and relasering if necessary, as well as endoscopic review of any other important aspects of the amniotic cavity or fetuses.

Step 1: diagnostic fetoscopy

A diagnostic endoscope is inserted into the amniotic cavity through the trocar sheath and directed towards the placenta. Arteries are identified endoscopically as they cross over veins, and may also have a darker hue. By definition, the vascular equator lies at the terminal end of the communicating vessels. A systematic documentation of all vascular anastomoses is done first. Deep vascular anastomoses are easily identified by noting that the perfusing artery and vein belong to different fetuses. In some cases, it may be necessary to follow the artery or the vein back to the umbilical cord of the corresponding twin to confirm the alternate origin of the vessels. As mentioned in Chapter 5, deep communications may involve a single artery and vein from each twin (simple AV anastomosis), or a three-vessel or four-vessel cotyledon (Figure 9.10 a–c). In a three-vessel cotyledon, one twin has an artery and vein perfusing the cotyledon, while a third vessel, either an artery or vein from the other twin, is also involved. In a four-vessel cotyledon, both fetuses perfuse a common cotyledon with an

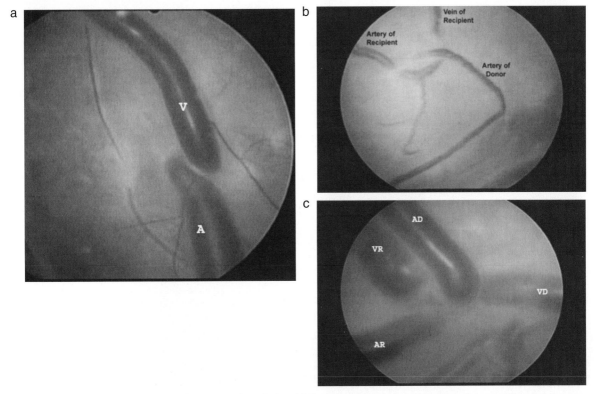

Figure 9.10 (a) Simple cotyledon. (b) Three-vessel cotyledon. (c) Four-vessel cotyledon. AD, artery of donor; VD, vein of donor; AR, artery of recipient; VR, vein of recipient.

artery and a vein of each. Deep anastomoses are classified as AVDR if the artery corresponds to the donor twin, or AVRD if the artery belongs to the recipient twin. The size of the anastomoses ('hair', small, medium, large, or very large) is also noted. Superficial anastomoses are identified as being arterioarterial (AA) or venovenous (VV) (Figures 9.11a,b), and can be easily seen running uninterrupted between the two fetal circulations. AA anastomoses are more easily detected, as they cross over veins. Superficial anastomoses may be branched or unbranched.[16] Typically, the direction of flow in VV anastomoses cannot be determined endoscopically. AA anastomoses may behave as functional AVDRs or AVRDs, depending on where blood drains (to a vein of the donor or to a vein of the recipient twin, respectively), but can only be seen endoscopically if a significant color difference exists between the two arterial circulations. Once all the anastomoses are documented, the diagnostic endoscope is removed and exchanged for the operating endoscope. In cases where surgery needs to proceed expeditiously, the diagnostic step is undertaken with the operating endoscope and the anastomoses are lasered as they are found.

Step 2: laser photocoagulation of the communicating vessels

The operating endoscope is loaded with the YAG laser fiber. The fiber is kept inside the operating

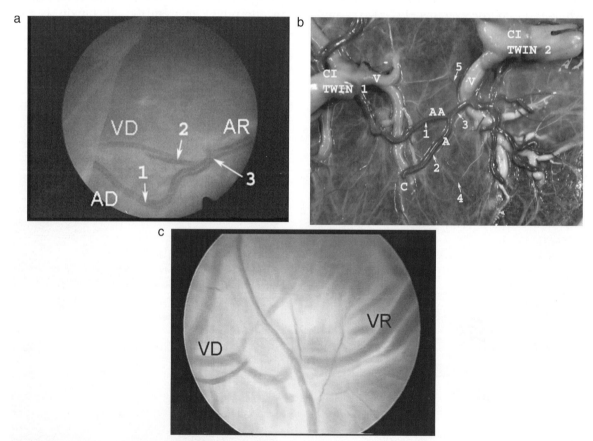

Figure 9.11 (a) Artery to artery anastomosis. (VD = vein of donor; AR = artery of recipient; AD = artery of donor; VR, vein of recipient numbers 1 to 3 denote potential laser sites.) (b) A large artery to artery (AA) anastomosis. Note that the vessel crosses over a large vein (V) of each twin. Effective interruption of the blood flow exchange with maximum preservation of placental tissue is discussed in the text. (CI=cord insertion; numbers 1 to 5 = potential laser sites; C=cotyledon.) (c) Vein to vein anastomosis. (Figures 9.11(a) and (c) reproduced with permission from[17]. Figure 9.11b reproduced courtesy of Enrico Lopriore MD, Leiden University Medical Center, The Netherlands.)

channel to prevent fetal or placental injury upon insertion of the operating endoscope into the amniotic cavity. The YAG laser machine is typically set at 15–20 watts. For large vessels, 25–30 watts may be necessary. The endoscope is placed over the target vessel, and the laser fiber is advanced beyond the tip of the endoscope, enough to see the junction of the laser fiber tip and the fiber. The site of photocoagulation is chosen, close to the terminal end of the vessel. The vessel is then photocoagulated by applying the energy on to the center of the width of the vessel. If the vessel is deemed large or very large, aiming the laser energy at the center may not be advisable, as it may result in rupture of the vessel and bleeding. Instead, the laser energy is directed to the edges of the vessel ('inching technique'), until the whole width of the vessel is obliterated (Figure 9.12). Lasering should be continued until the vessel is completely blanched out. Because the laser is used in continuous mode, the surgeon must decide when to stop firing to avoid perforation of the vessel. Since the only way to gauge effect is through endoscopy, a practical way to avoid vessel rupture is to stop coagulating once a blanching effect is seen. We refer to this technical tip as 'effect-stop'. The vessel is reassessed, and the photocoagulation process continued until the entire vessel diameter has been obliterated. The process is repeated for each anastomosis, until all the communications have been interrupted.

The sequence in which the vessels are lasered depends on how smoothly surgery has proceeded until this point. If bleeding from the anterior uterine wall has not occurred, particularly with movement of the endoscope within the cavity, the anastomoses may be lasered in the same sequence as they were identified. If bleeding is associated with movements of the endoscope, the anastomoses are lasered in reverse sequence as they were identified, thus moving the endoscope the least. If bleeding occurs as soon as the trocar has been inserted and continues despite corrective maneuvers, the anastomoses are lasered as they are identified without prior diagnostic fetoscopy.

Lasering of AV anastomoses

AV anastomoses can be interrupted by lasering the artery, the vein, or both. In theory, lasering of the vein still allows for blood to be lost into the cotyledon, and may be responsible for development of intraoperative fetal anemia. Therefore, when possible, we prefer to laser the artery first. Most placentas will have both AVDRs and AVRDs. Whenever possible, we prefer to laser AVDRs first followed by AVRDs, as this may allow for an intraoperative transfusion of the donor twin (sequential technique, or SQLPCV).

Lasering of superficial anastomoses

Lasering of AA and VV anastomoses requires that the surgeon decide where, along the path of the vessel, the interruption needs to be made

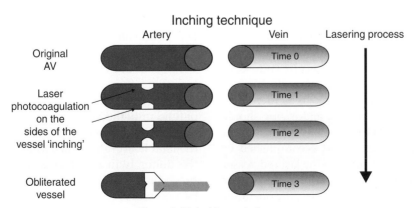

Figure 9.12 Inching technique.

(Figure 9.11a and b). This is based on the principle of maximum preservation of placental territory for both twins, as determined by the location of the draining or feeding branches (AA and VV, respectively). Figure 9.11a shows an AA anastomosis with an arterial branch to the donor twin. Effective interruption of the vascular communication could be achieved in different ways: a) Lasering at sites 1 and 2. This eliminates all blood exchange at this level. However, it deprives the donor twin from a cotyledon. b) Lasering at site 3. This interrupts the AA anastomosis and allows the donor twin perfuse the placenta at site 2. Figure 9.11b also shows a complex AA anastomosis. Interruption of the blood exchange through this vessel could be accomplished by a) Lasering at site 1 and 2. This choice significantly hinders the ability of twin 1 to perfuse the cotyledon (C). b) Lasering at site 3, while technically more challenging, (it is very close to the branching of the AA and to the underlying vein of twin 2) preserves the cotyledon (C) for twin 1. Separation would be completed by lasering at sites 4 and 5. Occasionally, interruption of the AA anastomosis cannot be performed where it would anatomically make most sense. In these cases, it is important to follow the vessel along its length to assure that a new functional AV anastomosis is not generated. As an example in Figures 9.11a and 9.11b, lasering only at site 1 creates an AV anastomosis (at site 2 and C, respectively).

Step 3: review

The last step in the lasering process involves careful review of all lasered vessels. This step assures that the vessels are completely obliterated and have not simply undergone a spastic closure. This step may also be used to identify and laser any other vessel that may have been overlooked in the two prior steps. The diagnostic endoscope is again used, as it provides maximum diagnostic power. If a patent anastomosis is identified, relasering with the operating endoscope should be done with care not to cause bleeding from the coagulated tissue. This is best accomplished by not targeting proximal areas of the lasered vessel. Once all lasered communications have been reviewed and relasered if necessary, the operating

scope is removed and the endoscopic aspect of the surgery is considered complete.

Post-laser amniodrainage

Surprisingly, the topic of how much fluid should be removed during a therapeutic amniocentesis has received relatively little attention.[18] Descriptive terms such as 'aggressive' or 'radical' have been used to describe the philosophical objective of the procedure. Objectively, goals range from decreasing the amniotic fluid volume to the level of oligohydramnios or to low-normal levels, using either MVP (maximum vertical pocket) or AFI (amniotic fluid index) as the measuring parameter.[19–22] Most centers advocate reducing the MVP to a level of 5–6 cm. Presumably, the lower the amniotic fluid volume at the end of the amniocentesis, the less frequent the number of procedures that will be required to reach viability and a successful outcome. Anecdotally, placental abruption has been reported as a potential complication of large-volume amnioreduction.[21]

A therapeutic amniocentesis is also performed at the end of laser surgery. We normally perform this with the suction–irrigation trumpet to which wall-suction tubing is attached at 300 mmHg. In contrast to patients treated solely with therapeutic amniocentesis, there is no need to drain the amniotic cavity of the recipient twin to inordinately low levels because the disease has now been effectively treated. Instead, the amniotic fluid volume is reduced to upper-normal or low polyhydramnios range, to avoid the potential complication of placental abruption. We have noted the development of bradycardia in some stuck donor twins during amniodrainage, presumably as a result of cord compression, which resolves with partial restoration of the amniotic fluid volume. In our current post-laser amniodrainage technique, fluid is removed in 500 ml increments for the first 1000 ml, followed by judicious removal of fluid until the MVP has reached approximately 9–10 cm, with constant ultrasound monitoring of the fetal heart rate of the twins. If bradycardia of the donor twin is detected, the amniodrainage procedure is halted and an amnioinfusion may be necessary. If bradycardia of the donor does not develop, the amniodrainage is continued until an MVP of 8–10 cm is reached.

Removal of the trocar

Once the desired level of amniotic fluid volume in the sac of the recipient twin is reached, the suction–irrigation trumpet is removed and the patient is alerted to the removal of the trocar. Trocar removal is monitored with ultrasound to detect bleeding from the anterior uterine wall or membrane detachment. If neither occurs, the incision is covered with a band-aid, steri-strips or dermabond to conclude the surgery.

Bleeding from the anterior uterine wall may occur at any point during surgery, but most commonly after removal of the trocar. Bleeding is typically short-lived, and can usually be contained with external digital pressure over the incision site of approximately 5 minutes. Occasionally, bleeding may be of greater magnitude, requiring either longer compression time (10–15 minutes), or rarely a laparotomy and surgical myometrial hemostasis. Lateral tilting of the patient may also be helpful in managing bleeding from the anterior uterine wall.

SPECIAL TECHNICAL CONSIDERATIONS

A translational step is required to take the fundamental concept on how to identify and photocoagulate placental vascular anastomoses to perform SLPCV in each and every specific clinical situation. In the ideal case, the placenta is posterior, access to the amniotic cavity of the recipient twin is not impeded, the anastomoses are all within the sac of the recipient twin and both twins have an adequate amount of individual placental mass to continue the pregnancy independently. Obviously, this is not nearly always the case. We have developed different specific techniques to address each and every anatomical variation.

Anastomoses within the sac of the donor twin

Vascular communications may be found within the sac of the donor twin in approximately one-thrid of patients with TTTS. In these patients, the anastomoses may take one of several forms:

- Terminal end visible. In these patients, the terminal end of the vessels and, thus, the actual site of the anastomosis, can be seen. Branching prior to the anastomosis may or may not exist, but does not interfere with access to the terminal end.
- Terminal end not visible. In these patients, the terminal end of the vessel is not visible, whether because of extensive branching of the recipient vasculature within the sac of the donor, or because of donor interference.

Depending on the presenting form, anastomoses within the sac of the donor may be photocoagulated in one of three ways:

1. Lasering within the sac of the recipient twin. This is done, provided that photocoagulation within the sac of the recipient twin does not compromise any individually perfused areas of the recipient twin. This is usually reserved for patients in situations where the terminal end is visible and there are no branches within the sac of the donor before the anastomosis (Figure 9.13a).
2. Lasering within the sac of the donor twin. This is done if lasering within the sac of the recipient twin would result in photocoagulation of recipient-perfused areas within the sac of the donor twin. This would typically occur in cases of numerous anastomoses within the sac of the donor or with extensive branching and inaccessibility to the actual terminal end. For this, an amnioinfusion of the sac of the donor twin is first done, followed by trocar insertion into the sac of the donor twin. We prefer to use a similar-size trocar and endoscope, to allow full disclosure of the anastomoses. Since the anastomoses have been identified and mapped from within the sac of the donor, a dual camera approach can be used with an assistant to monitor the process (Figure 9.13b,c).
3. Selective photothermolysis. In this technique, with the endoscope in the sac of the recipient twin, the laser beam is aimed at the visible terminal end of the vessel in the sac of the

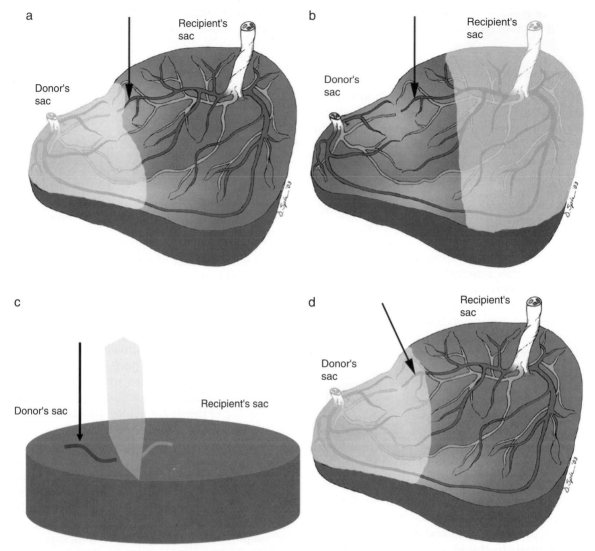

Figure 9.13 (a) Lasering simple anastomosis within the recipient sac. (b) Lasering within the donor's sac, by entering the donor's sac (anatomical). (c) Lasering within the donor's sac, by entering the donor's sac (schematic). (d) Lasering through the dividing membrane.

donor twin and the YAG laser is fired through the membrane against the vessel (Figure 9.13d). Photocoagulation of the vessel takes place without injury to the membrane. The physical principle of this technique is the absorbance of YAG laser energy by color. Since the membranes are transparent, the laser beam goes through the membrane without being absorbed. It is important to note here that injury to the membrane may occur if bleeding within the sac of the donor has

occurred previously, as even hemosiderin deposits would be enough to produce absorption of the laser energy.

Trocar assistance

The relationship between the trocar and the endoscope varies from manufacturer to manufacturer. Most of the endoscopes available for operative fetoscopy follow the hysteroscopy design, in which the tip of the endoscope is flushed with the tip of the trocar and the back end of the endoscope locks with the trocar sheath. In our design, the trocar and endoscope are independent of each other, with the endoscope being purposely 4 cm longer than the trocar length. Fluid leakage is prevented not by a locking mechanism, but rather, by a rubber cap and a check-flow valve within the trocar.

With our specific trocar and endoscopic design, we have developed the concept of trocar assistance. Essentially, the trocar sheath can be used to expose the surgical field as would be accomplished with a second port. Basically, the trocar sheath is advanced to the target vessel while the endoscope remains 1–2 cm inside the trocar sheath. Once the target vessel is identified, laser photocoagulation of the vessel from within the trocar sheath can be accomplished. We have found trocar assistance to be quite useful in the treatment of patients with anterior placentas, or even in those with posterior placentas in which the vessels may be tangential to the angle of entry of the trocar. The vessel is identified and compressed beneath the trocar sheath, and the operating endoscope fired within the sheath to obliterate it (Figure 9.14a,b). Trocar assistance may also be useful to expose vessels within the sac of the donor twin, whether obscured by the donor twin or by the dividing membrane.

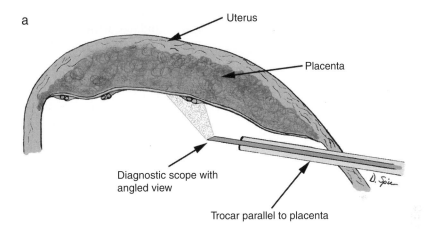

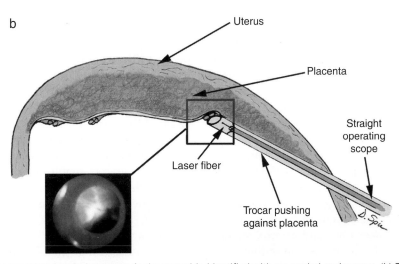

Figure 9.14 (a) Trocar-assisted technique step 1: the vessel is identified with an angled endoscope. (b) Trocar-assisted technique, step 2: the trocar sheath is placed against the vessel. The operating endoscope is retracted within the trocar sheath. The vessel is lasered at 90°.

Selective laser photocoagulation of communicating vessels in patients with an anterior placenta

An anterior placenta presents additional technical challenges in patients undergoing percutaneous SLPCV for severe TTTS. The challenges consist of finding a placenta-free area in the anterior uterine wall through which the trocar can be inserted and being able to assess all vascular communications from that entry site. Finding a placenta-free area in the anterior wall may be difficult, particularly if the placenta is widely extended. In addition, anterior placentas may also 'wrap around' the lateral walls, precluding free access to the amniotic cavity.

Approaches to the treatment of patients with anterior placentas that cannot be addressed with a straight operating endoscope have included performing a wide laparotomy with forward flipping of the uterus and entry into the amniotic cavity from the posterior wall (De Lia, pers comm); performing a mini-laparotomy and inserting a bent cannula;[23] use of flexible-steerable operating endoscopes. In 2001 we published on two techniques to address patients with anterior placentas.

Technique 1: flexible, steerable endoscope

Technique 1 uses a flexible endoscope through a single port. Under ultrasound guidance, a placenta-free area is identified in the anterior uterine wall. A 3 mm trocar is inserted percutaneously in the amniotic cavity of the recipient twin through a minimal skin incision. The placenta is surveyed with diagnostic endoscopes 2.7 mm in diameter, of varying angles of vision: 25° or 70° (angled-view endoscopes; Richard Wolf, Inc., Vernon Hills, IL) pointing the deflected angle of vision towards the placenta. All communicating vessels are identified as described above. The diagnostic endoscope is then exchanged for a 45 cm flexible-steerable 0° operating endoscope (Richard Wolf) with a 1 mm operating channel. The angle of flexion of the endoscope is 90° in two directions without the laser fiber and approximately 70° when a 400 μm laser fiber is within the operating channel. The previously identified vessels are photocoagulated by flexing the tip of the endoscope towards the placenta (see Figure 9.5).

The placenta is assessed again with the rigid 25° or 70° endoscope to evaluate adequacy of the photocoagulation procedure.

Technique 2: two-port, side-firing laser fiber

After the placenta has been surveyed with the angled-viewed endoscopes, a separate 2 mm port is inserted into the amniotic cavity of the recipient twin through an additional placenta-free area of the anterior uterine wall. Entry of this second port is monitored externally with ultrasound, and endoscopically from within the amniotic cavity. A 600 μm side-firing laser fiber (Surgical Laser Technologies, Montgomery, PA) which fires at a 70° angle is inserted through this port. The fiber is placed beneath the target vessels under endoscopic guidance with the angled-view endoscopes, and the vessels are photocoagulated (see Figure 9.8). Assessment of the photocoagulated areas is done with the angled-view endoscopes. Seventy-two patients were treated at our center from July 1997 to December 1999. Thirty-five patients (48.6%) had an anterior placenta. At least one fetus survived in 80% of patients with an anterior placenta (28 of 35) and 75.6% of those with a posterior placenta (28 of 37). This difference was not statistically significant ($p > 0.5$, df = 1, χ-square test, SPSS 9.0 for Windows, Chicago, IL), although the power of the study was low (power = 4%, nQuery Advisor 3.0, Statistical Solutions Inc., Dublin, Ireland). A total of 1450 patients would be necessary to rule out the null hypothesis with a power of 80% at the 0.05 level. Sixty percent (21 of 35) of patients were treated with technique 1 and 40% (14 of 35) with technique 2. At least one fetus survived in 76% (16 of 21) of patients treated with technique 1, and in 86% (12 of 14) of those treated with technique 2. This difference was also not statistically significant ($p = 0.67$, two-tailed Fisher exact test) (power 6%, with 285 patients required to rule out the null hypothesis with a power of 80% at the 0.05 level).

The mean operating time for patients with a posterior placenta in that study was 64.4 minutes (range 22–188, SD 35.51), compared with 81.14 minutes (range 20–172, SD 37.12). Patients with an anterior placenta had a significantly longer operating time than patients with a posterior placenta ($p = 0.02$, Student's t test).

Surgical pathology analysis of the placentas showed only 6 of 72 patients (8.3%) had patent vascular anastomoses, but 5 of those 6 patients belonged to the anterior placenta group. One of these 6 patients had persistent TTTS that required serial amniocenteses and delivery at 26 weeks with 1 fetus surviving, 2 had double intrauterine fetal demise, 1 miscarried, and 1 interrupted the pregnancy due to the development of ventriculomegaly in the donor twin. The remaining patient had resolution of the syndrome and delivered two healthy babies at 35 4/7 weeks' gestation; placental analysis in this patient showed a very small (filiform) patent anastomosis. [Currently, we rarely resort to techniques 1 or 2. Instead, we use the trocar-assisted technique as described above, for patients with anterior placentas that are not amenable to treatment simply with the straight operating endoscope (Figure 9.15a).]

Two additional particular issues may arise in patients with anterior placentas. First, the donor twin may be stuck against the anterior uterine wall between the chosen placenta-free area and the vascular equator (Figure 9.15b). In this case, circumventing the donor twin to reach the equator

may prove difficult or impossible, and another placenta-free area must be sought. A second potential issue may arise from vascular communications located between the site of trocar entry and the tip of the trocar, because the trocar sheath must advance a certain distance into the amniotic cavity in order to maintain access. Intraoperatively, it is possible to determine if an incomplete assessment of an anterior placenta has been done, because of the inability to follow all vessels to their terminal end. If the syndrome does not resolve in such cases, repeat laser, serial amniocenteses, or, in extreme cases, umbilical cord ligation may be offered to complete the therapy.

Supraselective laser photocoagulation of communicating vessels

SLPCV results in a functional or surgical dichorionization of a monochorionic placenta. Indeed, as a result of obliterating all vascular anastomoses, the remaining placental cotyledons are perfused individually by each twin (individual placental territory, or IPT). All shared cotyledons, with the exception of three-vessel or four-vessel cotyledons,

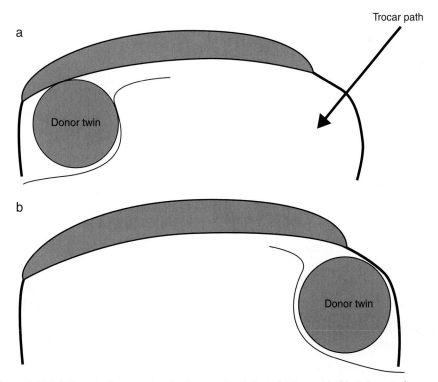

Figure 9.15 (a) Placenta-free area leading to sac of recipient. (b) Donor blocking placenta-free area.

are rendered non-functional. Survival of any one twin after SLPCV depends, at least partially, on whether the remaining IPT is enough to sustain in-utero life (see Chapter 5)

There are typically 20 cotyledons in a monochorionic placenta. What determines the percent of shared vs individual cotyledons in any given monochorionic placentation is not known, but at least theoretically, one of three permutations could potentially exist:

- Both fetuses have enough IPT to survive in utero after SLPCV. In this situation, the percent shared cotyledons is low, and each twin has an adequate IPT.
- Only one of the fetuses has enough IPT to survive after SLPCV. In this situation, one of the fetuses has an inadequate IPT as a result of unequal placental distribution.
- Neither twin has enough IPT to survive after SLPCV. In this situation, both fetuses are interdependent for their survival, with blood having to go through the other twin before it comes back oxygenated. We have dubbed this placental model 'circular pattern.'

Typically, the amount of IPT cannot be determined sonographically or endoscopically. However, if during the diagnostic fetoscopy step of SLPCV a circular pattern becomes obvious, dual in-utero demise after SLPCV can be predicted. Thus, a variation in the SLPCV technique must be performed. This can be done by targeting only one or a few (not all) of the AVDRs to decrease the amount of blood being lost by the donor twin, in an empiric attempt to balance the blood exchange between the fetuses. We have named this technique 'supraselective SLPCV, or SSLPCV.' Patients treated with SSLPCV continue to have patent vascular anastomoses. Although TTTS may resolve, patients treated with this technique are at risk for developing persistent or reverse TTTS, or any of the untoward consequences of spontaneous in-utero demise of one of the twins.

Selective laser photocoagulation of communicating vessels in triplet gestations

Triplet or higher-order multiple gestations may also develop TTTS, provided that a monochorionic

placentation exists. In the case of triplets, pregnancies may be either dichorionic or monochorionic. SLPCV in dichorionic triplets differs little from that of twins, other than the unaffected 'singleton' may interfere with trocar access to the amniotic cavity of the recipient twin.

In monochorionic triplets, one of three combinations may exist: one recipient–two donors, one donor–two recipients, and one donor–one recipient–one unaffected. Because vascular anastomoses will typically be present between all three fetuses, a seemingly unaffected triplet may serve as a go-between fetus between the other two. The goal of SLPCV in all monochorionic triplets is to identify and photocoagulate all of the anastomoses present, even in the '–unaffected' variety, to avoid persistent, reverse, or 'de novo' (in the case of –unaffected triplet) TTTS after surgery. Although some authors have suggested that all vascular anastomoses cannot be identified and photocoagulated in monochorionic triplets,[24] this is not our experience.

SLPCV in the one recipient–two donors variety is the simplest of the monochorionic triplets. The trocar is inserted into the amniotic cavity of the recipient twin and the anastomoses between the recipient and the two donors are identified. Anastomoses between the two donors are also easily seen, particularly if anhydramnios is present in the other two sacs. SLPCV in the case of one donor–two recipients is somewhat more difficult. If access to both recipients' sacs is possible through separate incisions, the anastomoses between each recipient and the donor can be easily obliterated. The anastomoses between the two recipients may be more difficult to see, because of obstruction by the dividing membrane. A dual-camera approach may be necessary in these cases, correlating the images seen through each port. Alternatively, the dividing membrane between the recipients may be flattened against the placenta by performing a combined amnioinfusion of one recipient and amniodrainage of the other sac through a 2 mm port. This transforms the case into a pseudo one recipient–two donors variety, allowing visualization of the anastomoses through the dividing membrane. Laser photocoagulation through selective photothermolysis completes the surgery.

Selective laser photocoagulation of communicating vessels in monoamniotic twins

Contrary to common belief, TTTS does occur in monoamniotic twins and is thought to occur in approximately 10% of monochorionic twins. Since monoamniotic twins represent approximately 1% of all monochorionic twins, TTTS would occur in 0.1% of monochorionic twins, or approximately 1:24 000 pregnancies. Monoamniotic twins may have any of the above placental distribution patterns, but, in particular, may be more prone to have extensive vascular anastomoses and a circular placental vascular pattern. In addition, the distance between the cords may be exceedingly short, with large AA or VV anastomoses. Cord entanglement may also be present, placing the fetuses at an increased risk of in-utero demise from this complication. Most cases, however, may simply show intertwining of the cords and not have a true knot.

SLPCV can be contemplated in monoamniotic twins provided cord entanglement is not present. If a circular pattern is suspected, SSLPCV may need to be performed instead. If a short intercord distance exists and large AA and/or VV anastomoses exist, trocar assistance and inching technique with high wattage may achieve vessel obliteration while trying to avoid thermal injury to the umbilical vein. If cord entanglement is present, serial amniocentesis or umbilical cord occlusion and transection may be the only alternatives left.

CONCLUSION

Laser surgery for TTTS is highly technologically and technically dependent. Over the years, we have developed both the appropriate instrumentation as well as the specific surgical techniques to address the surgical task in every specific instance. Attention to all technical details is pivotal in order to complete the surgery successfully in all cases. With the right equipment and surgical training, however, surgery is markedly facilitated and expedited. Success with SLPCV worldwide has resulted in increasingly more centers being involved with the laser treatment of TTTS. We hope the concepts discussed in this chapter will be of use to all of those performing or training to perform SLPCV for the treatment of TTTS.

REFERENCES

1. De Lia JE, Cruikshank DP, Keye WR Jr. Fetoscopic neodymium:YAG laser occlusion of placental vessels in severe twin–twin transfusion syndrome. Obstet Gynecol 1990; 75:1046–53.
2. De Lia J, Kuhlman R, Harstad T, et al. Twin–twin transfusion syndrome treated by fetoscopic neodymium: YAG laser occlusion of chorioangiopagus. Am J Obstet Gynecol 1993; 168 (1, part 2):308.
3. Ville Y, Hyett J, Hecher K, Nicolaides K. Preliminary experience with endoscopic laser surgery for severe twin–twin transfusion syndrome. N Engl J Med 1995; 332:224–7.
4. Quintero R, Morales W, Mendoza G et al. Selective photocoagulation of placental vessels in twin–twin transfusion syndrome: evolution of a surgical technique. Obstet Gynecol Surv 1998; 53:s97–103.
5. Quintero RA, Comas C, Bornick PW, Allen MH, Kruger M. Selective versus non-selective laser photocoagulation of placental vessels in twin–twin transfusion syndrome. Ultrasound Obstet Gynecol 2000; 16: 230–6.
6. Luks F, Deprest J, Marcus M, et al. Carbon dioxide pneumoamnios causes acidosis in fetal lamb. Fetal Diagn Ther 1994; 9:105–9.
7. Pelletier GJ, Srinathan SK, Langer JC. Effects of intraamniotic helium, carbon dioxide, and water on fetal lambs. J Pediat Surg 1995; 30:1155–8.
8. Quintero R. Diagnostic and operative fetoscopy: technical issues. In: Quintero R, ed. Diagnostic and operative fetoscopy. New York: The Parthenon Publishing Group, 2002:12–
9. Quintero RA, Bornick PW, Allen MH, Johnson PK. Selective laser photocoagulation of communicating vessels in severe twin–twin transfusion syndrome in women with an anterior placenta. Obstet Gynecol 2001; 97:477–81.
10. Absten GT. Basic laser physics for the gynecologist. In: McLaughlin D, ed. Lasers in gynecology. Philadelphia: Lippincott; 1991.
11. Absten GT. Physics of light and lasers. Obstet Gynecol Clin North Am 1991; 18:407–27.
12. Quintero R, Quintero L, Morales W, Allen M, Bornick P. Amniotic fluid pressures in severe twin–twin transfusion syndrome. Prenat Neonat Med 1998; 3:607–10.
13. Fisk NM, Giussani DA, Parkes MJ, Moore PJ, Hanson MA. Amniofusion increases amniotic pressure in pregnant sheep but does not alter fetal acid–base status. Am J Obstet Gynecol 1991; 165:1459–63.

14. Quintero R, Morales W. Operative fetoscopy: a new frontier in fetal medicine. Contemp Ob/Gyn 1999; 44: 45–68.

15. Epstein J, Arora A, Ellis H. Surface anatomy of the inferior epigastric artery in relation to laparoscopic injury. Clin Anat 2004; 17:400–8.

16. Bermudez C, Becerra CH, Bornick PW et al. Placental types and twin–twin transfusion syndrome. Am J Obstet Gynecol 2002; 187:489–94.

17. Quintero R. Selective laser photocoagulation of communicating vessels in twin–twin transfusion syndrome. In: Quintero R, ed. Diagnostic and operative fetoscopy. New York: The Parthenon Publishing Group, 2002: 43–54.

18. Abdel-Fattah SA, Carroll SG, Kyle PM, Soothill PW. Amnioreduction: how much to drain? Fetal Diagn Ther 1999; 14:279–82.

19. Saunders NJ, Snijders RJ, Nicolaides KH. Therapeutic amniocentesis in twin–twin transfusion syndrome appearing in the second trimester of pregnancy. Am J Obstet Gynecol 1992; 166:820–4.

20. Trespidi L, Boschetto C, Caravelli E et al. Serial amniocenteses in the management of twin–twin transfusion syndrome: when is it valuable? Fetal Diagn Ther 1997; 12:15–20.

21. Elliott JP, Sawyer AT, Radin TG, Strong RE. Large-volume therapeutic amniocentesis in the treatment of hydramnios. Obstet Gynecol 1994; 84:1025–7.

22. Elliott JP, Urig MA, Clewell WH. Aggressive therapeutic amniocentesis for treatment of twin–twin transfusion syndrome. Obstet Gynecol 1991; 77:537–40.

23. Deprest JA, Van Schoubroeck D, Van Ballaer PP et al. Alternative technique for Nd:YAG laser coagulation in twin-to-twin transfusion syndrome with anterior placenta. Ultrasound Obstet Gynecol 1998; 11:347–52.

24. Sepulveda W, Surerus E, Vandecruys H, Nicolaides KH. Fetofetal transfusion syndrome in triplet pregnancies: outcome after endoscopic laser surgery. Am J Obstet Gynecol 2005; 192:161–4.

10

Umbilical cord occlusion in twin–twin transfusion syndrome

Rubén A Quintero

Introduction • Methods • Results • Discussion

INTRODUCTION

As discussed in Chapter 9, the surgical treatment of twin–twin transfusion syndrome (TTTS) involves primarily laser obliteration of the anastomoses responsible for the syndrome. Occasionally, however, selective feticide of one of the fetuses must be contemplated. Indications for selective feticide in TTTS include a discordant anomalous twin or failed attempted laser therapy. The former are classified as being primary, the latter as being secondary selective feticides. Occasionally, patients may choose primary selective feticide after counseling, in accordance with their own personal opinions regarding potential outcomes.

Conventional methods for selective termination in non-monochorionic multiple gestations involve injection of potassium chloride into the vascular system of the target fetus. This is not appropriate in pregnancies complicated by TTTS, which by definition are monochorionic and have placental vascular communications.[1] Selective feticide in pregnancies complicated by TTTS must involve interruption of blood flow to one fetus while avoiding damage to the other fetus. Quintero et al described the first successful umbilical cord occlusion for the treatment of acardiac twins,[2] involving extracorporeal suture ligation of the umbilical cord of the target fetus. This technique was further expanded to the treatment of other complicated monochorionic twin pregnancies, including severe TTTS with a discordant lethal anomaly or with critically abnormal Doppler studies or hydrops. Other methods of umbilical cord occlusion (UCO) have been developed to achieve this end.[2–14] UCO typically requires access to the amniotic cavity of the target twin. In the case of the recipient twin, this is readily accomplished because of the presence of polyhydramnios. However, access to the donor's cord may be hindered by the presence of severe oligohydramnios. A study was conducted at our institution to compare the operative characteristics and clinical outcomes of UCO of the donor vs the recipient twin in complicated TTTS pregnancies.

METHODS

Standard sonographic diagnostic criteria for TTTS included polyhydramnios in the recipient twin (maximum vertical pocket [MVP] ≥ 8 cm), oligohydramnios in the donor twin (MVP ≤ 2 cm), single placenta, same gender, and thin-dividing membrane with absent λ or twin-peak sign. Each case was prospectively classified using the Quintero staging system,[15] as described in Chapter 7. Primary UCO was offered if there was (1) presence of a lethal discordant fetal anomaly, or (2) stage III/IV in a patient who elected this modality. All patients were informed of the potential risks and benefits of the proposed therapies, as well as the investigational nature of each. Patients choosing primary UCO were asked to reconsider other options such as selective laser photocoagulation of communicating vessels (SLPCV), but their final management decision was respected. The study was approved by the Institutional Review Board. All primary UCO cases were individually discussed and approved by the Ethics Committee as well.

All patients who elected to undergo a primary UCO were considered eligible for this study.

Surgical technique

The two methods of cord occlusion performed were umbilical cord ligation (UCL) or umbilical cord photocoagulation (UCP). UCL was performed via a 3.5 mm trocar inserted percutaneously into the amniotic cavity via 1–2 mm skin incision under continuous ultrasound guidance and general or local anesthesia. The cord of the target fetus was identified endoscopically with a 2.7–3.3 mm diagnostic or operating endoscope (Richard Wolf, Inc., Vernon Hills, IL, USA). A 3-0 Vicryl suture that had been previously threaded through a custom-designed knot-pusher was passed down the working channel of the endoscope with a semi-automatic grasper (Cook Ob/Gyn, Spencer, IN, USA), or through a second port, and was laid underneath the target umbilical cord. The suture was retrieved out of the amniotic cavity after looping it around the cord, where an extracorporeal knot was tied. The knot was delivered back into the amniotic cavity and tightened with the knot-pusher under continuous ultrasound guidance. Cessation of blood flow through the umbilical cord was documented by Doppler sonographically.

In those cases in which UCL was not feasible, UCP was performed. Once the umbilical cord of the abnormal twin was identified endoscopically, the cord was photocoagulated by using 20–40 watts of YAG laser energy with a 600 μm fiber through an operating endoscope until cessation of blood flow was documented sonographically.

RESULTS

Between July 1997 and June 2002, 252 patients with the diagnosis of TTTS underwent surgical treatment at our center. UCO was performed on 36 (14.3%) of these patients. Ten cases were excluded from the analysis because they had undergone secondary UCO after an attempted

SLPCV (technical success rate for TTTS 216/226, or 95.5%). One additional case was excluded because the ligated cord was that of a recipient twin that had died shortly before surgery. Thus, 25 cases of TTTS underwent primary UCO. Six (24%) had cord occlusion of the donor fetus (donor group) and 19 (76%) of the recipient fetus (recipient group). Six fetuses had the following discordant fetal malformations: 2 had neural tube defects (both donors), 1 had body-stalk anomaly (donor), 1 had pulmonary atresia (recipient), 1 had anencephaly (recipient), and 1 had intracranial hemorrhage (recipient). The two fetuses with stage I TTTS that underwent UCO had a lethal fetal anomaly (limb-body stalk anomaly, anencephaly). These data are summarized by stage in Table 10.1. There were no statistical differences between the donor vs the recipient groups in regards to stage of disease or fetal malformations.

There were no significant preoperative differences between the donor and recipient groups that underwent UCO (Table 10.2). Table 10.3 shows operative characteristics in the donor vs recipient groups. All 19 recipient fetuses underwent UCL. Four of six (66%) in the donor group had UCL while two (33%) had UCP. This difference in surgical approach between the two groups was statistically significant ($p = 0.05$). There was a significantly higher rate of two trocars required to complete the procedure in the donor

Table 10.1 Comparison of clinical characteristics of the donor vs recipient fetuses that underwent umbilical cord occlusion (Reproduced with permission from[16].)

	Total $n = 25$	Donor $n = 6$	Recipient $n = 19$	p
Staging				
Stage I	2	1	1	
Stage II	0	0	0	
Stage III	6	2	4	
Stage IV	17	3	14	NS
Fetal malformations				
Fetal anomaly + ICH	6	3	3	NS

ICH, intracranial hemorrhage; NS, not significant.

Table 10.2 Preoperative characteristics of the donor vs recipient fetuses that underwent umbilical cord occlusion (Reproduced with permission from[16].)

	Donor n = 6	Recipient n = 19	p
Placental location			
Anterior	3 (50%)	7 (36.8%)	NS
Posterior	3 (50%)	11 (57.9%)	
Lateral	0 (0.0%)	1 (5.3%)	
GA at surgery (weeks)			
Median	20.9	20.2	NS
Range	17.4–24.7	17.3–25	
Preoperative condition			
Amniodetachment	0 (0.0%)	4 (21.1%)	NS
Septostomy	1 (14.3%)	4 (21.1%)	NS
Preterm labor	2 (28.6%)	4 (21.1%)	NS

GA, gestational age; NS, not significant.

donor cord (83.4%) compared with the recipient cord (0.0%, $p < 0.001$). The median operating time in the donor group was almost twice as long as in the recipient group (75 vs 40 minutes, respectively). This difference was statistically significant ($p = 0.04$).

Clinical outcome data are summarized in Table 10.4. There was no difference in gestational age at delivery between the donor group (median 34.8 weeks) and recipient group (median 33.8 weeks). Twenty-two of 25 (88%) patients with TTTS who had undergone a primary UCO had liveborn infants. There were no significant differences in total survival rates between the two groups. Four patients (16%) had preterm premature rupture of membrane (PPROM) within 21 days of the procedure (median 2.0 days; range 0–12). Two had improvement of

group (50%) as compared to the recipient group (5.3%, $p = 0.03$). In all cases, the trocars entered the sac of the abnormal twin. There was a significantly higher rate of amnioinfusion for ligation of the

Table 10.3 Operative characteristics of the donor vs recipient fetuses that underwent umbilical cord occlusion (Reproduced with permission from[16].)

	Donor n = 6	Recipient n = 19	p
Procedure			
UCL	4 (66.7%)	19 (100.0%)	0.05
UCP	2 (33.3%)	0 (0.0%)	
Trocars			
One trocar	3 (50%)	18 (94.7%)	0.03
Two trocars	3 (50%)	1 (5.3%)	
Time of surgery (min)			
Median	75	40	0.04
Range	50–134	7–110	
Amnioinfusion at operation	5 (83.4%)	0 (0.0%)	<0.001
Membrane disruption at operation	2 (33.3%)	2 (10.5%)	NS

UCL, umbilical cord ligation; UCP, umbilical cord photocoagulation; NS, not significant.

Table 10.4 Clinical outcome of the donor vs recipient fetuses that underwent umbilical cord occlusion (Reproduced with permission from[16].)

	Donor n = 6	Recipient n = 19	p
Gestational age at delivery (weeks)			
Median	34.8	33.8	NS
Range	30.0–38.7	19.5–39.2	
Interval between procedure and delivery (days)			
Median	94.5	99	NS
Range	76–118	1–144	
Birthweight (g)			
Median	2191.5	2372	NS
Min–max	1616–3203	600–3335	
Survival rate per pregnancy	6/6 (100%)	16/19 (84.2%)	NS
IUFD	0 (0.0%)	3 (15.7%)	NS
NND	0 (0.0%)	0 (0.0%)	
Complications			
PROM <21 days	1 (16.6%)	3 (15.7%)	NS
Cord entanglement	0 (0.0%)	0 (0.0%)	
Infection	0 (0.0%)	0 (0.0%)	
Neurological morbidity	0 (0%)	0 (0%)	
Cardiovascular dysfunction	0 (0%)	0 (0%)	

IUFD, intrauterine fetal death; NND, neonatal death; PPROM, premature repture of the membranes; NS, not significant.

PPROM spontaneously and one underwent amniopatch by the method previously reported.[17] All three had liveborn infants. The fourth PPROM case miscarried at 20 weeks of gestation.

Cord insertions were classified as central, marginal, or velamentous at surgical pathology. The incidence of the different cord insertion types were as follows:

- donor – central 13 (52%), marginal 5 (20%), velamentous 7 (28%).
- recipient – central 18 (72%), marginal 5 (20%), velamentous 2 (8%).

There was no difference in the incidence of velamentous insertion between the donors or the recipients (7/25 donors, 2/25 recipients, $p = 0.13$ Fisher's exact test). There was no difference in the incidence of velamentous cord insertion of the occluded cord: 3/6 donors, 2/19 recipients ($p = 0.08$, Fisher's exact test). Perinatal survival relative to the placental insertion of the occluded cord was not statistically different: 15/17 central (88.2%), 2/3 marginal (66%), 5/5 (100%) velamentous, $p = 0.37$. There were no neurological or cardiac function abnormalities in any of the survivors.

The total number and percentage of UCO performed per year compared with the number of laser surgeries for TTTS are shown in Table 10.5. A nearly fourfold decrease in the percentage of total UCOs was noted during the 5-year span of the study.

Table 10.5 Number (n) and percentage (%) of SLPCV and total (primary plus secondary) UCL cases performed in each year of this study (Reproduced with permission from[16].)

| Year | SLPCV | | UCL (n) | | |
	n	%	n	%	Total
1997	2	66.7	1	33.3	3
1998	16	64.0	9	36.0	25
1999	45	80.4	11	19.6	56
2000	38	79.2	10	20.8	48
2001	73	96.1	3	3.9	76
2002	26	92.9	2	7.1	28
Total	200	84.7	36	15.3	236

SLPCV, selective laser photocoagulation of communicating vessels; UCL, umbilical cord ligation.

DISCUSSION

Selective feticide in TTTS involves occlusion of the umbilical cord of one of the fetuses with the hope that the co-twin will survive intact. By interrupting the vascular communications between the fetuses at the level of the umbilical cord, damage to the co-twin via feto–fetal hemorrhage may be avoided. The fundamental difference between SLPCV and UCO lies in that, although both methods interrupt the vascular communications between the two fetuses, SLPCV allows both twins a chance to survive. On the other hand, survival after SLPCV is unpredictable, sometimes resulting in the intrauterine demise of the 'healthier' twin, with survival of the seemingly most affected fetus. Patients are often distraught with the notion that the healthier fetus may die after SLPCV and, as a result, may request primary UCL. Parents may also request primary UCL in the case of twins discordant for a lethal anomaly. Secondary UCL, after a failed attempt at SLPCV, is rare in our experience, although always a counseling topic in any stage III or stage IV patient.

After our original description of UCL for the treatment of TRAP sequence, several UCO methods have been developed, to include, umbilical cord ligation (UCL),[18] laser photocoagulation of the umbilical vessels (UCP),[12,19] electrocoagulation of the umbilical cord,[13,14] and umbilical cord ultrasonic transection. Each technique is associated with varying degrees of invasiveness and operative skill. No surgical approach has been shown to have superior outcomes with regard to co-twin survival thus far.

At our center, UCO was offered to TTTS patients carrying a fetus with a lethal discordant fetal anomaly, or if stage III or IV disease was diagnosed and the patient desired UCO of the critically ill fetus, after extensive counseling regarding other possible therapeutic modalities. An overall 88% survival rate of the co-twin was noted in this study. UCL was the method of choice. This method allows for complete and instantaneous occlusion of all umbilical vessels, which may optimally prevent feto–fetal hemorrhage.

UCL requires adequate accessibility to the target umbilical cord. If access to the target cord is limited, our secondary approach is UCP. The advantage of laser occlusion of the umbilical cord is that this procedure may be performed even if access to the cord is limited. However, cord occlusion is not as rapid and simultaneous as UCL.

Selective feticide in pregnancies complicated by TTTS poses the additional operative challenge of varying approach based on if the target fetus is the donor or the recipient twin. In our study, no clinical or preoperative differences were noted between the two groups (see Tables 10.1 and 10.2). However, there were some operative differences, such as requirement for two trocars and amnioinfusion and operating time, which suggest that cord occlusion of the donor twin may be technically more demanding than that of the recipient twin (see Table 10.3). This is not unexpected in that additional operative maneuvers are required to allow for optimal visualization and access to the umbilical cord of the oligohydramniotic donor fetus. Also, because a major requirement of UCO is to enter the gestational sac of the target cord, direct access to the cord of the recipient within polyhydramnios is technically easier. Although in this study all target cord were handled within their own respective gestational sac, we now have experience with transmembranous laser photocoagulation (selective thermophotolysis). This latter technique may overcome many of the identified difficulties associated with UCL of the donor twin within its own sac.

Despite the technical differences described above, UCO via UCL/UCP resulted in similar outcome data in regards to survival of the co-twin, gestational age at delivery of the co-twin, birthweight, and PPROM rate of the donor vs the recipient fetus (see Table 10.4). The single survivor statistics for TTTS treated by cord occlusion via UCL/UCP appear similar to the results after SLPCV therapy,[20] and may be higher than those treated by serial amniodrainage if stage of disease is taken into account. For this reason, primary UCO is not recommended any longer for otherwise uncomplicated stage III or IV TTTS.

Outcome results of UCL/UCP appear favorable compared with other methods of selective feticide techniques performed in monochorionic multiples. Embolization using varying thrombogenic substances had relatively high rates of demise of the co-twin, presumably due to passage of the substance to the co-twin via incompletely obliterated vascular communications.[6–11]

A multicenter study of 50 consecutive umbilical cord occlusions via UCP and/or bipolar electrocoagulation for varying indications has recently been reported.[21] UCP done primarily and bipolar electrocoagulation done secondarily if necessary was performed in 37 cases, and primary bipolar electrocoagulation was performed in 13 cases. The overall survival rate was 75%, and overall PPROM rate was 52%. The relatively high PPROM rate in that study, particularly the 25% persistent PPROM that occurred before 30 weeks' gestation, is of concern. Newer techniques such as umbilical cord ultrasonic transection are currently under investigation, but are unlikely to provide any additional advantages.[14] Direct comparison of each technique in regards to co-twin survival must be performed to determine optimal surgical method.

Table 10.5 describes a decreasing percentage of primary and secondary UCOs compared with laser surgery over time for the treatment of TTTS at our center. This may be a reflection of surgeon experience as well as patient reassurance in regards to the comparable outcome results of SLPCV vs UCO. Indeed, the likelihood of at least one survivor is approximately 85% in both techniques, with the obvious difference that with SLPCV both fetuses may have a chance to survive. This is particularly important in view of the recent availability of bipolar coagulation, which is perceived as a simpler method of achieving separation of the circulations of both twins. Unfortunately, such technological advance may result in the unnecessary demise of many stage III or IV fetuses that could have otherwise had an opportunity to survive with SLPCV. Nonetheless, patients may sometimes request UCO as a primary therapeutic technique in TTTS stages III or IV, as laser occlusion of the vascular anastomoses cannot predict which of the two fetuses will survive. Our experience shows that of those stage III–IV patients with a single intrauterine fetal death (IUFD) after SLPCV, the demised fetus may be the one with normal preoperative Dopplers approximately 20% of the time. Considering the pros and cons of each approach, we currently do not advocate primary UCO for TTTS stages III or IV, unless there are additional complications, such as discordant anomalies or a terminally ill fetus, that may compromise the health of the co-twin in utero.

This chapter addresses the issues of umbilical cord occlusion in TTTS via UCL/UCP. Because the approach varies based on whether the target fetus is the donor or the recipient, different techniques must be utilized to successfully perform this procedure. This may include using more than one trocar and/or amnioinfusion to obtain access to the donor fetus. Operator experience with more than one cord occlusive method is required. In this study of TTTS patients that underwent primary UCO, we showed that donor cord occlusion may be technically more difficult, yet overall outcome results are similar between the donor and recipient twins.

REFERENCES

1. Machin G, Still K, Lalani T. Correlations of placental vascular anatomy and clinical outcomes in 69 monochorionic twin pregnancies. Am J Med Genet 1996; 61:229–36.

2. Quintero RA, Reich H, Puder KS et al. Brief report: umbilical-cord ligation of an acardiac twin by fetoscopy at 19 weeks of gestation. N Engl J Med 1994; 330:469–71.

3. Ginsberg N, Applebaum M, Rabin S et al. Term birth after midtrimester hysterotomy and selective delivery of an acardiac twin. Am J Obstet Gynecol 1992; 167:33–7.

4. Fries M, Goldberg J, Golbus M. Treatment of acardiac-acephalus twin gestations by hysterotomy and selective delivery. Obstet Gynecol 1992; 79:601–4.

5. Robie G, Payne G, Morgan M. Selective delivery of an acardiac, acephalic twin. N Engl J Med 1989; 320:512–13.

6. Hamada H, Okane M, Koresawa M et al. [Fetal therapy in utero by blockage of the umbilical blood flow of acardiac monster in twin pregnancy]. Nippon Sanka Fujinka Gakkai Zasshi 1989; 41:1803–9. [in Japanese]

7. Grab D, Schneider V, Keckstein J et al. Twin, acardiac, outcome. Fetus 1992; 2:11–13.

8. Porreco R, Barton S, Haverkamp A. Occlusion of umbilical artery in acardiac, acephalic twin. Lancet 1991; 337:326–7.

9. Roberts R, Shah D, Jeanty P, Beattie J. Twin, acardiac, ultrasound-guided embolization. Fetus 1991; 1:5–10.

10. Holzgreve W, Tercanli S, Krings W, Schuierer G. A simpler technique for umbilical-cord blockade of an acardiac twin. N Engl J Med 1994; 331:56–7.

11. Sepulveda W, Bower S, Hassan J, Fisk N. Ablation of acardiac twin by alcohol injection into the intra-abdominal umbilical artery. Obstet Gynecol 1995; 86:680–1.

12. Arias F, Sunderji S, Gimpelson R, Colton E. Treatment of acardiac twinning. Obstet Gynecol 1998; 91:818–21.

13. Deprest JA, Audibert F, Van Schoubroeck D, Hecher K, Mahieu-Caputo D. Bipolar coagulation of the umbilical cord in complicated monochorionic twin pregnancy. Am J Obstet Gynecol 2000; 182:340–5.

14. Lopoo JB, Paek BW, Maichin GA et al. Cord ultrasonic transection procedure for selective termination of a monochorionic twin. Fetal Diagn Ther 2000; 15:177–9.

15. Quintero RA, Morales WJ, Allen MH et al. Staging of twin–twin transfusion syndrome. J Perinatol 1999; 19:550–5.

16. Nakata M, Chmait RH, Quintero RA. Umbilical cord occlusion of the donor versus recipient fetus in twin–twin transfusion syndrome. Ultrasound Obstet Gynecol 2004; 23:446–50.

17. Quintero RA, Morales WJ, Allen M et al. Treatment of iatrogenic previable premature rupture of membranes with intra-amniotic injection of platelets and cryoprecipitate (amniopatch): preliminary experience. Am J Obstet Gynecol 1999; 181:744–9.

18. Quintero RA, Romero R, Reich H et al. In utero percutaneous umbilical cord ligation in the management of complicated monochorionic multiple gestations. Ultrasound Obstet Gynecol 1996; 8:16–22.

19. Hecher K, Hackeloer BJ, Ville Y. Umbilical cord coagulation by operative microendoscopy at 16 weeks' gestation in an acardiac twin. Ultrasound Obstet Gynecol 1997; 10:130–2.

20. Quintero RA, Dickinson JE, Morales WJ et al. Stage-based treatment of twin–twin transfusion syndrome. Am J Obstet Gynecol 2003; 188:1333–40.

21. Lewi L, Gratacos E, Van Schoubroeck D et al. Fifty consecutive cord coagulations in monochorionic multiplets. Am J Obstet Gynecol 2003; 187:s61.

11

Treatment of twin–twin transfusion syndrome: an evidence-based analysis

Eftichia V Kontopoulos and Rubén A Quintero

Introduction • **Expectant management** • **Medical treatment** • **Septostomy** • **Serial amniocentesis** • **Laser therapy** • **Laser therapy versus amniocentesis** • **Selective feticide** • **Conclusion**

INTRODUCTION

Management of twin–twin transfusion syndrome (TTTS) has encompassed a wide spectrum of options, including expectant management, medical therapy, and surgery, as well as pregnancy termination. Over the past few years, significant emphasis has been given to the development of clinical practice guidelines that are derived from evidence-based medicine. Levels of evidence have been classified by the US Preventive Services Task Force according to their strength (Table 11.1). The purpose of this chapter is to review the available literature on the management of TTTS with regard to the level of evidence of each management alternative.

EXPECTANT MANAGEMENT

The best article summarizing expectant management was published by Saunders et al.[1] In this publication, 8 articles with a total of 106 patients managed expectantly were identified. Only 5/106 (4.7%) patients managed expectantly were associated with fetal survival. Fifteen articles with a total of 96 patients managed with serial amniocentesis were identified. Survival with serial amniocentesis was 33/96 (34%). This difference is statistically significant ($p < 0.001$). The authors managed an additional 21 patients. One patient had a voluntary termination of pregnancy and another miscarried within a week of expectant management. Eight of the remaining 19 (42%) patients treated with serial

amniocentesis were associated with at least one survivor. Overall, in this report, 5/107 (4.6%) managed expectantly compared unfavorably with 41/115 (35%) of patients managed with serial amniocentesis ($p < 0.001$). Level of evidence: III.

More recently, Van Gemert has summarized the experience with expectant management for 1990–2000. Table 11.2 shows the contributing reports, with an overall survival rate of 36.9% (69/187). Interestingly, survival rate with expectant management in this collective series was as high as that with serial amniocentesis as reported by Saunders. As can be seen, of the 11 series reported, only one used the current sonographic definition of TTTS as a maximum vertical pocket

Table 11.1 Evaluation of evidence (US Preventive Services Task Force Classification)	
Level I	At least one properly designed RCT
Level II-1	Well-designed non-randomized CT
Level II-2	Well-designed cohort or case-control studies from more than one center or research group
Level II-3	Multiple time series with or without the intervention or dramatic results in uncontrolled experiments
Level III	Opinions of respected authorities, descriptive studies or reports of expert committees

RCT, randomized controlled trial; CT, controlled trial.

Table 11.2 Expectant management of twin–twin transfusion syndrome

Author	N	GA	Polyhydramnios	Oligohydramnios	Survival				per No. fetuses	NM
					0	1	2	>0		
Gonsoulin (1990)[41]	9	<28	NS	Stuck					6/18	
Urig (1990)[42]	5	<24	NS	Stuck	5	0	0	0	0/10	NS
Radestad (1990)[43]	18	<34	Increase in fundal height 3 cm in 1 week	NS	9	6	3	9	11/18	NS
Mahony (1990)[44] (included in Reisner, 1993)[45]	5	<25	MVP >12 cm	Stuck	3	2	0	2	2/10	1
Steinberg (1990)[46]	12	NS	NS	NS	10	2	0	2	2/24	
Bromley (1992)[47]	9	<26	NS	Stuck	3	0	6	6	12/18	NS
Saunders (1992)[1]	1	NS	NS Distended bladder	Stuck Non-visible bladder	1	0	0	0	0/2	NS
Reisner (1993)[45]	5	<30	AFI >25 (<20 wks) AFI >30 (>20 wks) MVP >12 cm	Stuck	2	2	1	3	4/10	0
Dennis (1997)[21]	6	<26.4	Polyhydramnios	Oligohydramnios	3	0	3	3	6/12	NS
Lachapelle (1997)[48] (one case was treated with amniocentesis, not specified)	5	<27.8	MVP ≥8 cm	MVP ≤2 cm	1	1	3	4	7/10	NS
Zondervan (1999)[49]	25	NS	Polyhydramnios	Oligohydramnios (stuck)	8	NS	NS	17	21/50	14% (3/21)
Total								44/86 (51%)	69/172 (40%)	

N, number of patients; GA, gestational age; NM, neurological morbidity; MVP, maximum vertical pocket; AFI, amniotic fluid index. Modified from Van Gemert et al.[2]

(MVP) ≥8 cm in the sac of the recipient and ≤2 cm in the sac of the donor twin.[2] Moreover, the gestational age (GA) at treatment included patients up to 34 weeks' gestation, which is beyond the 26-week mark typically used in analyzing outcomes of laser therapy. Therefore, historical data on expectant management cannot be used for comparison with other current approaches. Level of evidence: III.

MEDICAL TREATMENT

Medical treatment of TTTS has included only isolated case reports involving the use of digoxin[3–5] or indomethacin.[6–8] The rationale for the use of digoxin is to treat a recipient twin in heart failure. Relatively high maternal serum levels of digoxin must be achieved in order to reach therapeutic levels in TTTS, as the mean feto–maternal gradient is 0.56.[9] Fetal levels are also directly related to GA. Of the three articles describing the use of digoxin, only one patient was treated successfully with this medication alone. Of the three articles describing the use of indomethacin, no obvious benefit from the use of this medication was found. These findings are not surprising, considering the opposite hemodynamic status of the recipient and the donor twin. Based on the limited evidence available, medical treatment of TTTS, at least as a first-line therapy, is currently not recommended. Level of evidence: III.

SEPTOSTOMY

The rationale on the use of septostomy or dividing-membrane amniorrhexis for the treatment of TTTS was to equilibrate the amniotic pressures on both sides of the membrane.[10,11] Prior to its proposal, a difference in amniotic fluid pressures in the two sacs was never demonstrated. On the contrary, Quintero and others showed that, in fact, the pressure in both sacs is similar.[12,13] Notwithstanding, a randomized controlled trial was carried out to compare septostomy versus amnioreduction.[14] The study was terminated at the planned interim analysis stage after 73 women were enrolled. This was because the rate of survival of at least 1 infant was similar in the amnioreduction group compared with the septostomy group (78% vs 80% of pregnancies, respectively; RR = 0.94, 95% CI 0.55–1.61; $p = 0.82$). Patients undergoing septostomy were more likely to require a single procedure for treatment (64% vs 46%; $p = 0.04$). Level of evidence: I.

While the data clearly show no benefit of septostomy over serial amniocentesis, its complications have not been emphasized enough. Passive transfer of amniotic fluid from the sac of the donor to the recipient eliminates the possibility of monitoring improvement of the donor in terms of urine production. Septostomy may also make subsequent amniocenteses or laser difficult, as the dividing membrane interferes with the procedure (a finding perhaps reflected in the randomized clinical trial, but with a different explanation). Finally, septostomy may result in pseudo-monoamniotic pregnancy, with demise of one or both fetuses from cord entanglement. Therefore, septostomy should not be used to treat TTTS.

SERIAL AMNIOCENTESIS

Prior to 2001, several small-number case series had been published regarding the use of serial amnioreduction as originally suggested by Saunders et al.[1] The rationale for the use of amniocentesis was to decrease the likelihood of miscarriage and preterm labor associated with polyhydramnios in the sac of the recipient twin. In addition, improved placental perfusion to the donor twin was also thought to result from this intervention. A wide-range of survival rates from 33 to 83% had been reported. In an effort to compile the available experience at the time, Mari et al set up an international registry of TTTS patients treated with serial amnioreduction.[15] A total of 223 patients, from 20 centers, treated before 28 weeks' gestation were analyzed. It is unclear from the study if the cases included patients that were previously published, unpublished, or both. The definition of TTTS was left to the discretion of the each investigator. As a result at least 17% of patients did not have a stuck twin. Complications from the procedure within 48 hours included ruptured membranes 6%, spontaneous delivery 3%, fetal distress 2.2%, fetal death 1.7%, and placental abruption 1.3%, with an overall risk of complications of 15%. The median interval from amniocentesis to delivery was 17.5 days. At least one fetus survived in 70.8% of patients, and both twins survived in 48% of cases. The incidence of postnatal abnormal intracranial imaging was 18%. Logistic regression showed that poor prognostic factors included early gestational age (<22 weeks), more than 1 liter of fluid removed per week, absent end-diastolic velocity in the umbilical artery of the donor twin, and hydrops.[15]

Although this study was the largest series at the time, it was a retrospective analysis without a clear sonographic definition of the syndrome that included patients up to 28 weeks of gestation. In addition, the relatively few number of patients, considering the large number of centers involved, also point to a limited experience by most centers or the potential for bias by a single center that would concentrate management. The actual number of patients per center was not provided. Nonetheless, the results confirmed that serial amniocentesis was superior than historical controls managed expectantly. However, the relatively short time, in terms of pregnancy prolongation, gained after the procedure and the high incidence of neonatal neurological morbidity were apparent. The study pointed out risk factors associated with poor perinatal outcome, and constituted the basis for the design of a randomized clinical trial comparing serial amniocentesis with laser therapy.

Table 11-3 shows the experience with serial amniocentesis as reported in the literature for 1990–2005. The table does not include the amniocentesis registry to avoid overlap, because, as mentioned above, many prior reports could have been included in the registry. Also, the table does not include series comparing amniocentesis with laser. Of the 24 studies available, only 5 used a standard sonographic definition of TTTS similar to the polyhydramnios MVP ≥8 cm, oligohydramnios MVP ≤2 cm criteria used today,[16–20] and only 3 studies used a gestational age of 26 weeks as the upper limit for inclusion.[18,21,22] Only 13 studies reported on neurological morbidity. The overall survival rate for at least one fetus was 68% (243/355), with an associated neurological morbidity of 22.9% (103/449).

Despite the lack of use of a standard definition of TTTS and the potential for bias for inclusion of non-TTTS patients, the overall perinatal survival rate of TTTS in these studies is somewhat similar to that reported in studies using standardized criteria (see below). A common finding in these studies is the high rate of neurological morbidity. Level of evidence: II-3.

LASER THERAPY

The rationale for the use of laser therapy is to eliminate the syndrome altogether by obliterating the vascular anastomoses responsible for the syndrome.[23] Although relatively simple in concept, the actual endoscopic technique to differentiate vascular anastomoses from individually perfused placental cotyledons was not described until 1998 (selective laser photocoagulation of communicating vessels, or SLPCV).[24] Thus, comparison of laser series needs to account for this evolutionary step. In one study, patients treated with a selective technique had an improved likelihood of at least one fetus surviving than those treated with a non-selective technique (83% vs 61%, p = 0.04)

(Table 11.4).[25] This conclusion is supported by combining patients treated with a non-selective technique (prior to 1998, including 18 patients in the Quintero study from 2000) with those treated with a selective technique (126/176, 71.5% vs 162/198, 81.8%, p = 0.018). It is important to note that most studies used a similar definition of TTTS. Moreover, the incidence of neurological morbidity was quite low in reference to amniocenteses series, regardless of the laser technique used. Level of evidence: II-2.

LASER THERAPY VERSUS AMNIOCENTESIS

The most important controversial therapeutic issue has involved the comparison of outcomes of amniocentesis vs laser-treated patients. Two controlled non-randomized trials comparing serial amniocentesis with laser photocoagulation showed less favorable results for amniocentesis compared with laser (Table 11.5).[26,27] Both series used similar diagnostic criteria and therapeutic approach, such that combined analysis of the series is possible (78/121, 64.4% vs 137/168, 81.5%, amniocentesis vs laser, respectively, p = 0.001). Moreover, survival in amniocentesis-treated patients decreased with advancing stage (stage I, bladder of the donor visible; stage II, bladder of the donor not visible; stage III, critically abnormal Doppler studies – absent end-diastolic velocity in the umbilical artery, pulsatile umbilical venous flow, reverse flow in the ductus venosus; stage IV, hydrops),[28] but not in laser-treated patients.[27] Level of evidence: II-1.

Finally, a randomized controlled trial performed by the Eurofetus group compared serial amniocentesis vs selective laser therapy.[29] Randomization was performed using a 1:1 ratio. A total of 172 patients were estimated to be required to show a 15% difference between amniocentesis (55%) and laser (70%), using a two-tailed analysis, a p value of 0.05, and 80% power. The patients included were less than 26 weeks' gestation and most had severe disease (>90% stages II–III Quintero in both groups). The study was stopped early after 70 patients had been randomized to the amniocenteses group and 72 to the laser group, as an interim analysis showed 51% (36/70) survival in the amniocentesis group vs 76% (55/72) survival in the laser group (p = 0.009). This difference

Table 11.3 Perinatal outcomes associated with serial amniocentesis

Author	N	GA	Polyhydramnios	Oligohydramnios	Survival					NM
					0	1	2	>0	per No. fetuses	
Gonsoulin (1990)[41]	10	<28	NS	Stuck	10	1	7	8	4/22	
Radestadt (1990)[43]	18	<32	Increase in FH 3 cm	NS	NS	1	7	8	23/36	NS
Cincotta (2000)[50]	17 (5 not treated)	<28	NS	Stuck twin	4	3	10	13	23/34	5/23
Van Gemert (2000)[51]	6	<27	Polyhydramnios	MVP <2 cm	3	2	1	3	4/12	NS
Denbow (1998)*[52]	17	<29	Polyhydramnios	MVP <1 cm	NS	NS	NS			18/34 (58%)
Lopriore et al (2003)[16]	29	<28	MVP >8 cm	MVP <1 cm	12	5	12	17	29/58	5/19 (26%)
Urig (1990)[42]	9	<29	NS	Stuck	5	0	4	4	8/18	NS
Saunders (1992)[1]	19	<30	NS	NS	10	4	5	9	14/38	NS
Mahony (1990)[44] (included in Reisner 1993[45])	8	<28.5	MVP >12	Stuck	2	1	5	6	11/16	4/11 (36%)
Reisner (1993)[45]	27		AFI >25 (<20 weeks) AFI >30 (>20 weeks) MVP >12 cm	Stuck	5	5	17	22	39/54	7/39 (18%)
Dennis (1997)[21]	11	<26	Polyhydramnios	Oligohydramnios	1	2	8	10	18/22	NS
Zondervaan (1999)[49]	27	<28	Polyhydramnios	Oligohydramnios	4	NS	NS	23	33/54	7/33
Elliot (1994)[53]	36	NS	MVP >8 cm, AFI >25	NS	NS	NS	NS	NS	NS	NS
Pinette (1993)[17]	13	<29.9	>8	<2	0	5	8	9	21/26	1/21
Bruner (1993)[54]	9	<27.9	Polyhydramnios	Oligohydramnios, stuck	NS	2	NS	NS	NS	
Fries (1993)[55]	5	<28	Polyhydramnios	Oligohydramnios	1	3	1	4	5/10	1/5
Weiner (1994)[56]	12	<27	NS	Oligohydramnios	NS	NS	NS	NS	11/22	NS

(Continued)

Table 11.3 Perinatal outcomes associated with serial amniocentesis—cont'd

Author	N	GA	Polyhydramnios	Oligohydramnios	Survival				per No. fetuses	NM
					0	1	2	>0		
Dickinson (1995)[57]	10	<34	AFI >25	Oligohydramnios, stuck	3	1	6	7	13/20	NS
Kilby (1997)[58]	9	<25	>12	<1, no bladder	4	0	5	5	10/18	2/10
Trespidi (1997)[18]	23	<26	>8	<1	8	6	9	15	26/46	4/26
Fesslova (1998)[19]	17	<28	>8	<1	6	2	9	11	20/34	NA
Mari (2000)[20]	31	<33	>8 (<20), >10 (>20)	<1, Stuck	NS	NS	NS	NS	40/61	8/51
Bajoria (1998)[50]	23	<28	Poly, AFI >30	Oligohydramnios	5	9	9	18	27/46	5/29
Dickinson (2000)[22]	92	<25.6	AF	Stuck	27	24	41	65	106/184	36/148
Total									243/355 (68%)	474/815 (58%)
Total with MVP >8 cm and <2 cm									57/91 (62%)	146/243 (60%)

N, number of patients; GA, gestational age; NM, neurological morbidity; MVP, maximum vertical pocket; AFI, amniotic fluid index; FH, fundal height.
* Only surviving cases were included.

Table 11.4 Laser therapy studies										
						Survival				
Author	N	GA	Polyhydramnios	Oligohydramnios	0	1	2	>0	NM
De Lia (1995)[60]	26	<24	MVP >9 cm / AFI ≥30 and fundal height >29 cm	NS	8	9	9	18	3.6%
Ville (1998)[61]	132	<27	Polyhydramnios + enlarged bladder	Oligohydramnios + collapsed bladder	35	50	47	97	4.2%
Hecher (2000)[62]	127	<26	MVP ≥8 cm	MVP ≤1 cm	24	34	69	103	5.6%
Quintero (2000)[25]	71	<25.6	MVP ≥8 cm	MVP <2 cm	28	31	12	59	1.2%

N, number of patients; GA, gestational age; NM, neurological morbidity; MVP, maximum vertical pocket; AFI, amniotic fluid index.

persisted even at 6 months of age ($p = 0.002$). The GA at delivery was also significantly different (29 weeks vs 33.3 weeks, $p = 0.003$). Superior results were apparent, regardless of TTTS stage. The incidence of neurological complications was significantly higher in the amniocentesis group (14% vs 6%, amniocentesis vs laser, respectively, $p = 0.02$) with only 31% of babies alive at 6 months without neurological complications in the amniocentesis group vs 52% in the laser group ($p = 0.003$). Level of evidence: I.

SELECTIVE FETICIDE

Spontaneous intrauterine fetal demise of a monochorionic twin is associated with risk of death or injury of the co-twin.[30,31] The pathophysiological mechanism responsible for the adverse effects on the second twin is through perimortem feto–fetal hemorrhage from the living twin to the dying or dead co-twin.[32] Thus, the rationale for selective feticide in monochorionic twins with TTTS is to prevent death or injury of a healthier twin resulting from the spontaneous death of a sicker co-twin. The fundamental technique evolved from the successful treatment of TRAP (twin-reversal arterial perfusion) syndrome with umbilical cord occlusion.[33] Clinical experience with this technique had shown that umbilical cord occlusion of a twin did not result in any immediate adverse effects to the surviving twin. Since then, several techniques for feticide have been proposed, such as cord

ligation, monopolar and bipolar coagulation, and radiofrequency ablation.[34–37] The target umbilical cord should be that of the sicker fetus, although some authors have always chosen the cord of the donor twin.[38,39] In a series of 25 patients by Nakata et al, there were no differences in co-twin survival (100% vs 84.2%), median GA at delivery (34.8 vs 33.8 weeks), and preterm premature rupture of membranes rate (16.6% vs 15.7%) whether the donor or recipient twin, respectively, was the subject of primary umbilical cord occlusion (see Chapter 10). However, a higher incidence of two-trocar access (50% vs 5.3%; $p = 0.03$), amnioinfusion (83.3% vs 0%; $p < 0.001$), and a longer operating time (75 vs 40 minutes, $p = 0.04$) were noted in occlusion of the donor twin's cord. Thus, umbilical cord occlusion of the donor twin is technically more challenging than that of the recipient twin. Level of evidence: II-2

Umbilical cord occlusion is rarely performed today in centers with ample experience in the laser treatment of TTTS. Current indications for umbilical cord occlusion in TTTS include an anomalous or moribund co-twin, because demise of either twin can occur after SLPCV. Thus, patients with TTTS and an anomalous twin can potentially be faced with demise of the healthier fetus and survival of the anomalous twin after SLPCV. Other than for such an indication, umbilical cord occlusion is rarely used as first-line treatment in the treatment of TTTS.

Table 11.5 Laser therapy verus amniocentesis

Author	N Amnio/laser	GA	Polyhydramnios MVP	Oligohydramnios MVP	Survival amino				NM Amnio	Survival laser				NM laser
					0	1	2	>0		0	1	2	>0	
Hecher (1999)[26]	43/73	<25	>8 cm	<1 cm	17	8	18	26	NS	15	27	31	58	NS
Quintero (2003)[27]	78/95	<25.6	>8 cm	<2 cm	26	14	38	52	24.4%	16	36	43	79	4.2%
Senat (2004)[29]	70/72	<26	(≤20 weeks) >8 cm (≥20 weeks) >10 cm	<2 cm	34	18	18	36	14.3%	17	29	26	55	5.6%

N, number of patients; GA, gestational age; NM, neurological morbidity; MVP, maximum vertical pocket.

CONCLUSION

The use of evidence-based medicine in developing practice guidelines for the management of TTTS has encompassed many years and different forms of treatment. Current results suggest that laser treatment should be the first line of therapy, regardless of gestational age or Stage. This constitutes an important paradigm shift in a positive direction, as the evidence shows improved results with improved surgical technique and technology. As a consequence, laser therapy, should be considered 'standard of care' in the management of patients with TTTS, despite being less available and requiring more skills and equipment than serial amniocentesis. Recognition of this new standard is important as it pertains to the negative implications that other forms of management (expectant, serial amniocentesis, septostomy) may have on laser therapy.[40] The future in the management of TTTS will depend on standardization of surgical techniques, improved technology, correction of identified limitations, and patient and physician education.

REFERENCES

1. Saunders NJ, Snijders RJ, Nicolaides KH. Therapeutic amniocentesis in twin–twin transfusion syndrome appearing in the second trimester of pregnancy. Am J Obstet Gynecol 1992; 166:820–4.
2. van Gemert MJ, Umur A, Tijssen JG, Ross MG. Twin–twin transfusion syndrome: etiology, severity and rational management. Curr Opin Obstet Gynecol 2001; 13:193–206.
3. De Lia J, Emery M, Sheafor S et al. Twin transfusion syndrome: successful in utero treatment with digoxin. Int J Gynecol Obstet 1985; 23:197.
4. Arabin B, Laurini RN, van Eyck J, Nicolaides KH. Treatment of twin–twin transfusion syndrome by laser and digoxin. Biophysical and angiographic evaluation. Fetal Diagn Ther 1998; 13:141–6.
5. Zosmer N, Bajoria R, Weiner E et al. Clinical and echographic features of in utero cardiac dysfunction in the recipient twin in twin–twin transfusion syndrome. Br Heart J 1994; 72:74–9.
6. Jones J, Sbarra A, Dilillo L et al. Indomethacin in severe twin-to-twin transfusion syndrome. Am J Perinatol 1993; 10:24.
7. Nicolaides K, Pettersen H. Fetal therapy. Curr Opin Obstet Gynecol 1994; 6:468–71.
8. Nores J, Athanassiou A, Elkadry E et al. Gender differences in twin–twin transfusion syndrome. Obstet Gynecol 1997; 90:580–2.
9. Pfeiffer KA, Plath H, Reinsberg J, Fahnenstich H, Schmolling J. [Maternal and fetal digoxin level in fetofetal transfusion syndrome (FFTS)]. Z Geburtshilfe Neonatol 2000; 204:26–30. [in German]
10. Saade GR, Belfort MA, Berry DL, et al. Amniotic septostomy for the treatment of twin oligohydramnios–polyhydramnios sequence. Fetal Diagn Ther 1998; 13:86–93.
11. Hubinont C, Bernard P, Pirot N, Biard J, Donnez J. Twin-to-twin transfusion syndrome: treatment by amniodrainage and septostomy. Eur J Obstet Gynecol Reprod Biol 2000; 92:141–4.
12. Quintero R, Quintero L, Morales W, Allen M, Bornick P. Amniotic fluid pressures in severe twin–twin transfusion syndrome. Prenat Neonat Med 1998; 3:607–10.
13. Hartung J, Chaoui R, Bollmann R. Amniotic fluid pressure in both cavities of twin-to-twin transfusion syndrome: a vote against septostomy. Fetal Diagn Ther 2000; 15:79–82.
14. Moise KJ Jr, Dorman K, Lamvu G et al. A randomized trial of amnioreduction versus septostomy in the treatment of twin–twin transfusion syndrome. Am J Obstet Gynecol 2005; 193:701–7.
15. Mari G, Roberts A, Detti L et al. Perinatal morbidity and mortality rates in severe twin–twin transfusion syndrome: results of the International Amnioreduction Registry. Am J Obstet Gynecol 2001; 185:708–15.
16. Lopriore E, Nagel HT, Vandenbussche FP, Walther FJ. Long-term neurodevelopmental outcome in twin-to-twin transfusion syndrome. Am J Obstet Gynecol 2003; 189:1314–19.
17. Pinette MG, Pan Y, Pinette SG, Stubblefield PG. Treatment of twin–twin transfusion syndrome. Obstet Gynecol 1993; 82:841–6.
18. Trespidi L, Boschetto C, Caravelli E et al. Serial amniocenteses in the management of twin–twin transfusion syndrome: when is it valuable? Fetal Diagn Ther 1997; 12:15–20.
19. Fesslova V, Villa L, Nava S, Mosca F, Nicolini U. Fetal and neonatal echocardiographic findings in twin–twin transfusion syndrome. Am J Obstet Gynecol 1998; 179:1056–62.
20. Mari G, Detti L, Oz U, Abuhamad AZ. Long-term outcome in twin–twin transfusion syndrome treated with serial aggressive amnioreduction. Am J Obstet Gynecol 2000; 183:211–17.
21. Dennis LG, Winkler CL. Twin-to-twin transfusion syndrome: aggressive therapeutic amniocentesis. Am J Obstet Gynecol 1997; 177:342–7; discussion 7–9.
22. Dickinson JE, Evans SF. Obstetric and perinatal outcomes from the Australian and New Zealand Twin–Twin

Transfusion Syndrome Registry. Am J Obstet Gynecol 2000; 182:706–12.

23. De Lia JE, Cruikshank DP, Keye WR Jr. Fetoscopic neodymium:yttrium–aluminum–garnet laser occlusion of placental vessels in severe twin–twin transfusion syndrome. Obstet Gynecol 1990; 75:1046–53.

24. Quintero R, Morales W, Mendoza G et al. Selective photocoagulation of placental vessels in twin–twin transfusion syndrome: evolution of a surgical technique. Obstet Gynecol Surv 1998; 53:s97–103.

25. Quintero RA, Comas C, Bornick PW, Allen MH, Kruger M. Selective versus non-selective laser photocoagulation of placental vessels in twin–twin transfusion syndrome. Ultrasound Obstet Gynecol 2000; 16:230–6.

26. Hecher K, Plath H, Bregenzer T, Hansmann M, Hackeloer BJ. Endoscopic laser surgery versus serial amniocenteses in the treatment of severe twin–twin transfusion syndrome. Am J Obstet Gynecol 1999; 180:717–24.

27. Quintero RA, Dickinson JE, Morales WJ et al. Stage-based treatment of twin–twin transfusion syndrome. Am J Obstet Gynecol 2003; 188:1333–40.

28. Quintero R, Morales W, Allen M et al. Staging of twin–twin transfusion syndrome. J Perinatol 1999; 19:550–5.

29. Senat MV, Deprest J, Boulvain M et al. Endoscopic laser surgery versus serial amnioreduction for severe twin-to-twin transfusion syndrome. N Engl J Med 2004; 351:136–44.

30. Dudley D, D'Alton M. Single fetal death in twin gestation. Semin Perinatol 1986; 10:65–72.

31. Fusi L, Gordon H. Twin pregnancy complicated by single intrauterine death. Problems and outcome with conservative management. Br J Obstet Gynaecol 1990; 97:511–16.

32. Okamura K, Murotsuki J, Tanigawara S, Uehara S, Yahima A. Funipuncture for evaluation of hematologic and coagulation indices in the surviving twin following co-twin's death. Obstet Gynecol 1994; 83:975–8.

33. Quintero RA, Reich H, Puder KS et al. Brief report: umbilical-cord ligation of an acardiac twin by fetoscopy at 19 weeks of gestation. N Engl J Med 1994; 330:469–71.

34. Deprest JA, Audibert F, Van Schoubroeck D, Hecher K, Mahieu-Caputo D. Bipolar coagulation of the umbilical cord in complicated monochorionic twin pregnancy. Am J Obstet Gynecol 2000; 182:340–5.

35. Tan TY, Sepulveda W. Acardiac twin: a systematic review of minimally invasive treatment modalities. Ultrasound Obstet Gynecol 2003; 22:409–19.

36. Sydorak RM, Feldstein V, Machin G et al. Fetoscopic treatment for discordant twins. J Pediatr Surg 2002; 37:1736–9.

37. Tsao K, Feldstein VA, Albanese CT et al. Selecti⋅ reduction of acardiac twin by radiofrequency ablatio Am J Obstet Gynecol 2002; 187:635–40.

38. Nicolini U, Poblete A, Boschetto C, Bonati F, Roberts A. Complicated monochorionic twin pregnancies: experience with bipolar cord coagulation. Am J Obstet Gynecol 2001; 185:703–7.

39. Taylor MJ, Shalev E, Tanawattanacharoen S et al. Ultrasound-guided umbilical cord occlusion using bipolar diathermy for Stage III/IV twin–twin transfusion syndrome. Prenat Diagn 2002; 22:70–6.

40. Quintero RA, Kontopoulos EV, Chmait R, Bornick PW, Allen M. Management of twin–twin transfusion syndrome in pregnancies with iatrogenic detachment of membranes following therapeutic amniocentesis and the role of interim amniopatch. Ultrasound Obstet Gynecol 2005; 26:628–33.

41. Gonsoulin W, Moise KJ, Kirshon B et al. Outcome of twin–twin transfusion diagnosed before 28 weeks of gestation. Obstet Gynecol 1990; 75:214–6.

42. Urig M, Clevell W, Elliot J. Twin–twin transfusion syndrome. Am J Obstet Gynecol 1990; 163:1522–6.

43. Radestad A, Thomassen PA. Acute polyhydramnios in twin pregnancy. A retrospective study with special reference to therapeutic amniocentesis. Acta Obstet Gynecol Scand 1990; 69:297–300.

44. Mahony BS, Petty CN, Nyberg DA et al. The "stuck twin" phenomenon: ultrasonographic findings, pregnancy outcome, and management with serial amniocentesis. Am J Obstet Gynecol 1990; 163:1513–22.

45. Reisner DP, Mahony BS, Petty CN et al. Stuck twin syndrome: outcome in thirty-seven consecutive cases. Am J Obstet Gynecol 1993; 169:991–5.

46. Steinberg LH, Hurley VA, Desmedt E, Beischer NA. Acute polyhydramnios in twin pregnancies. Aust N Z J Obstet Gynaecol 1990; 30:196–200.

47. Bromley B, Frigoletto FD Jr, Estroff JA, Benacerraf BR. The natural history of oligohydramnios/polyhydramnios sequence in monochorionic diamniotic twins. Ultrasound Obstet Gynecol 1992; 2:317–20.

48. Lachapelle MF, Leduc L, Cote JM, Grignon A, Fouron JC. Potential value of fetal echocardiography in the differential diagnosis of twin pregnancy with presence of polyhydramnios–oligohydramnios syndrome. Am J Obstet Gynecol 1997; 177:388–94.

49. Zondervan HA, Stoutenbeek P, Arabin B et al. [Third circulation: twin transfusion syndrome]. Ned Tijdschr Geneeskd 1999; 143:1022–7. [in Dutch]

50. Cincotta RB, Gray PH, Phythian G, Rogers YM, Chan FY. Long term outcome of twin–twin transfusion syndrome. Arch Dis Child Fetal Neonatal Ed 2000; 83:F171–6.

51. van Gemert MJ, Vandenbussche FP, Schaap AH et al. Classification of discordant fetal growth may contribute to risk stratification in monochorionic twin pregnancies. Ultrasound Obstet Gynecol 2000; 16:237–44.

52. Denbow ML, Battin MR, Cowan F et al. Neonatal cranial ultrasonographic findings in preterm twins

complicated by severe fetofetal transfusion syndrome. Am J Obstet Gynecol 1998; 178:479–83.

53. Elliott JP, Sawyer AT, Radin TG, Strong RE. Large-volume therapeutic amniocentesis in the treatment of hydramnios. Obstet Gynecol 1994; 84:1025–7.

54. Bruner JP, Rosemond RL. Twin-to-twin transfusion syndrome: a subset of the twin oligohydramnios–polyhydramnios sequence. Am J Obstet Gynecol 1993; 169:925–30.

55. Fries MH, Goldstein RB, Kilpatrick SJ et al. The role of velamentous cord insertion in the etiology of twin–twin transfusion syndrome. Obstet Gynecol 1993; 81:569–74.

56. Weiner CP, Ludomirski A. Diagnosis, pathophysiology, and treatment of chronic twin-to-twin transfusion syndrome. Fetal Diagn Ther 1994; 9:283–90.

57. Dickinson JE. Severe twin–twin transfusion syndrome: current management concepts. Aust N Z J Obstet Gynaecol 1995; 35:16–21.

58. Kilby MD, Howe DT, McHugo JM, Whittle MJ. Bladder visualisation as a prognostic sign in oligohydramnios–polyhydramnios sequence in twin pregnancies treated using therapeutic amniocentesis. Br J Obstet Gynaecol 1997; 104:939–42.

59. Bajoria R. Chorionic plate vascular anatomy determines the efficacy of amnioreduction therapy for twin–twin transfusion syndrome. Hum Reprod 1998; 13:1709–13.

60. De Lia JE, Kuhlmann RS, Harstad TW, Cruikshank DP. Fetoscopic laser ablation of placental vessels in severe previable twin–twin transfusion syndrome. Am J Obstet Gynecol 1995; 172:1202–8; discussion 1208–11.

61. Ville Y, Hecher K, Gagnon A et al. Endoscopic laser coagulation in the management of severe twin-to-twin transfusion syndrome. Br J Obstet Gynaecol 1998; 105:446–53.

62. Hecher K, Diehl W, Zikulnig L, Vetter M, Hackeloer BJ. Endoscopic laser coagulation of placental anastomoses in 200 pregnancies with severe mid-trimester twin-to-twin transfusion syndrome. Eur J Obstet Gynecol Reprod Biol 2000; 92:135–9.

12

The role of Doppler assessment in twin–twin transfusion syndrome

Josep M Martínez and Rubén A Quintero

Introduction • Pre-operative Doppler • Intraoperative Doppler • Postoperative Doppler • Future developments • Conclusions

INTRODUCTION

Twin–twin transfusion syndrome (TTTS) occurs in 10–15% of monochorionic multiple pregnancies. Untreated, it is associated with a high risk of perinatal mortality and morbidity, particularly in the form of severe neurological sequelae.[1–5] The disease is thought to occur from chronic unbalanced blood transfusion between twins across placental vascular communications, resulting in a donor and a recipient twin.[6,7] Since TTTS is associated with such hemodynamic disturbance in the cardiovascular status of either twin, Doppler studies may have a significant role in the diagnosis and management of the disease.[8]

The donor twin, who is thought to become hypovolemic, is therefore more likely to show Doppler abnormalities in the arterial system, developing oliguria, oligohydramnios, together with a minimal or non-visible bladder during most of the examination, and a variable degree of growth restriction. The recipient twin, who is thought to become hypervolemic and eventually present cardiac failure, is therefore more likely to show Doppler abnormalities in the venous system, developing polyuria and polyhydramnios, together with a persistently distended bladder.[9] Very recently, direct assessment of blood flow through the placental anastomosis by intra-amniotic Doppler assessment has been proposed to validate this theory, although it is still not possible owing to technological limitations.[10]

PRE-OPERATIVE DOPPLER

The diagnosis of TTTS is exclusively performed by ultrasound.[11] The currently accepted diagnostic criteria are: oligo–polyhydramnios sequence in a monochorionic pregnancy at less than 26 weeks of gestation. Polyhydramnios occurs in the recipient twin and is defined as a maximum vertical pocket (MVP) of amniotic fluid of ≥8 cm, whereas oligohydramnios occurs in the donor twin and is defined by an MVP of amniotic fluid of ≤2 cm. Monochorionicity is established by the presence of a single placenta, same gender, and thin dividing membrane with absence of lambda or twin peak sign.[11] Doppler evaluation is not required to diagnose TTTS.

TTTS is essentially a hemodynamic derangement that may result in significant Doppler changes in one or both fetuses. During the decade of the 1990s, the finding of an abnormal Doppler study had already been identified as a sign of poor prognosis.[1,5,9] In 1999 Quintero made an important contribution to the knowledge and management of the disease, proposing a sonographic staging classification of TTTS[12] that allows an assessment of the severity of the disease. Stage III is defined by the presence of critically abnormal Doppler studies in either twin, namely absent or reversed end-diastolic velocity in the umbilical artery, reversed flow in the ductus venosus, or pulsatile umbilical venous flow (Figure 12.1). Although donors typically show abnormalities in the umbilical artery and

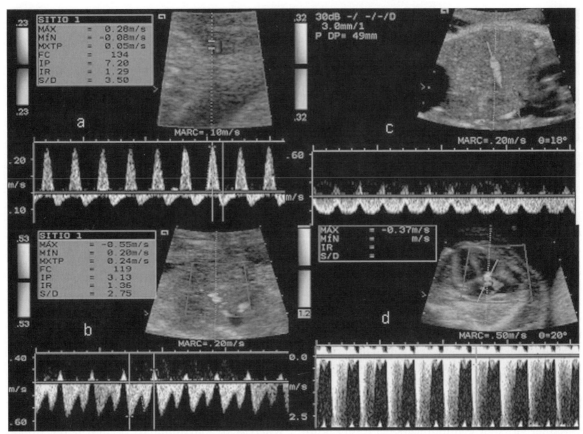

Figure 12.1 Critically abnormal Doppler flow velocity waveforms (a, b, or c define stage III). (a) Reversed end-diastolic flow in the umbilical artery. (b) Reversed flow in the ductus venosus during the atrial contraction. (c) Pulsatile umbilical vein flow. (d) Tricuspid valve regurgitation.

recipients in the venous system, either twin may show alterations in one or both systems. Since Quintero's staging report, Doppler assessment of the twins is considered mandatory upon diagnosing TTTS.

Abnormal umbilical artery Doppler studies are typically seen in the donor twin. Although unequal placental mass sharing could be caused, the finding of absent or reversed end-diastolic flow in the umbilical artery of the donor twin is more likely due to its hypovolemic and vasoconstriction status. Doppler studies of the middle cerebral artery and venous system are usually normal in the donor twin. This notion is indirectly supported by the reappearance of diastolic flow in the umbilical artery in about 25–50% of fetuses after laser therapy.[8,13,14]

The recipient twin is more likely to show abnormal Doppler studies in the venous return system. In advanced stages (stages III and IV), the ductus venosus usually shows increased pulsatility indices with absent or reverse flow during atrial contraction while the umbilical vein may show a typical pulsatile flow pattern. Other common ultrasound and Doppler features reflecting right heart overload are tricuspid regurgitation and hypertrophic right ventricle with increased thickness of the myocardium, eventually leading to progressive pulmonary valve stenosis. An increased blood flow volume in the umbilical vein of recipient twins in comparison with donors and even normal fetuses matched by gestational age has also been reported.[14,15] All these Doppler parameters indicate a likely progression from cardiac overload, as a consequence of chronic hypervolemia, to severe cardiac insufficiency, eventually development of hydrops fetalis, and even death if left untreated.

We and others have found that the parameter most predictive of intrauterine fetal death (IUFD) of the donor twin is absent or reverse end-diastolic velocity in the umbilical artery of the donor twin, both in patients treated with amnioreduction[16,17] or with laser.[5,8,13,14] This Doppler pattern has been found to be present in up to 12–46% of the donors in laser series, and is associated with an increased risk of perinatal death of the donor (61–75%). Other preoperative Doppler parameters do not seem to predict IUFD in either twin,[8] although Hecher reported a higher risk of IUFD of the recipient twin when this pattern was present in this twin, before or after therapy.[13] Pulsatile umbilical venous flow, and absent or reverse ductus venosus flow during the atrial contraction, and tricuspid regurgitation, are frequently found (30–50%) in the recipient twin, but have not been associated with increased risk of IUFD of this twin after laser.[8,13,14]

INTRAOPERATIVE DOPPLER

Selective fetoscopic laser photocoagulation of the communicating vessels is undoubtedly the treatment of choice for TTTS.[11] Intraoperative Doppler is essential to complete the procedure.[18]

During the immediate preoperative evaluation, color Doppler is useful to identify the insertion of the umbilical cords. This step is used to predict the site of the anastomoses and to choose the trocar insertion site. A short distance between the cords may harbinger the presence of a large number and large caliber anastomoses. Color Doppler, and in particular power Doppler, is used to detect maternal vessels in the uterine wall that need to be avoided during the trocar insertion.[5,18] During the surgery, the fetal heart rates are closely monitored by pulsed Doppler. Finally, color Doppler is used to control the removal of the trocar to detect uterine bleeding.

POSTOPERATIVE DOPPLER

Post-operative Doppler studies are used to assess the twins' well-being by exploring the arterial, venous, and intracardiac systems in the same manner as before the procedure.

In general, Doppler studies have a limited role in predicting postoperative IUFD in TTTS patients treated with laser therapy. In our study performed in Tampa on patients undergoing laser therapy for the treatment of TTTS, Doppler waveform analysis of the umbilical artery, middle cerebral artery, ductus venosus, umbilical vein, and tricuspid valve were performed in both twins 6–24 hours before surgery and within 16–24 hours after surgery. The only Doppler parameter found to have a predictive value was the umbilical artery of the donor twin. No other Doppler parameter was significantly associated with a greater likelihood of IUFD in the donor or in the recipient twin.[8] These results may have important implications in our understanding of the effect of surgery on the hemodynamic status of the fetuses as well as other potential factors that may determine in-utero survival.

Because laser therapy essentially renders the original monochorionic twin pregnancy into a 'functional dichorionic' gestation, one could hypothesize that Doppler could be used to predict the individual outcome and risk of IUFD of the fetuses. This argument is based on the fact that interruption of the vascular communications between the fetuses avoids the untoward effects of IUFD of one of the twins on the surviving co-twin. However, several issues must be pointed out. First, the fetuses and their Doppler status are interdependent prior to surgery; Doppler signals may reflect the interaction between the fetuses and not just the individual status of each twin. Thus, abnormal Doppler studies due to the presence of vascular communications. Secondly, surgery may exert a profound effect in the hemodynamic status of the fetuses that could translate into the postoperative Doppler studies. Because neither the preoperative fetal interaction nor the postoperative surgical effect can be predicted before surgery, the limited value for Doppler in predicting IUFD after laser therapy is not surprising.[8]

Laser surgery cannot 'add' any additional placenta to either twin, except maybe in the case of a 3-vessel cotyledon. As a corollary, postoperative appearance of diastolic blood flow in fetuses with preoperative absent or reversed flow suggests, that the Doppler pattern did not result from placental insufficiency, but rather, from hypotension.[8]

Postoperative reverse flow in the ductous venosus was not found by us to be associated with an increased risk of IUFD of the donor.[8] However, other authors have found that few if any increased pulsitility index of the ductous venous and even transient hydropic changes may be found in surviving donor twins.[13–15, 19] These hemodynamic changes are thought to be the consequence of a transient state of hypervolemia and an adaptation response of the donor after successful laser intervention.[13–15] Because our study looked at reverse ductal flow and not pulsitility index, this may explain the differences found with other studies. An advantage of using categorical rather than continuous variables to reflect Doppler changes is that it eliminates the confounding effect of gestational age. Since the parameters represent the extreme of the spectrum in Doppler changes, it follows that the sensitivity of the Doppler parameter may be decreased, but the specificity is improved. In agreement with these hypotheses, donor fetuses had a significant increase in umbilical venous blood flow after laser therapy, both in general and by estimated fetal weight.[14,15]

Recipient twins frequently show abnormal venous return Doppler velocimetry. Most recipients demonstrate improvement of the cardiac overload after laser therapy, with a decreased ductus venosus pulsatility index, resolution of absent or reversed flow during atrial contraction, and disappearance of tricuspid regurgitation (50–60% of cases). This may occur as early as 24 hours after surgery.[13–15] In contrast to donors, recipient twins demonstrate decreased umbilical venous blood flow.[14,15] Furthermore, total umbilical vein blood flow in recipient fetuses was significantly higher than in donor fetuses before laser therapy but not after surgery, suggesting that laser therapy is corrective of the syndrome.[14,15]

Progressive postoperative worsening of venous return Dopplers and development of hydrops in the recipient could portent a poor perinatal outcome for the recipient,[13–15] although this has not been our experience.[8] Demise of a recipient twin with abnormal venous system Doppler could result from surgery being performed beyond the point of no return in a terminally ill fetus. Alternatively, further hemodynamic overload of the recipient may result from intraoperative transfusion secondary to laser obliteration of recipient-to-donor before donor-to-recipient arteriovenous communications. Although proof of either of these hypotheses is virtually impossible, the latter concept may be used to manage stage III cases with critically abnormal venous return of the recipient twin, by severing the donor-to-recipient arteriovenous communications first, followed by the recipient-to-donor arteriovenous communications. This may prevent intraoperative overload of the recipient twin.[8]

Doppler waveform analysis of the middle cerebral artery has been reported as a useful method for the differential diagnosis between selective growth retardation and TTTS in monochorionic twins. The middle cerebral artery pulsatility index is lower in IUGR fetuses compared to fetuses with TTTS.[20] Our results, show that 25% of donors and 50% of recipients had a pulsatility index below the 5th percentile. Furthermore, this parameter did not have any influence on fetal outcome.[8] Others have also reported a decreased cerebral pulsatility index in recipient twins.[9] We speculate that chronic blood exchange and imbalanced hemodynamic status may elicit a 'brain-sparing effect' as a compensating mechanism, but without the classical meaning and poor prognosis that has been reported in intrauterine growth retardation from placental insufficiency.[8]

Doppler assessment of the MCA for the detection of fetal anemia has been recently proposed in single twin demise. An increased PSV suggestive of fetal anemia has been used as an indication for fetal transfusion to prevent death or sequelae in the surviving twin.[21–23]

FUTURE DEVELOPMENTS

Measurement of the actual blood flow in the communicating vessels to demonstrate the hypothesis of unbalanced blood flow between fundamental hypothesis of TTTS has not been possible. Our group has recently attempted to assess individual blood flow through placental vascular anastomoses using intra-amniotic small-caliber ultrasound catheters[24] with color and pulsed Doppler. Contrary to our expectations, the calculated net blood flow was from recipient to donor in both cases.[10] Despite this disappointing result, we believe this approach can be perfected to provide irrefutable evidence in support of the hypothesis of unbalanced blood flow exchange between two monochorionic twins as the etiology of TTTS. Our experience has demonstrated that these measurements are indeed possible, although the accuracy of the measurements is still suboptimal.[10] We look forward to further improvements in ultrasound catheter technology and Doppler measurements.

CONCLUSIONS

Doppler studies in the assessment of patients with TTTS add a new dimension to the management of the disease. Doppler studies may help predict and understand postoperative outcomes and may point to the potential contribution of concomitant factors in the incidence of intrauterine fetal demise, such as placental insufficiency in donors or cardiac overload in recipients. Our studies may also suggest the possibility of considering individualization of the firing sequence during laser therapy, to decrease the likelihood of intraoperative transfusion and its potential deleterious effects on either of the twins. Because from 25 to 50% of donor twins with preoperative absent or reversed end-diastolic flow in the umbilical artery may show improvement and survive after laser therapy, we would caution about resorting to umbilical cord occlusion of this fetus as a primary management choice for these patients.

REFERENCES

1. De Lia J, Fisk N, Hecher K et al. Twin-to-twin transfusion syndrome: debates on the etiology, natural history and management. Ultrasound Obstet Gynecol 2000; 16:210–13.
2. Blickstein I. The twin–twin transfusion syndrome. Obstet Gynecol 1990; 76:714–22.
3. Gonsoulin W, Moise KJ, Kirshon B et al. Outcome of twin–twin transfusion diagnosed before 28 weeks of gestation. Obstet Gynecol 1990; 75:214–16.
4. Saunders NJ, Snijders RJ, Nicolaides KH. Therapeutic amniocentesis in twin–twin transfusion syndrome appearing in the second trimester of pregnancy. Am J Obstet Gynecol 1992; 166:820–4.
5. Ville Y, Hecher K, Gagnon A et al. Endoscopic laser coagulation in the management of severe twin-to-twin transfusion syndrome. Br J Obstet Gynaecol 1998; 105(4):446–53.
6. Diehl W, Hecher K, Zikulnig L, Vetter M, Hackeloer BJ. Placental vascular anastomoses visualized during fetoscopic laser surgery in severe mid-trimester twin–twin transfusion syndrome. Placenta 2001; 22:876–81.
7. Bermudez C, Becerra CH, Bornick PW et al. Placental types and twin–twin transfusion syndrome. Am J Obstet Gynecol 2002; 187:489–94.
8. Martinez JM, Bermudez C, Becerra CH et al. The role of Doppler studies in predicting individual intrauterine fetal demise after laser therapy for twin–twin transfusion syndrome. Ultrasound Obstet Gynecol 2003; 22:246–51.
9. Hecher K, Ville Y, Snijders R, Nicolaides K. Doppler studies of the fetal circulation in twin–twin transfusion syndrome. Ultrasound Obstet Gynecol 1995; 5:318–24.
10. Nakata M, Martínez JM, Díaz C, Chmait RH, Quintero RA. Intra-amniotic Doppler measurement of blood flow in placental vascular anastomoses in twin–twin transfusion syndrome. Ultrasound Obstet Gynecol 2004; 24:102–3.
11. Senat MV, Deprest J, Boulvain M et al. Endoscopic laser surgery versus serial amnioreduction for severe twin-to-twin transfusion syndrome. N Engl J Med 2004; 351:136–44.
12. Quintero R, Morales W, Allen M et al. Staging of twin–twin transfusion syndrome. J Perinatol 1999; 19:550–5.
13. Zikulnig L, Hecher K, Bregenzer T, Baz E, Hackeloer BJ. Prognostic factors in severe twin–twin transfusion syndrome treated by endoscopic laser surgery. Ultrasound Obstet Gynecol 1999; 14:380–7.
14. Gratacos E, Van Schoubroeck D, Carreras E et al. Impact of laser coagulation in severe twin–twin transfusion syndrome on fetal Doppler indices and venous blood flow volume. Ultrasound Obstet Gynecol 2002; 20:125–30.
15. Ishii K, Chmait RH, Martínez JM, Nakata M, Quintero RA. Ultrasound assessment of venous blood flow before and after laser therapy: an approach to understanding the pathophysiology of twin–twin transfusion syndrome. Ultrasound Obstet Gynecol 2004; 24:164–8.
16. Taylor MJ, Denbow ML, Duncan KR, Overton TG, Fisk NM. Antenatal factors at diagnosis that predict outcome in twin–twin transfusion syndrome. Am J Obstet Gynecol 2000; 183:1023–8.
17. Mari G, Roberts A, Detti L et al. Perinatal morbidity and mortality rates in severe twin–twin transfusion

syndrome: results of the International Amnioreduction Registry. Am J Obstet Gynecol 2001; 185:708–15.

18. Quintero R, Morales W, Mendoza G et al. Selective photocoagulation of placental vessels in twin–twin transfusion syndrome: evolution of a surgical technique. Obstet Gynecol Surv 1998; 5312:s97–s103.

19. Gratacos E, Van Schoubroeck D, Carreras E et al. Transient hydropic signs in the donor fetus after fetoscopic laser coagulation in severe twin–twin transfusion syndrome: incidence and clinical relevance. Ultrasound Obstet Gynecol 2002; 19:449–53.

20. Suzuki S, Ishikawa G, Sawa R et al. Iatrogenic monoamniotic twin gestation with progressive twin–twin transfusion syndrome. Fetal Diagn Ther 1999; 14:98–101.

21. Senat MV, Loizeau S, Couderc S, Bernard JP, Ville Y. The value of middle cerebral artery peak systolic velocity in the diagnosis of fetal anemia after intrauterine death of one monochorionic twin. Am J Obstet Gynecol 2003; 189:1320–4.

22. Mari G, Deter RI, Carpenter RL et al. Noninvasive diagnosis by Doppler ultrasonography of fetal anemia due to maternal red-cell alloimmunization. Collaborative Group for Doppler Assessment of the Blood Velocity in Anemic Fetuses. N Engl J Med 2000; 342:9–14.

23. Quintero RA, Martínez JM, Bermúdez C, López J, Becerra C. Fetoscopic demonstration of perimortem feto-fetal hemorrhage in twin–twin transfusion syndrome. Ultrasound Obstet Gynecol 2002; 20:638–9.

24. Quintero RA, Bermudez C, Becerra CH, Bornick PW, Allen M. Intra-amniotic ultrasound. Ultrasound Obstet Gynecol 2001; 18:681–2.

13

Outcomes and complications of the surgical treatment of twin–twin transfusion syndrome

Walter J Morales

Introduction • Outcomes • Complications • Conclusions

INTRODUCTION

Twin–twin transfusion syndrome (TTTS) occurs in approximately 10–15% of monochorionic twin pregnancies. If untreated, this condition will almost always result in perinatal mortality or long-term neurological handicap of surviving infants.[1,2] Various procedures have been proposed in the treatment of this syndrome, including selective feticide,[3] serial decompressing amniocentesis,[4] and intentional septostomy.[5] These procedures have met with limited success, particularly in those cases presenting with early diagnosis (20 weeks), abnormal Doppler studies (stage III), or fetal hydrops (stage IV).

In an attempt to improve the outcome in patients with TTTS, laser photocoagulation of the placental vascular communication responsible for this condition was initially introduced in 1990.[6] The surgical techniques have gradually evolved to the present approach of selective laser photocoagulation of communicating vessels (SLPCV) conducted under local anesthesia.[7] This chapter describes the outcomes and complications of patients with TTTS treated with SLPCV at our center in Tampa from 1997 through 2003.

OUTCOMES

During the study period 1997 through 2003, 448 patients diagnosed with TTTS were referred for endoscopic SLPCV therapy. Of these, 42 patients were deemed not to be candidates for surgery for a number of reasons, including incorrect diagnosis of TTTS, significantly detached amniotic membranes or placental hematoma from prior therapeutic amniocentesis, or advanced cervical dilatation due to incompetent cervix. The remaining 404 patients, including 17 with triplet gestation, underwent endoscopic surgery under Institutional Review Board approved protocols. Of these patients, 369, including 16 with triplets, were treated by means of SLPCV, and the remaining 35 underwent umbilical cord occlusion (UCO). The outcomes of the twin and triplet pregnancies are summarized in Tables 13.1 and 13.2.

Patients with either twin or triplet gestation and treated by means of SLPCV had a favorable outcome, with 87% achieving at least one surviving infant with a mean gestational age of 32.8 weeks. Dual survivors occurred in 55% of the pregnancies, with only 5% of these delivering at less than 28 weeks. In addition, when the

Table 13.1 Outcomes of twins with TTTS

	Procedure	
	SLPCV (n = 353)	UCO (n = 34)
Gestational age at therapy, weeks	20.5	20.5
Gestational age at delivery, weeks	31.7	31.4
Interval, weeks	11.2	10.9
Dual survivor, No. (%)	192 (54)	–
At least one survivor, No. (%)	307 (87)	26 (77)
Gestational age of survivors, weeks	33.1	34.3
Survivors at 28 weeks, No. (%)	42 (9)	3 (9)

SLPCV, selective laser photocoagulation of communicating vessels; UCO, umbilical cord occlusion.

Table 13.2 Outcomes of triplets with TTTS

	Procedure	
	SLPCV (n = 16)	UCO (n = 1)
Gestational age at therapy, weeks	21.4	20.4
Gestational age at delivery, weeks	31.5	30.5
Interval, weeks	10.1	10.1
Dual survivor, No. (%)	10 (62)	–
At least one survivor, No. (%)	15 (94)	1 (100)
Gestational age of survivors, weeks	32.5	30.5
Survivors at 28 weeks, No. (%)	4 (16)	–

SLPCV, selective laser photocoagulation of communicating vessels; UCO, umbilical cord occlusion.

outcome data were analyzed by severity of the disease defined by a staging classification,[8] there were no significant differences in outcomes of patients of different stages treated with SLPCV (Table 13.3).

Of the 369 patients treated by means of SLPCV, the surgery was successful in achieving the desired clinical goal of interrupting the progression of the TTTS. Only 11 (3%) of these patients required additional therapeutic amniocentesis to treat the persistent polyhydramnios sequence, and two patients needed a second SLPCV procedure to treat persistent patent communicating vessels. Post-delivery evaluation of placentas by a single experienced pathologist

confirmed that in over 95% of the specimens the surgical procedure had interrupted flow in the communicating vessels.

The data summarized in Tables 13.1 and 13.2 indicate no improved outcomes by the UCO procedure. Thus, with the exception of technically unfeasible cases or in pregnancies involving a structurally abnormal fetus, SLPCV should be the preferred approach.

COMPLICATIONS

Complications arising from endoscopic fetal surgery include preterm rupture of membranes (PROM), membrane detachment with or without

Table 13.3 Outcomes by severity of TTTS treated by SLPCV

	Stage I (n = 51)	Stage II (n = 105)	Stage III (n = 175)	Stage IV (n = 38)
Gestational age at therapy, weeks	20.2	20.5	20.3	22.0
Gestational age at delivery, weeks	32.6	32.3	31.2	31.7
Interval, weeks	12.4	11.8	10.9	9.7
At least one survivor, No. (%)	47 (92)	94 (89)	149 (85)	32 (84)
Dual survivor, No. (%)	37 (73)	69 (68)	77 (44)	19 (49)
Gestational age of survivors, weeks	33.5	33.5	32.6	32.4
Survivors at 28 weeks, No. (%)	6 (7)	7 (4)	24 (11)	5 (10)

SLPCV, selective laser photocoagulation of communicating vessels.

Table 13.4 Complications in patients with TTTS

| | Twins | | Triplets | |
	SLPCV procedure	UCO procedure	SLPCV procedure	UCO procedure
No.	353	34	16	1
No. with complications	58 (16%)	8 (23%)	1 (6%)	–
No. with one complication	23 (6%)	4 (12%)	–	–
Type of complication:				
PROM	24 (7%)	4 (12%)	1 (6%)	–
Membrane detachment	35 (10%)	2 (6%)	–	–
Bleeding	15 (4%)	4 (12%)	–	–
PTL	2 (1%)	–	–	–
Maternal complication	3 (1%)	1 (3%)		

SLPCV, selective laser photocoagulation of communicating vessels; UCO, umbilical cord occlusion; PROM, preterm rupture of membranes; PTL, preterm labor.

accumulation of extraovular fluid, intra-amniotic bleeding or placental hematoma associated with a decrease of over 2 g of hemoglobin from the preoperative level, preterm labor defined as persistent regular uterine contractions requiring tocolytic therapy for over 24 hours after the surgical procedure, or a significant maternal complication related to the surgical procedure.

Overall, 65 (16%) of the 404 patients treated for TTTS experienced a complication, with 27 (6.6%) of patients experiencing more than one complication. The different complications identified in the 404 patients with TTTS treated surgically by either SLPCV or UCO are summarized in Table 13.4. Of the 369 patients treated by means of SLPCV, 59 (16%) experienced a complication. PROM and membrane detachment were the two most common complications, being diagnosed in 24 (7%) and 35 (9%) of patients, respectively.

The outcomes of the group of 59 pregnancies experiencing a complication were compared to the group without complications (Table 13.5). Although both groups underwent the SLPCV procedure at the same gestational age (20.5 weeks), and had similar numbers of patients with severe disease, stage III or IV, the group with complications delivered at a significantly earlier gestational age, 27.6 vs 32.8 weeks, had a higher proportion of pregnancies delivered at less than 28 weeks, 52% vs 14%, lower number with dual survivors, 29% vs 60%, and lower number of

pregnancies with at least one surviving infant, 56% vs 92%.

When the outcome of pregnancies was broken down by the type of complication, those with rupture of membranes experienced the worst outcome, with none having a dual survivor and only 29% achieving one surviving infant (Table 13.6). A group of 25 patients experienced membrane detachment and in 13 (52%) patients the membrane defect was successfully resealed using an amniopatch consisting of an intra-amniotic injection of platelets and cryoprecipitate.[9] The group

Table 13.5 Effect of complications in pregnancy outcome of patients with TTTS treated with SLPCV

| | Complications | |
	No (n = 310)	Yes (n = 59)
Patients with stage III–IV, No. (%)	180 (58)	33 (56)
Gestational age at procedure, weeks	20.5	20.5
Gestational age at delivery, weeks	32.8	27.6
Interval, weeks	12.3	7.1
Dual survivor, No. (%)	185 (60)	17 (29)
At least one survivor, No. (%)	284 (92)	33 (56)
Delivery at 28 weeks, No. (%)	43 (14)	31 (52)

SLPCV, selective laser photocoagulation of communicating vessels.

Table 13.6 Pregnancy outcomes by type of complication

	No. of complications (n = 310)	PROM* (n = 14)	Membranes detached[†] (n = 25)	PROM and membranes detached[#] (n = 10)	Bleeding (n = 12)
Gestational age at procedure, weeks	20.5	21.2	20.2	20.1	20.7
Gestational age at delivery, weeks	32.8	24.0	31.0	24.7	29.9
Interval, weeks	12.3	3.8	10.8	4.6	9.2
Dual survivor, No. (%)	185 (60)	–	10 (40)	2 (20)	7 (58)
At least one survivor, No. (%)	284 (92)	4 (29)	22 (88)	3 (30)	10 (83)
Delivery at <28 weeks, No. (%)	43 (14)	13 (93)	8 (32)	7 (70)	3 (25)

PROM, preterm rupture of membranes.
*1 patient spontaneously resealed membranes.
[†]8 of 13 patients (62%) had a successful blood patch.
[#]2 of 5 patients (40%) had a successful blood patch.

undergoing an amniopatch procedure had a significantly longer extension of the pregnancy compared to those not treated with amniopatch therapy after membrane detachment, 13.3 vs 8.0 weeks.

Different presurgical conditions were examined for risks of complications and adverse pregnancy outcomes. Patients with anterior placenta had an increased incidence of complications, 20% vs 12%. Patients presenting with a diagnosis of incompetent cervix requiring an emergent cerclage immediately following the SLPCV procedure experienced a significant incidence of pregnancy delivered at less than 28 weeks, 38% vs 18%. During the period of study, 62 (17%) of the 369 patients required the placement of two trocars to complete the procedure. The group in which two trocars was used experienced a higher rate of complications, 27% vs 14%.

The rate of complications was not affected by the severity of the disease. The incidences of complications associated with stages I–IV were 10%, 18%, 14%, and 22%, respectively. The rate of complications also was not increased when the recipient was the presenting twin 18% vs 15%. Although there was a higher rate of complications in 53 patients undergoing more than one therapeutic decompression amniocentesis, 24% vs 14%, the difference did not achieve statistical significance. However, this data does not include 16 patients with TTTS who were excluded from

SLPCV therapy due to extensive membrane detachment, accidental septostomy, or intra-amniotic bleeding following decompression amniocentesis.

Finally, three patients experienced serious maternal complications. One patient suffered profound intractable bleeding during the surgical procedure under general anesthesia, requiring emergent intraoperative laparotomy and abdominal hysterectomy. Despite aggressive medical therapy, the patient ultimately died from complications due to amniotic fluid embolus. A second patient experienced severe bleeding from placental abruption and required emergent hysterectomy. This patient had an uneventful postoperative course and was discharged home 4 days after surgery. A third patient underwent a mini-laparotomy to allow surgical ligation of localized uterine bleeding without loss of pregnancy. These three patients who experienced severe maternal complications were treated during the first 3 years of the program and no serious events have occurred in the 273 patients with TTTS treated since June 2000.

CONCLUSIONS

The outcome data presented in this chapter provide a persuasive argument for treating patients with TTTS by means of endoscopic SLPCV. The procedure is, however, clearly not free of complications, and patients and referring physicians must be made aware of these facts. Nonetheless, despite the invasive and delicate nature of this procedure, no serious complications have occurred over the last 3 years of the study, during which time 73% of the patients underwent SLPCV therapy. The obvious learning curve associated with any new technique has resulted in refinement in the technique, with improved maternal and neonatal outcomes. The procedure is currently being carried out under local as opposed to general anesthesia, almost exclusively with one trocar insertion, and with a median operative time of 48 minutes over the last 3 years. In addition, improvements in the endoscopic equipment have allowed treatment of patients with anterior placentas with almost equal efficacy and safety as those with posterior placental insertions.[10]

Other correctable presurgical factors such as avoiding decompression amniocentesis in patients with advanced disease, and carefully monitoring patients for incompetent cervix with surgical treatment as needed, are expected to improve outcomes. In addition, the use of blood amniopatch in correcting post-surgical membrane detachment due to collection of extraovular amniotic fluid will likewise result in improved pregnancy outcomes.

REFERENCES

1. Urig MA, Clewell WH, Elliott JP. Twin–twin transfusion syndrome. Am J Obstet Gynecol 1990; 163:1522–6.

2. Lopriore E, Nagel HT, Vandenbussche FP, Walther FJ. Long-term neurodevelopmental outcome in twin-to-twin transfusion syndrome. Am J Obstet Gynecol 2003; 189:1314–19.

3. Deprest JA, Audibert F, Van Schoubroeck D, Hecher K. Bipolar coagulation of the umbilical cord in complicated monochorionic twin pregnancy. Am J Obstet Gynecol 2000; 182:340–5.

4. Elliott JP, Urig MA, Clewell WH. Aggressive therapeutic amniocentesis for treatment of twin–twin transfusion syndrome. Obstet Gynecol 1991; 77:537–40.

5. Pistorius LR, Howarth GR. Failure of amniotic septostomy in the management of 3 subsequent cases of severe previable twin–twin transfusion syndrome. Fetal Diagn Ther 1999; 14:337–40.

6. De Lia JE, Cruikshank DP, Keye WR Jr. Fetoscopic neodymium:YAG laser occlusion of placental vessels in severe twin–twin transfusion syndrome. Obstet Gynecol 1990; 75:1046–53.

7. Quintero RA, Morales WJ, Mendoza G, Allen M. Selective photocoagulation of placental vessels in twin–twin transfusion syndrome: evolution of a surgical technique. Obstet Gynecol Surv 1998; 53(Suppl):S97–103.

8. Quintero RA, Morales WJ, Allen MH, et al. Staging of twin–twin transfusion syndrome. J Perinatol 1999; 19:550–5.

9. Quintero RA, Morales WJ, Allen M et al. Treatment of iatrogenic previable premature rupture of membranes with intra-amniotic injection of platelets and cryoprecipitate (amniopatch): preliminary experience. Am J Obstet Gynecol 1999; 181:744–9.

10. Quintero RA, Bornick PW, Allen MH, Johnson PK. Selective laser photocoagulation of communicating vessels in severe twin–twin transfusion syndrome in women with anterior placenta. Obstet Gynecol 2001; 97:477–81.

14

Echocardiography in twin–twin transfusion

James Huhta

Introduction • Etiology • Echocardiography techniques • Postnatal results

INTRODUCTION

Twin–twin transfusion syndrome (TTTS) is now being defined and treated in an aggressive fashion and it is appropriate to examine the methods of echocardiography to ask how it may contribute to the pre- and post-treatment assessment.

ETIOLOGY

Twin pregnancy may be associated with monochorionicity and the potential for discordance of the amniotic fluid volume in each sac, also the growth of the fetuses may be altered to create the larger/smaller twin situation. The smaller twin functions from a cardiovascular point of view as a growth-restricted fetus might: placental insufficiency leads to relative hypoxemia and nutritional deficiency. This increased placental resistance may be reflected in a high pulsatility index in the umbilical artery in the smaller twin. In the first trimester, the larger twin is essentially normal, having the majority of the placenta and a normal heart and vascular system. The presence of intravascular communications[1] between the two placental areas leads, in the minority, to 'transfusion' of blood to the larger. At the new steady state, there is volume overload of the larger twin, and relative hypovolemia of the smaller twin. The hypovolemia in the small twin triggers reflexes that are designed to conserve salt and water and to raise blood pressure. The renin–angiotensin system is activated and endothelin-1 and brain natriuretic peptide production are activated.[2] These hormones have little effect on the hypovolemic, growth-restricted smaller twin, but they pass also to the larger twin through vascular communications to affect the circulation of the larger twin. This larger 'sentinel twin', although intrinsically normal, then manifests retention of salt and water and vasoconstriction. This results in severe hypervolemia and hypertension and a marked increase in cardiac output and urine production. The latter causes a marked increase in the amniotic fluid volume, resulting in the classical oligo–polyhydramnios presentation of TTTS.[3] Rarely (5%), there can be reversal of the transfusional gradient and phenotype, suggesting the possibility of an additional anomaly such as a genetic syndrome or structural defect.[4]

The result of the hypertension in the recipient twin, albeit from the combined causes of increased volume and vasoconstricting substances, is the development of cardiac biventricular hypertrophy, one of the first manifestations of the twin–twin cardiac discordance.[5] This myocardial hypertrophy can have several detrimental consequences, including hypertrophic cardiomyopathy that results in diastolic dysfunction, changes in the right ventricular outflow tract (see pulmonary stenosis), and compromised cardiac output. The hypertension associated with this sequence may also be part of the etiology of brain injury in the larger recipient twin in TTTS. This hypertension can occur in the first trimester and can result in infarction in the heart, brain, or other organs. Adverse neurodevelopmental outcome in TTTS survivors with standard therapy is common (26%), especially after the intrauterine fetal demise of a co-twin.[6] Dense echogenic changes in the walls of the pulmonary artery and aorta have been described recently and this type of vasculopathy is most likely the result of blood pressure that is inordinately high at early stages of great artery remodeling.[7]

The progression of cardiomyopathy can eventually lead to reduction in the cardiac output. Normally, the peak velocity in the recipient twin should be 30–50% greater than normal for gestational age. If this is not the case, it is due to decreased cardiac output and may be a harbinger of decreased cardiac output and the development of acidosis.

Congenital heart disease, particularly pulmonary stenosis, has been associated with injury to the right ventricle in the recipient twin. This pulmonary stenosis may be so severe as to simulate pulmonary atresia and can be associated with severe right ventricular hypoplasia with hypertrophy.[8]

ECHOCARDIOGRAPHY TECHNIQUES

The echocardiography contribution to the assessment of twins consists of applying modern methods to determining the cardiovascular physiology and the extent of the compromise of the myocardial function of each twin. There is also the mandate to identify any congenital cardiac defect that could alter the natural history of either twin. Recognition of discordance of the placental impedances is manifested by changes in the umbilical artery Doppler findings (Figure 14.1).

The first manifestation of abnormality in the recipient twin that is indicative of hypertension is myocardial hypertrophy. This may be assessed with Doppler interrogation of the venous system.

Venous Doppler

Pulsed Doppler in the veins of the twins allows assessment indirectly of the presence of elevated central venous pressure. Near the heart, a loss of the normal E wave in the normally

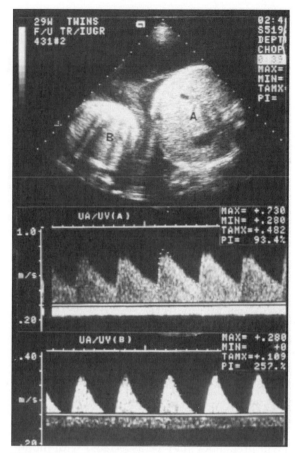

Figure 14.1 Twin–twin transfusion syndrome with a larger recipient twin (A) and a smaller donor twin (B) (upper panel). The discordance in the umbilical artery (UA) Doppler patterns is shown with normal pattern for A and absent end-diastolic flow in B (lower panel). In this example, note that both umbilical venous (UV) Doppler patterns are normal and flat without pulsations below the baseline.

triphasic waveform with a large A reversal is indicative of increased end-diastolic pressure in the right ventricle (Figure 14.2). Venous Doppler abnormalities will then manifest farther from the heart as the cardiac output drops and the filling pressures in the heart increase. Progression to atrial reversal in the ductus venosus is an ominous sign and was noted by Hecher and co-workers to be associated with impending acidosis in the following 48–72 hours in fetuses with growth restriction. With worsening of the heart failure, venous pulsations at the atrial rate

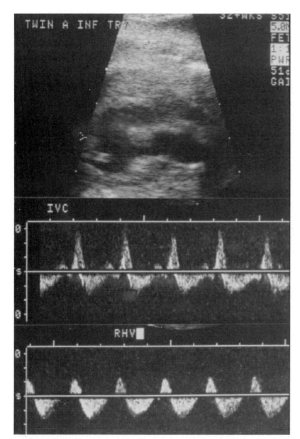

Figure 14.2 Echocardiography of a larger recipient twin in twin–twin transfusion syndrome. There is severe biventricular hypertrophy (upper panel), with abnormal inferior vena caval (IVC) Doppler with a large atrial reversal (middle panel). The right hepatic vein (RHV) shows a biphasic pattern with large atrial reversal, and loss of the early diastolic wave indicating increased central venous pressure (lower panel).

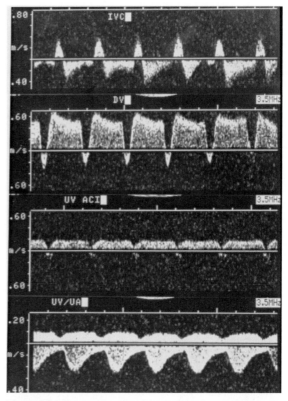

Figure 14.3 Venous Doppler abnormalities in a recipient twin gestation with severe congestive heart failure. Sampling sequentially from the inferior vena cava (IVC), to the ductus venosus (DV), to the umbilical cord in the free loop in the umbilical vein and artery (UV/UA). There is atrial reversal in the IVC and DV. The pulsations extend back to the umbilical vein at the cord insertion (ACI) in the free loop of the cord. The finding of umbilical venous pulsations is the most significant venous Doppler finding as a sign of heart failure (lower panel) and is a deduction of 2 points from the CV profile score.

appear in the umbilical vein (Figure 14.3). This sign has been correlated with poor outcome in hydrops fetalis, growth restriction, and other cardiac conditions. Elevated central venous pressure is probably the finding that leads eventually to hydrops fetalis in the recipient twin.

Cardiac dysfunction

The recipient twin shows signs of heart failure in the heart in addition to the early manifestation of ventricular hypertrophy. Traces of tricuspid valve regurgitation that were not there originally can progress to holosystolic regurgitation.

Later progression is indicated by the finding of mitral regurgitation. The jet of valvular regurgitation can be assessed by pulsed Doppler to determine the duration of the jet and thereby roughly quantitate its importance. With holosystolic regurgitation, the peak velocity of the jet (V_{max}) and its upstroke speed can be used to determine the blood pressure and to indirectly assess the myocardial function. With tricuspid regurgitation, for example, the examiner switches to continuous wave Doppler to allow high velocities to be measured. Any peak velocity V_{max} >4 m/s is consistent with severe hypertension at any time in gestation (Figure 14.4). The estimated right ventricular (RV) pressure is measured by squaring the peak transcuspid valve regurgitation (TR) velocity (V_{max}^2) and multiplying by 4 to give the RV to right atrial (RA) gradient:

$$Pressure\ gradient = 4 \times V_{max}^2\ (mmHg) \qquad (1)$$

This is the Bernoulli equation. RV pressure would then be that figure in mmHg + the estimated RA pressure (usually 5 mmHg in a well fetus).

The rate of rise of the TR jet (the dP/dt) is calculated from the waveform of the jet by measuring the time from the point on the curve at 1 m/s to the point on the curve at 3 m/s. That time in milliseconds divided into 32 gives the dP/dt in mmHg/s. Any result less than 400 is associated with poor ventricular function.

$$dP/dt = 32\ mmHg/time\ (milliseconds \\ from\ 1\text{–}3\ m/s) \qquad (2)$$

A normal value is >800 mmHg/s.

Fetal heart failure assessment

Perhaps no group of fetuses have taught us as much about incipient and full-blown fetal congestive heart failure as the recipient twins in untreated TTTS. The progression of abnormalities identified by fetal echocardiography has been documented in several articles and is used in staging patients for fetal intervention[11] (Table 14.1 and Figure 14.5). The venous Doppler plays an important role in reflecting the increases in intracardiac pressures that occur prior to the development of hydrops fetalis.

The cardiovascular profile score is used to communicate the combination of hemodynamic abnormalities presenting at any moment in time and to attempt to stratify the group of twins that is at risk of fetal demise. Using five categories and 2 points for each, a 10-point score is used to describe the degree of deterioration that has developed (Table 14.2 and Figure 14.6). Typically, the heart size is increased and there may be tricuspic valve regurgitation (Figure 14.5).

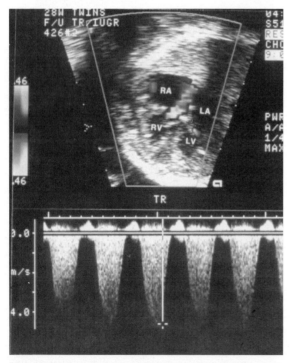

Figure 14.4 Recipient twin echocardiography showing tricuspid valve regurgitation (TR) by color Doppler (upper panel) from the right ventricle (RV) to the right atrium (RA). Continuous wave Doppler is able to quantitate the peak velocity of the jet at 4.5 m/s, predicting a pressure in the RV of >85 mmHg by the Bernoulli equation. Note that rapid rate of rise of the early systolic portion of the waveform, consistent with a normal dP/dt.

Table 14.1 Sequence of events in the development of and deterioration of the recipient twin in twin–twin transfusion syndrome
• Monochorionic twinning with diamniotic or monoamniotic sacs • Discordant commitment of placental mass • Donor twin has a small amount placental mass and shows increased placental resistance • Discordant umbilical artery pulsatility indices (increased donor and normal recipient) • Recipient polyhydramnios/donor oligohydramnios • Recipient myocardial hypertrophy • Recipient tricuspid valve regurgitation • Recipient abnormal venous Doppler (atrial reversal in the ductus venosus or umbilical venous pulsations) • Recipient mitral regurgitation

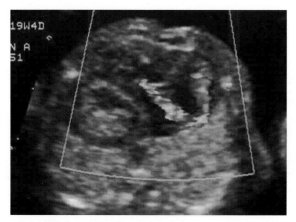

Figure 14.5 Twin–twin recipient echocardiography at 19 weeks' gestation showing tricuspid valve regurgitation by color Doppler from the RV to the RA. Note the marked increase in heart size with the heart area >40% of the chest area.

POSTNATAL RESULTS

Laser treatment for twin–twin transfusion is now accepted as the treatment of choice.[9-13] The fetal cardiac presentation may be used to predict the outcome of laser treatment.[11]

Neonatal hypertension

Postnatal problems are common in the immediate post delivery 24–48 hours. One uncommonly recognized problem is the acute onset of severe systemic hypertension with rapid fall in cardiac output, acidosis, and a sudden drop in blood pressure. There is limited experience with this entity but there are some signs that predispose to this postnatal course (Table 14.2). All of those neonates developing severe systemic hypertension had myocardial hypertrophy identified in utero and many had increased

atrial reversal in the inferior vena cava. After birth, the myocardial thickening was severe in some cases (Figure 14.7).

Few studies have been performed on the surviving recipient twins. One would expect that they may be predisposed to systemic hypertension, but little is known about their cardiovascular health later in life. Early exposure to increased work load may result in increased degrees of hyperplasia in the myocardium the number of cardiac myocytes may actually be increased!

Neurodevelopmental Outcome

Either twin may survive with cerebral damage and the timing of these insults may be difficult to determine.[12]

ACKNOWLEDGMENTS

I wish to thank my coworkers at Pennsylvania Hospital and Thomas Jefferson University JE Tolosa, J Mateus, VK Bhutani, R Romero, DC Wood, S Abassi, E Sivieri, and C Zoppini for the use of their data on cardiac wall thicknesses and right ventricular pressure estimates in recipient twins. Dr Rubén A Quintero has generously allowed me to study those twins most affected by this abnormal physiology. I thank Aleta Casbohm RDMS for expert sonography in the fetus and after birth in these babies. Eric Tucker at the University of South Florida aided with manuscript editing. Dr Huhta is supported by the Daicoff-Andrews Chair in Perinatal Cardiology from the Foundations of All Children's Hospital and the University of South Florida College of Medicine.

Table 14.2 Fetal/neonatal echocardiography data in 10 TTT syndrome gestations

	TR>4 m/s	CTAR>0.4	MH	UVP	NSH	NPT
Recipient	4/10	5/10	10/10	4/10	5/10	3/10
Donor	0/10	0/10	0/10	0/10	0/10	0/10

CTAR = cardiac-to-thoracic area ratio, MH = myocardial hypertrophy (left ventricular wall thickness >2 SD), NSH = neonatal systemic hypertension (>95th percentile systolic and diastolic), NPT = nitroprusside therapy postnatally, TTT = twin–twin transfusion, TR = tricuspid valve regurgitation peak velocity in meters per second, UVP = umbilical vein pulsations. Mortality was 4/10 in both recipients and donors.

Donor score sheet score = 9/10
Cardiovascular profile score 10 Points = Normal

	Normal	−1 point	−2 points
Hydrops	None (2 pts)	Ascites *or* Pleural *or* Pericardial effusion	Skin edema
Venous Doppler (umbilical vein) (ductus venosus)	UV DV (2 pts)	UV DV	UV pulsations
Heart size (heart area/chest area)	< 0.35 (2 pts)	0.35–0.50	> 0.50 or <0.20
Cardiac function	Normal TV & MV RV/LV S.F. >0.28 Biphasic filling (2 pts)	Holosystolic TR *or* RV/LV S.F. <0.28	Holosystolic MR *or* TR *dP/dt* <400 *or* Monophasic filling
Arterial Doppler (umbilical artery)	UA (2 pts)	UA (AEDV)	UA (REDV)

Recipient CV profile score = 4/10
Cardiovascular profile score 10 Points = Normal

	Normal	−1 point	−2 points
Hydrops	None (2 pts)	Ascites *or* Pleural *or* Pericardial effusion	Skin edema
Venous Doppler (umbilical vein) (ductus venosus)	UV DV (2 pts)	UV DV	UV pulsations
Heart size (Heart area/chest area)	≤ 0.35 (2 pts)	0.35–0.50	> 0.50 or <0.20
Cardiac function	Normal TV & MV RV/LV S.F. >0.28 Biphasic filling (2 pts)	Holosystolic TR *or* RV/LV S.F. <0.28	Holosystolic MR *or* TR *dP/dt* < 400 *or* Monophasic filling
Arterial Doppler (umbilical artery)	UA (2 pts)	UA (AEDV)	UA (REDV)

Figure 14.6 Use of the cardiovascular profile score for the assessment of fetal heart failure in twin-twin transfusion. The work sheet is used to score both twins.

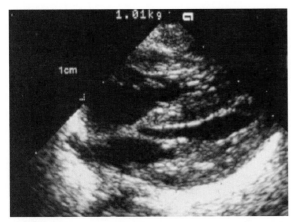

Figure 14.7 Postnatal echocardiography of the left and right ventricles. Note the thickness of the interventricular septum is nearly 7 mm in this 1000 g birthweight neonate.

REFERENCES

1. Murakoshi T, Quintero RA, Bornick PW, Allen MH. In vivo endoscopic assessment of arterioarterial anastomoses: insight into their hemodynamic function. J Matern Fetal Neonatal Med 2003; 14:247–55.
2. Bajoria R, Ward S, Chatterjee R. Brain natriuretic peptide and endothelin-1 in the pathogenesis of polyhydramnios–oligohydramnios in monochorionic twins. Am J Obstet Gynecol 2003; 189:189–94.
3. Quintero RA, Morales WJ, Allen MH et al. Staging of twin–twin transfusion syndrome. J Perinatol 1999; 19:550–5.
4. Wee LY, Taylor MJ, Vanderheyden T et al. Reversal of twin–twin transfusion syndrome: frequency, vascular anatomy, associated anomalies and outcome. Prenat Diagn 2004; 24:104–10.
5. Mahieu-Caputo D, Salomon LJ, Le Bidois J et al. Fetal hypertension: an insight into the pathogenesis of the twin–twin transfusion syndrome. Prenat Diagn 2003; 23:640–5.
6. Lopriore E, Nagel HT, Vandenbussche FP, Walther FJ. Long-term neurodevelopmental outcome in twin-to-twin transfusion syndrome. Am J Obstet Gynecol 2003; 189:1314–19.
7. Inamura N, Nakajima T, Kayatani F, Kawata H, Takeuchi M. Idiopathic arterial calcification in infancy with twin–twin transfusion syndrome. Pediatr Int 2003; 45:481–3.
8. Karatza AA, Wolfenden JL, Taylor MJO et al. Influence of twin–twin transfusion syndrome on fetal cardiovascular structure and function: prospective case-control study of 136 monochorionic twin pregnancies. Heart 2002; 88:271–7.
9. Crombleholme TM. The treatment of twin–twin transfusion syndrome. Semin Pediatr Surg 2003; 12:175–81.
10. Morine M, Maeda K, Higashino K et al. Transient hydrops fetalis of the donor fetus in twin–twin transfusion syndrome after therapeutic amnioreduction. Ultrasound Obstet Gynecol 2003; 22:182–5.
11. Martinez JM, Bermudez C, Becerra C et al. The role of Doppler studies in predicting individual intrauterine fetal demise after laser therapy for twin–twin transfusion syndrome. Ultrasound Obstet Gynecol 2003; 22:246–51.
12. Banek CS, Hecher K, Hackeloer BJ, Bartmann P. Long-term neurodevelopment outcome after intrauterine laser treatment for severe twin–twin transfusion syndrome. Am J Obstet Gynecol 2003; 188:876–80.
13. Gardiner HM, Taylor MJ, Karatza A et al. Twin–twin transfusion syndrome: the influence of intrauterine laser photocoagulation on arterial distensibility in childhood. Circulation 2003; 107:1906–11.

15

Organization of nursing responsibilities

Patricia W Bornick and Mary H Allen

Introduction • Preoperative phase • Intraoperative phase • Postoperative care • Conclusion

INTRODUCTION

The organization of a fetal therapy program for laser treatment of twin–twin transfusion syndrome (TTTS) requires significant nursing involvement. Patient education, counseling, and integration of different patient care services are necessary. Studies regarding the risks and benefits of laser surgery for TTTS are ongoing; therefore, research procedures and the follow-up of the patients also constitute major areas of nursing responsibilities.[1,2] This chapter describes our patient care algorithms and protocols, as an aid for other centers interested in caring for and studying patients affected with TTTS.

PREOPERATIVE PHASE

Patient selection

Most patients are diagnosed at another facility and are referred by their perinatologist or obstetrician to the fetal therapy center. The patient and her physician provide obstetrical and ultrasound information via a referral questionnaire (Figure 15.1). Selection criteria for fetal surgery are reviewed, and if met, an evaluation for possible surgery is scheduled. Even at this stage other confounders are identified and incorporated into the care plan prior to travel to our center. These include, but are not limited to diabetes, preterm labor, shortened cervix, heart disease, and maternal weight.

Patient education

Families affected with TTTS face the difficulty of dealing not only with the pathophysiological disease process but also with the psychological and emotional issues to be addressed which include potential loss of the pregnancy,[3] and are better able to cope with the procedure if they are adequately prepared and supported by the nurse. Ideally, this begins before the family travels for evaluation. The family's preparation begins when the physician recommends possible laser surgery for TTTS and discusses its risks and benefits. The nurse coordinator telephonically reviews with the patient the timetable of events for the evaluation and procedure. She assesses the patient's understanding of the instructions and reinforces the explanations if necessary. The nurse coordinator is readily available via phone or email to answer additional questions and concerns. Patients with access to the Internet find it a valuable resource. Our center provides a website with a TTTS patient education page, overview of the hospital stay, and travel and lodging information. Former TTTS patients have established websites on the Internet which provide patients with information on the disease, and treatment options, as well as emotional support. Patients with access to the Internet usually arrive with a better understanding of the disease process (Table 15.1).

After the patient's arrival and confirmation of the diagnosis, the fetal surgeon and the nurse coordinator hold counseling sessions with the

TWIN TWIN TRANSFUSION SYNDROME (TTTS) / SELECTIVE INTRAUTERINE GROWTH RETARDATION (SIUGR) REFERRAL QUESTIONNAIRE

Date_____

PATIENT_____AGE_____LMP _____Maternal Weight_____

PHYSICIAN_____EDC_____EGA_____Twins___Triplets____

PHYSICIAN PHONE NO. _____ FAX_____

PHYSICIAN ADDRESS_____

CITY/STATE_____ INSURANCE CO_____

TTTS is defined as a monochorionic twin pregnancy with a Maximum Vertical Pocket <2 cm in the Donor and >8 cm in the Recipient. The Donor may or may not have a visible bladder. Size discordance is no longer considered a criteria.

SIUGR is defined as one fetus being less than the 10th percentile while the other fetus is appropriately grown (AGA). Although amniotic fluids may be discordant, they do not meet the criteria for TTTS (<2 cm and >8 cm). Our protocol for laser surgery for SIUGR requires absent or reverse flow in the umbilical artery.

PLACENTA LOCATION PRIMARILY   _____Anterior _____ Posterior

CHORIONICITY   _____Mono/Di   _____Mono/Mono   _____Di/Di   _____Unknown

AMNIOTIC FLUID   Maximum Vertical Pocket in each sac

Recipient _____ cm	
Donor _____ cm	

WEIGHT DISCORDANCE   Fetal Weight Measurements

Recipient _____ grams
Donor _____ grams

FETAL BLADDER

The urinary bladder in the Donor fetus appeared to be: _____ Filling   _____ Not Filling

FETAL ANOMALIES   Yes____ No____ Comments_____

ABNORMAL INTRACRANIAL U/S FINDINGS	RECIPIENT	DONOR
Does either fetus have evidence of: Intraventricular hemorrhage	_____Yes ____ No	_____Yes ____ No
Porencephalic cysts	_____Yes ____ No	_____Yes ____ No
Ventriculomegaly	_____Yes ____ No	_____Yes ____ No
FETAL HYDROPS		
Does either fetus have evidence of: Abdominal ascites	_____Yes ____ No	_____Yes ____ No
Scalp edema	_____Yes ____ No	_____Yes ____ No
Pleural effusion	_____Yes ____ No	_____Yes ____ No
DOPPLER STUDIES – Umbilical artery : AEDV	_____Yes ____ No	_____Yes ____ No
REDV	_____Yes ____ No	_____Yes ____ No
Ductus Venosus – Reverse Flow	_____Yes ____ No	_____Yes ____ No
Pulsatile Umbilical Vein	_____Yes ____ No	_____Yes ____ No

CERVICAL LENGTH REQUIRED

Via transvaginal scanning, the cervical length appeared to measure _____cm Funneling? _____Yes _____No

If cervix measures < 2.5 cm a cerclage is required prior to laser therapy.

Figure 15.1 Twin–twin transfusion syndrome referral questionnaire is used to assess whether a patient meets the criteria for laser therapy and can safely travel to the fetal surgery center.

TRIPLE SCREEN

If this test has been done is there an increased risk for:

Down's syndrome? ___Yes ____No   Neural tube defect? ____Yes ___No

AMNIOCENTESIS

Has the patient under gone any amniocentesis procedures? ____Genetic ____ Therapeutic _____ None

If a genetic amniocentesis has been performed, please state the fetal karyotype : ____46, XX ____ 46, XY

If a therapeutic (decompression) amniocentesis has been performed, please complete the following information :

Date of Proc	Amount Removed	Fluid Color	Placenta Penetrated	Outer Membrane Detachment	Disruption of dividing membrane (Septostomy)	Gross Rupture of Membranes (PROM)	Chorio-Amnionitis	Placental Abruption
			Yes	Yes	Yes	Yes	Yes	Yes
			No	No	No	No	No	No
			Yes	Yes	Yes	Yes	Yes	Yes
			No	No	No	No	No	No
			Yes	Yes	Yes	Yes	Yes	Yes
			No	No	No	No	No	No

INCOMPETENT CERVIX

Does this patient have a history of an incompetent cervix ?   _____Yes   _____ No

Has a cerclage suture been performed with this pregnancy ?   _____ Yes   _____ No

PRETERM LABOR

Has this patient experienced any symptoms of preterm labor ?   _____ Yes   _____ No

Have any medications for preterm labor been administered ?   _____ Yes   _____ No

List:_____

MEDICAL HISTORY

Please list any pertinent maternal medical conditions (i.e. diabetes, hypertension, lupus, CHD, etc.)

PLEASE FAX QUESTIONAIRE TO:

DATE RECEIVED _____	DIAGNOSIS _____
RECOMMEDATION _____	FOLLOW UP _____

Figure 15.1 Cont'd

Table 15.1 Internet resources for twin–twin transfusion syndrome	
Websites for patients	Websites for physicians
www.fetalhopefoundation.org	http://fetalmd.hsc.
www.tttsfoundation.org	usf.edu
www.tripletconnection.org	www.webmd.com
	www.thefetus.net
www.twin2twin.org	www.nlm.nih.gov/
http://ttts.8k.com/main.htm	medlineplus
http://www.twin-twin.org/	www.obgyn.net

patient, her significant other, and their family members, if present. The surgeon presents the treatment options, possible outcomes, and surgical risks. An educational packet with information is provided. The packet contains an overview of the hospital, an explanation of the patient's stay in the hospital, TTTS patient education, previous issues of the fetal therapy newsletter, and published articles pertinent to the surgery. Also included are contact numbers of key team members to answer any questions or concerns and emergency care while residing in our city. The nurse reviews the content of the packet with the patient and her significant other. Family members are invited to be present during the ultrasound assessment, counseling, and education sessions if the patient so chooses. Having a family member present may comfort the patient and involves another in her care. The nurse explains what the patient will hear, see, and feel during the procedure and in the immediate postop period. A patient who is anxious while undergoing laser surgery experiences more discomfort during the procedure. Therefore, the nurse's role in creating a relaxed atmosphere is vital.[4] All patient education regarding laser treatment of TTTS is approved by the hospital's Institutional Review Board (IRB). If the patient wishes to proceed with the procedure, she is asked to sign the hospital consent form for surgery and the IRB-approved informed consent after all questions are answered.[5]

Initial assessment and preoperative care

Upon arrival, the obstetrical sonographer and fetal surgeon assess the patient. A comprehensive ultrasound assessment of the pregnancy is performed as well as a detailed history and physical examination. After confirmation of the diagnosis, the patient presents to the preadmission testing department to continue the assessment. The anesthesiologist will evaluate the patient and discuss the plan for anesthesia. Blood samples will be drawn for complete blood count, type and screen, coagulation profile, electrolytes, liver enzymes, blood urea nitrogen, and creatinine. Patients with a shortened cervix or complaints of contractions are assessed for uterine activity in the obstetrical triage area or labor and delivery (LDR).

The patient reports to the preoperative area 90 minutes prior to the scheduled surgery time. Intravenous fluids (IV) are initiated for hydration due to the NPO (nothing by mouth) status of the patient. Pulmonary edema has been reported in fetal surgery patients[6] and other hospitalized obstetrical patients. IV fluid boluses are thus administered with caution. Conversely, the adverse effects of dehydration, hypotension, and preterm labor may compromise the surgery, the mother, and the fetus. If nursing assessment notes dehydration, the fetal surgeon is notified and an order obtained for an IV fluid bolus. While IV fluids are administered, strict intake and output is recorded. Antibiotics – cefazolin 1.0 g and gentamicin 80 mg are administered in the preoperative area. If there is a penicillin allergy, clindamycin 900 mg is substituted. The fetal surgeon and the nurse coordinator visit the patient in the preop area prior to surgery to answer any last-minute questions. The obstetrical nurse also visits the patient and obtains a baseline obstetrical assessment and incorporates these findings into the care plan and coordinates with the obstetrical nursing staff. She provides additional information on tocolysis and obstetrical care to the patient. The family remains with the patient until it is time for surgery.

INTRAOPERATIVE PHASE

The team

The surgical team consists of the surgeon, the surgeon assistant, the anesthesiologist/certified registered nurse anesthetist (CRNA), the circulating nurse, the surgical technician/nurse, the laser safety operator, and the sonographer. The laser safety operator assists the circulating nurse when the laser is not in use. The sonographer participates as a member of the surgical team. She scrubs her hands and is gowned and gloved for the procedure: while maintaining an aseptic technique with the hand that is holding the ultrasound transducer on the operative field, she uses the other hand to control the ultrasound equipment.

Equipment

The room is arranged (Figure 15.2) to allow all the members of the team to view the surgery from various positions in the operating room (OR). There are two video towers with monitors. The primary video tower is equipped with a video mixer that is capable of combining two imaging techniques, endoscopy and ultrasound. This gives the surgeon the choice of viewing the ultrasound and endoscopy images together or separately. A fluid delivery system (Hydroflex, Controller) equipped with a fluid monitor (AquaSens Fluid Monitoring System; Davol, Inc., Cranston, RI) is used to irrigate and replace

the fluid in the amniotic cavity. The neodynium: YAG laser (SLT CLMD/Dual 40–60 watts; PhotoMedex, Montgomeryville, PA) is used with a 600 μm fiber at settings of 15–40 watts depending on the surgical task. The footswitch is positioned next to the surgeon's right foot. There are two endoscopic cameras utilized during the procedure. One camera is dedicated to the diagnostic endoscope necessary for the assessment of the placenta. The other camera is dedicated to the operative endoscope. The lights are dimmed in the room during the entire procedure to allow the surgeon and the rest of the team a clear visualization of the ultrasound and endoscopic images on the monitor. A small monitor is also placed near the patient to allow her to observe the procedure and ask questions if she wishes.

Instruments

Table 15.2 shows the contents of the typical operative fetoscopy surgical tray. A standard 3.8 mm trocar is used for the 3.3 mm diagnostic

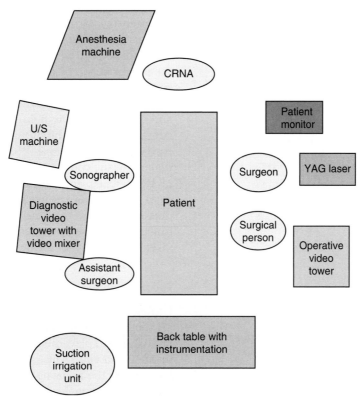

Figure 15.2 Arrangement of surgical suite for operative fetoscopy.

and operative endoscopes. An additional 2.0 mm or 3.8 mm trocar is also available for cases with difficult access that necessitate the use of an additional port. After the procedure, extreme care and attention are directed to the maintenance of the expensive, delicate instruments used in the procedure. The fragile endoscopes, as well as the accessory instruments, require meticulous cleaning, drying, and storing.[7]

Intraoperative management

The team prepares the room for an emergency cesarean section when the fetuses have reached the age of viability (>24 weeks). The infant care center in a corner of the OR is prepared. A Mayo stand is draped and the necessary cesarean section instruments are placed on it. Prior to bringing the patient into surgery, the LDR and neonatal intensive care unit (NICU) are alerted to the possibility of a premature delivery.

The circulating nurse greets the patient in the preop area and checks the identification band. She confirms the surgical procedure with the patient and the chart. Initial assessment is done in the preop area, including any known allergies and physical limitations. Before leaving the preop area for surgery, fetal heart rate (FHR) is obtained via ultrasound by the sonographer or surgeon. Ultrasound is used to obtain FHR, as opposed to hand-held Doppler, because it is difficult to obtain reliable FHR of twin fetuses with altered circulation at an early gestational age. The circulating nurse and the anesthesia care provider transport the patient to the OR. With the assistance of the nurse anesthetist (CRNA), the circulating nurse transfers the patient to the OR bed, covering her with a warm blanket. In supine position, the nurse places a pillow under the patient's knees to relieve pressure on the back and the safety strap is fastened 2 inches above the knee. The CRNA places the bed in a lateral tilt to prevent aortic or vena caval compression. The surgery is performed with IV sedation and local anesthesia to maintain adequate pain control and minimize maternal complications. After IV sedation, the nurse inserts a Foley catheter and then preps the patient's abdomen with Betadine (povidone-iodine). The scrub person assists the surgeon with draping using a cesarean section drape with a fluid collection pouch with an adhesive barrier that adheres to the skin around the aperture opening. This drape is used because the fluid can collect in the pouch to keep the patient dry. The surgeon, with the aid of the circulator, drapes the ultrasound transducer with a sterile probe cover and an articulating arm drape and secures it on the field. The scrub nurse and circulator connect the tubings, light and camera cords to the towers and the pump. The sonographer scans the patient, taking an initial assessment of the fetuses, the placenta, and the amniotic cavity. The FHRs are checked by ultrasound and documented on the operative record. At this time, the surgeon evaluates the best site for trocar insertion and the surgical procedure begins.

The procedure

Ultrasound provides a panoramic view of the placenta, the amniotic cavity, and the fetuses, allowing safe placement of surgical instruments inside the cavity.[8] The surgeon makes a 2–3 mm incision on the maternal abdomen with a No.11 blade and inserts the trocar into the uterus under

---

Table 15.2 Basic fetoscopy instrument tray

N	Endoscopes	
2*	Diagnostic, 25°, 30 cm length, 3.3 mm diameter	
2*	Diagnostic, 70°, 30 cm length, 3.3 mm diameter	
1	Operative, 0°, 40 cm length, 3.3 mm diameter	

N	Trocar	Trocar sleeve
1	3.8 mm	10 cm
1	3.8 mm	15 cm
1	3.8 mm	20 cm
1	2.0 mm	15 cm

N	Other instruments	
3**	Knot pusher	
1	Blunt probe	
1	3.0 mm suction irrigator	
2	Water adapter	

N, number of described instruments in the tray.
*1 standard light placement and 1 reverse light placement for anterior placentas.
**1 short, 1 medium, 1 long.

ultrasound guidance. The diagnostic endoscope is inserted. If there is discoloration of the amniotic fluid caused by blood from a previous amniocentesis, excess vernix, or meconium, the endoscope is removed. The surgeon inserts the 3 mm suction irrigator and, under ultrasound guidance, suctions and irrigates the uterine cavity with normal saline until the amniotic fluid is clear. The endoscope is reinserted and the procedure continues. After the assessment of the placenta is completed, the diagnostic endoscope is exchanged for the operative endoscope with the laser fiber inserted into the operative channel. The vascular communications are systematically ablated in accordance with the placental mapping. Intraoperative assessment of the immediate surgical results prior to the removal of the instruments is essential to assure all vascular communications between the fetuses have been obliterated. When the procedure is satisfactorily completed, the surgeon removes the endoscope. Excess amniotic fluid is suctioned until the volume returns to an acceptable level. No stitches are necessary due to the small size (2–3 mm) of the incision.

POSTOPERATIVE CARE

At the completion of the surgical procedure, the sonographer again assesses the FHRs of both fetuses via ultrasound. FHRs, amniotic fluid suction and irrigation amounts, and urine output are all documented on the operative record. The patient's abdomen is cleansed of any residual Betadine and Steri-Strips are applied. Prior to transfer to the post anesthesia care unit (PACU), the sheets and gown are changed if necessary to keep the patient dry and warm.

The patient is admitted to the PACU for approximately 60–90 minutes. Although rare, complications may include pain, bleeding, preterm labor, premature rupture of membranes, infection, and pulmonary edema.[6,8–16] Care of the patient includes keeping her recumbent, tilted to either side, comfortable, monitoring her blood pressure and pulse, and observing for adverse reactions. Increased abdominal pain, paleness, nausea, or change of vital signs should be reported to the physician. Recovery is usually uneventful and often uterine activity is minimal and ceases

quickly.[7] However because prompt recognition of preterm labor is essential, an obstetrical nurse works in conjunction with the PACU nurse to evaluate uterine activity and determine appropriate tocolysis. Uterine activity is monitored via tocodynamometry. Occasionally, increased uterine activity or other complications indicate that the patient be admitted to LDR for intravenous tocolysis and continuous uterine monitoring. FHRs are not routinely monitored.

The patient is transferred to the high-risk obstetrical department as soon as she is stabilized. The tocodynamometer is discontinued, but can be reapplied if the patient complains of uterine cramping or contractions. The patient remains on bed rest for 4 more hours. After this time, the catheter is removed and the patient is allowed bathroom privileges only. The fetal surgeon orders medications for pain, nausea, and sleep as needed. Pain is minimal with this procedure due to the small size of the incision. On the first postoperative day an ultrasound is performed to evaluate the status of the fetuses.

The hospital stay is usually 24 hours, which increases the challenge to provide education and support that is needed for the patient. The nursing staff reviews postoperative discharge instructions. Level of activity following discharge is determined by her postoperative physical condition and the results of her ultrasound evaluation. The patient is instructed to notify her healthcare provider if she experiences vaginal bleeding, severe lower abdominal pain, premature rupture of membranes, uterine contractions, or fever. Due to the high-risk nature of these pregnancies, there is always a possibility of a demise of the fetus(es). A packet of bereavement information is made available to the parents who experience a loss. Social services and pastoral care are available for additional support.[17–20] Unless complications arise, patients are typically discharged to a hotel in the local area. Approximately 48 hours after surgery, they return home to the care of their referring obstetrician and perinatologist. Coordination of care and the educational process continues at home through phone calls and email. The team members are always available to answer questions or concerns from patients and their physicians. Patients remain candidates for vaginal delivery following surgery.

Ultimately, the goal of intermingling clinical expertise and research is to improve perinatal outcome.[1] The nursing team, along with the sonographers and physicians, perform systematic data collection during the preoperative, intraoperative, postoperative, and delivery phases of the pregnancy. TTTS patients treated at our institution are asked to ship their placenta to our pathology department for surgical pathology analysis. To this end, a container with instructions is provided. Of utmost importance is the follow-up after delivery. All data are analyzed by the principal investigator/fetal surgeon to better understand the relationship between the maternal/placental/fetal factors, treatment, and outcomes. Results of studies are published in peer-reviewed literature.

CONCLUSION

Nurses are important members of the fetal surgery team, trained to assist in researching, coordinating, and performing endoscopy to treat TTTS. Nursing personnel provide continuity of care for these families from diagnosis through treatment to delivery as well as obtaining follow-up information on maternal and neonatal outcomes. It is a logical extension of these roles that allows nurses to provide care to patients from all areas of the United States and abroad, receiving treatment for a condition once considered hopeless, giving hope to these families, and more often than not, the joy of being able to celebrate the birth of their children.

ACKNOWLEDGMENT

We would to acknowledge Nenita S Garabelis RN, for her assistance in the preparation of this chapter.

REFERENCES

1. Howell LJ. The unborn surgical patient. A nursing frontier. Nurs Clin North Am 1994; 29(4):681–94.
2. Collins JE. Fetal surgery: changing the outcome before birth. J Obstet Gynecol Neonatal Nurs 1994; 23(2):166–9.
3. Blizzard D. A trying experience: fetoscopy and maternal decision making. Clin Obstet Gynecol 2005; 48(3):562–73.
4. de Jong P, Doel F, Falconer A. Outpatient diagnostic hysteroscopy. Br J Obstet Gynaecol 1990; 97(4):299–303.
5. McCullough LB, Coverdale JH, Chervenak FA. A comprehensive ethical framework for responsibly designing and conducting pharmacologic research that involves pregnant women. Am J Obstet Gynecol 2005; 193(3 Pt 2):901–7.
6. DiFederico EM, Harrison M, Matthay MA. Pulmonary edema in a woman following fetal surgery. Chest 1996; 109(4):1114–17.
7. Prather C, Wolfe A. The nurse's role in office hysteroscopy. J Obstet Gynecol Neonatal Nurs 1995; 24(9): 813–16.
8. Quintero R. Diagnostic and operative fetoscopy. New York: Parthenon; 2002.
9. DiFederico EM, Burlingame JM, Kilpatrick SJ, Harrison M, Matthay MA. Pulmonary edema in obstetric patients is rapidly resolved except in the presence of infection or of nitroglycerin tocolysis after open fetal surgery. Am J Obstet Gynecol 1998; 179(4):925–33.
10. Quintero R, Morales W. Operative fetoscopy: a new frontier in fetal medicine. Contemp Ob/Gyn 1999; 44:45–68.
11. Gratacos E, Deprest J. Current experience with fetoscopy and the Eurofoetus registry for fetoscopic procedures. Eur J Obstet Gynecol Reprod Biol 2000; 92(1):151–9.
12. Allen MH, Garabelis NS, Bornick PW, Quintero RA. Minimally invasive treatment of twin-to-twin transfusion syndrome. AORN J 2000; 71(4):796, 801–10; quiz 811–12, 815–18.
13. Fowler SF, Sydorak RM, Albanese CT et al. Fetal endoscopic surgery: lessons learned and trends reviewed. J Pediatr Surg 2002; 37(12):1700–2.
14. Sydorak RM, Albanese CT. Minimal access techniques for fetal surgery. World J Surg 2003; 27(1):95–102.
15. Danzer E, Sydorak RM, Harrison MR, Albanese CT. Minimal access fetal surgery. Eur J Obstet Gynecol Reprod Biol 2003; 108(1):3–13.
16. Bussey JG, Luks F, Carr SR, Plevyak M, Tracy TF Jr. Minimal-access fetal surgery for twin-to-twin transfusion syndrome. Surg Endosc 2004; 18(1):83–6.
17. Harrigan R, Naber MM, Jensen KA, Tse A, Perez D. Perinatal grief: response to the loss of an infant. Neonatal Netw 1993; 12(5):25–31.
18. Bryan EM. The death of a twin. Palliat Med 1995; 9(3):187–92.
19. Cuisinier M, de Kleine M, Kollee L, Bethlehem G, de Graauw C. Grief following the loss of a newborn twin compared to a singleton. Acta Paediatr 1996; 85(3):339–43.
20. Swanson PB, Pearsall-Jones JG, Hay DA. How mothers cope with the death of a twin or higher multiple. Twin Res 2002; 5(3):156–64.

16

Ethical challenges in the management of twin–twin transfusion syndrome

Daniel W Skupski, Frank A Chervenak and Laurence B McCullough

Introduction • Therapy for twin–twin transfusion syndrome • Non-directive and directive counseling in the informed consent process • Ethically justified decision-making pathway • Conclusion

INTRODUCTION

Twin–twin transfusion syndrome (TTTS) is a complex and poorly understood disease that has traditionally led to almost universal perinatal mortality if left untreated.[1–3] It occurs exclusively in monozygotic pregnancies, and almost exclusively in monochorionic pregnancies.[4,5] Although it can be classified as a rare disease, the incidence may have increased in recent years on the basis of the increased rate of assisted reproductive techniques that has led to an increase in both monochorionic and dichorionic twin gestations.[6,7] Thus, it is with increasing frequency that the clinician is faced with this perplexing problem. The diagnosis and treatment of TTTS have some unique and complicating features that make this disease fruitful for ethical analysis. The ethics of the clinical management of TTTS is unique because of the distinctive sequence of non-directive and directive counseling in the decision-making process. The aim of this chapter is to highlight the importance of ethics in the decision-making process regarding management options in TTTS and to provide an ethically justified decision pathway for both physicians and patients that guides the informed consent process by identifying the roles and timing of both non-directive and directive counseling.

THERAPY FOR TWIN–TWIN TRANSFUSION SYNDROME

Therapies have been developed that target (1) the polyhydramnios that is known to lead to preterm labor, and (2) the vascular connections within the placenta. These therapies are, respectively, amniotic fluid volume reduction or amniodrainage, and laser ablation. All therapies that are currently known or thought to be effective are invasive and lead to some risk, including pregnancy loss if performed before viability, preterm birth if performed at or shortly after viability, difficulty in monitoring the disease due to amnion–chorion separation, the production of a pseudomonoamniotic gestation with possible cord entanglement and fetal demise, production of a donor fetal 'sling' or 'cocoon,' and maternal morbidity.[8–11] In addition, two other options for therapy need to be considered: termination of pregnancy and selective termination (by laser or cord occlusion).[12–17] Many patients may choose to end a previable pregnancy when faced with the prospect of 25–50% mortality for their fetuses and treatments that are intensive and fraught with some risk to maternal health. This decision should be respected. The option of selective termination before viability is unique in the setting of TTTS, is based on the identification of severe disease or a moribund state in one of the fetuses, and has its own unique ethical issues that also need to be addressed.

The diagnosis and management of TTTS is challenging and has been the subject of much scientific investigation throughout the world. Excellent studies and reviews have been published about the current state of treatment and ongoing investigation. An additional challenge to the obstetrical profession concerns appropriate counseling of pregnant women about their management options.

NON-DIRECTIVE AND DIRECTIVE COUNSELING IN THE INFORMED CONSENT PROCESS

The physician has important responsibilities in the informed consent process.[18,19] These responsibilities include identifying all medically reasonable alternatives: i.e. those for which there is evidence of clinical efficacy, not just those that are technically feasible. Medically reasonable alternatives should then be presented to the patient along with a clear and careful discussion of their clinical benefits and risks. When evidence supports one of these medically reasonable alternatives as clinically superior, the physician should recommend it. This is ethically justified directive counseling.

Non-directive counseling means that the physician should present all medically reasonable alternatives but make no recommendation among them. When the evidence for efficacy among alternative therapies is not decisive, non-directive counseling should be followed.[19]

In obstetrics, non-directive counseling should also be followed regarding the options of terminating or continuing a pregnancy before viability. The ethical justification for non-directive counseling is the pregnant woman's right to determine the previable fetus' moral status as a patient. Because the previable fetus cannot be said with certainty to possess independent moral status, the pregnant woman is free to withhold from, confer onto, or withdraw from the previable fetus the moral status of being a patient.[19]

The ethical justification for directive counseling in obstetrics is the evidence that a clinical intervention is reliably expected to protect and promote the health-related interests of a pregnant woman or her fetal patient. This applies to the previable or viable fetus when the pregnant woman decides to continue her pregnancy to viability and thus to term, in effect conferring the moral status of being a patient on her previable fetus.[19]

Directive or non-directive counseling assumes the mother is eligible for any treatment option. However, fetal therapy for TTTS, or any other fetal condition, is elective surgery. As such, extra careful consideration needs to be given for patients at very high risk for adverse outcomes due to other unrelated problems such as complete placenta previa. Because the risk of intra-operative or post-operative hemorrhage during laser photocoagulation for TTTS is omnipresent, the option of blood transfusion is important to allow for optimal outcomes. Thus, we also feel it may not be prudent to perform fetal therapy for patients who will not consider blood transfusion based on personal or religious reasons.

ETHICALLY JUSTIFIED DECISION-MAKING PATHWAY

Decision making about the management of a pregnancy complicated by TTTS involves an identifiable sequence of non-directive and directive counseling both before and after viability. This sequence for decision making both before and after viability is displayed in Figure 16.1.[20] The medical community can be fairly precise in the diagnosis of TTTS, in the discussion of prognosis, and in the prediction of moribund status of either fetus in large part due to the excellence and volume of published trials. The reference list includes only a few of these trials.[13–15,21–26] The decision pathway shown in Figure 16.1 has as its foundation this excellent scientific information.

As in all clinical decisions with patients, the first step in this pathway involves expert evaluation. In the case of TTTS this includes both diagnosis and staging. Results of this evaluation should then be presented to the pregnant woman or the couple. Counseling about the disposition of her pregnancy should be rigorously non-directive, because whether the previable fetus should be regarded as a patient is a decision beyond the competence of physicians and is therefore solely a function of the pregnant woman's autonomy. She is free to confer or withhold the moral status

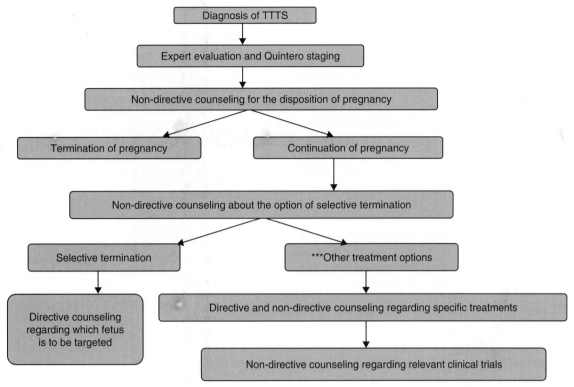

Figure 16.1 Decision-making pathway for pregnancies diagnosed with twin–twin transfusion syndrome (TTTS). ***Point where decision making begins after viability. (Reproduced from Skupski et al,[20] with permission of Karger Publishing.)

of being a patient according to her own values and beliefs. In order to be truly non-directive in counseling the physician must prevent personal moral bias from influencing what information is presented and how it is presented. If the woman elects termination of her pregnancy at this point in the decision-making process, the physician should make an appropriate referral if he or she does not perform termination of pregnancy.

If she elects to continue her previable pregnancy, the next decision concerns selective termination. This decision also involves non-directive counseling. This is a decision governed by the pregnant woman's autonomous decision to confer the moral status of being a patient on one fetus but withholding or withdrawing this moral status from the other fetus.[19,27]

If the woman elects selective termination, the physician should make an appropriate referral if he or she does not perform the procedure. An important dimension of this decision is the role

of directive counseling regarding the fetus to be targeted: namely, the less-healthy fetus as identified by ultrasound evaluation. This limited role for directive counseling in TTTS is distinguished from decision making in genetic counseling, which should be systematically non-directive in presentation of information and about the disposition of pregnancy.

If the woman elects to continue her pregnancy, directive and non-directive counseling should be undertaken regarding treatment. Where each of these types of counseling fit into the picture depends on the specific aspects of the particular patient. The non-directive component is that the physician should discuss all medically reasonable alternatives, which, in general, include therapeutic amniocentesis or laser ablation. Based on the currently available evidence and the details of the particular patient, the physician should be directive concerning the alternative or alternatives that are reliably judged to be the best. When there is evidence-based uncertainty about the relative efficacy of different therapeutic options, counseling should be non-directive.

Clinical trials are available for some interventions. By definition, clinical investigation should not be understood or presented as the standard of care. There is no ethical obligation for a woman – on behalf of the fetal patient – to enroll in a clinical trial. Thus, counseling should be non-directive about seeking out and enrolling in clinical trials. A comprehensive ethical framework for fetal research should apply to research in TTTS, such as one previously proposed.[28]

The decision-making pathway for fetuses after viability begins with point *** in Figure 16.1 and proceeds with the relative roles of non-directive and directive counseling determined by the specific aspects of the particular patient.

CONCLUSION

The wealth of scientific information in recent clinical trials on the topic of TTTS can be used to a maximum advantage by placing this information at the disposal of the patient in the framework of informed consent using both directive and non-directive counseling as described in this chapter. In the management of pregnancies complicated by TTTS, ethics is an essential component of decision making for pregnant women and their obstetricians. The decision-making pathway that we have described in Figure 16.1 is adequate to the current complexity and future development of therapies for TTTS and is consistent with the ethical obligations of physicians in the informed consent process.

REFERENCES

1. Urig MA, Clewell WH, Elliott JP. Twin–twin transfusion syndrome. Am J Obstet Gynecol 1990; 163:1522–6.
2. Mahoney BS, Petty CN, Nyberg DA et al. The "stuck twin" phenomenon: ultrasonographic findings, pregnancy outcome, and management with serial amniocenteses. Am J Obstet Gynecol 1990; 163:1513–22.
3. Saunders NJ, Snijders RJM, Nicolaides KH. Therapeutic amniocentesis in twin–twin transfusion syndrome appearing in the second trimester of pregnancy. Am J Obstet Gynecol 1992; 166:820–4.
4. Robertson EG, Neer KJ. Placental injection studies in twin gestation. Am J Obstet Gynecol 1983; 147:170–5.
5. Strong SJ, Corney G. The placenta in twin pregnancy. Oxford: Pergamon Press; 1966.
6. Platt MJ, Marshall A, Pharoah PO. The effects of assisted reproduction on the trends and zygosity of multiple births in England and Wales 1974–99. Twin Res 2001; 4:417–21.
7. Alikani M, Cekleniak NA, Walters E, Cohen J. Monozygotic twinning following assisted conception: an analysis of 81 consecutive cases. Hum Reprod 2003; 18:1937–43.
8. Al-Kouatly H, Skupski DW. Intrauterine sling: an unusual manifestation of the stuck twin syndrome. Ultrasound Obstet Gynecol 1999; 14:419–21.
9. De Lia JE, Worthington D. Intrauterine sling with umbilical cord entanglement in diamniotic twins. Ultrasound Obstet Gynecol 2000; 15:447.
10. Quintero RA, Chmait RH. The cocoon sign: a potential sonographic pitfall in the diagnosis of twin–twin transfusion syndrome. Ultrasound Obstet Gynecol 2004; 23:38–41.
11. De Lia JE, Kuhlmann RS, Emery MG. Maternal metabolic abnormalities in twin-to-twin transfusion syndrome at mid-pregnancy. Twin Res 2000; 3:113–17.
12. Gallot D, Laurichesse H, Lemery D. Selective feticide in monochorionic twin pregnancies by ultrasound-guided umbilical cord occlusion. Ultrasound Obstet Gynecol 2003; 22:484–8.
13. Taylor MJ, Shalev E, Tanawattanacharoen S et al. Ultrasound-guided umbilical cord occlusion using bipolar diathermy for Stage III/IV twin–twin transfusion syndrome. Prenat Diagn 2002; 22:70–6.
14. Nicolini U, Poblete A, Boschetto C, Bonati F, Roberts A. Complicated monochorionic twin pregnancies: experience with bipolar cord coagulation. Am J Obstet Gynecol 2001; 185:703–7.
15. Deprest JA, Audibert F, Van Schoubroeck D, Hecher K, Mahieu-Caputo D. Bipolar coagulation of the umbilical cord in complicated monochorionic twin pregnancy. Am J Obstet Gynecol 2000; 182:340–5.
16. Deprest JA, Van Ballaer PP, Evrard VA et al. Experience with fetoscopic cord ligation. Eur J Obstet Gynecol 1998; 81:157–64.
17. Quintero RA, Romero R, Reich H et al. In utero percutaneous umbilical cord ligation in the management of complicated monochorionic multiple gestations. Ultrasound Obstet Gynecol 1996; 8:16–22.
18. Faden RR, Beauchamp TL. A history and theory of informed consent. New York: Oxford University Press; 1986.
19. McCullough LB, Chervenak FA. Ethics in obstetrics and gynecology. New York: Oxford University Press; 1994.
20. Skupski DW, Chervenak FA, McCullough LB. An ethically justified decision-making pathway for the management of pregnancies complicated by twin-to-twin transfusion syndrome. Fetal Diagn Therapy, in press.

21. De Lia JE, Kuhlmann RS, Harstad TW, Cruikshank DP. Fetoscopic laser ablation of placental vessels in severe previable twin–twin transfusion syndrome. Am J Obstet Gynecol 1995; 172:1202–8.

22. Ville Y, Hyett J, Hecher K, Nicolaides K. Preliminary experience with endoscopic laser surgery for severe twin–twin transfusion syndrome. N Engl J Med 1995; 332:224–7.

23. Ville Y, Hecher K, Gagnon A et al. Endoscopic laser coagulation in the management of severe twin-to-twin transfusion syndrome. Br J Obstet Gynaecol 1998; 105:446–53.

24. Quintero RA, Dickinson JE, Morales WJ et al. Stage-based treatment of twin–twin transfusion syndrome. Am J Obstet Gynecol 2003; 188:1333–40.

25. Senat MV, Deprest J, Boulvain M et al. Endoscopic laser surgery versus serial amnioreduction for severe twin-to-twin transfusion syndrome. N Engl J Med 2004; 351:136–44.

26. Moise KJ Jr, Dorman K, Lamvu G et al. A randomized trial of septostomy versus amnioreduction in the treatment of twin oligohydramnios–polyhydramnios sequence. Am J Obstet Gynecol 2005; 193:701–7.

27. Chervenak FA, McCullough LB. An ethical justification of reduction and selective termination of multifetal pregnancy. Israel J Obstet Gynecol 1997; 8:49–51.

28. Chervenak FA, McCullough LB. A comprehensive ethical framework for fetal research and its application to fetal surgery for spina bifida. Am J Obstet Gynecol 2002; 187:10–14.

17

Neurological outcomes after therapeutic interventions for twin–twin transfusion syndrome

Jan E Dickinson

Introduction • Neurological outcomes in monochorionic twin gestations • Neonatal cranial imaging in twin–twin transfusion syndrome • Neurological outcomes in children treated with amnioreduction therapies • Neurological outcomes in children treated with endoscopic laser surgery

INTRODUCTION

As therapeutic interventions for twin-twin transfusion syndrome (TTTS) have enhanced the perinatal survival rates for this complication of monochorionic twinning, medical attention has shifted from mortality to morbidity for surviving children. Although there remains a dearth of high-quality long-term outcome data, some recent publications have improved knowledge of both the incidence and pattern of neurological morbidity for survivors of severe TTTS. Despite the recognition of the adverse impacts of intrauterine stress on extrauterine functioning, long-term morbidity data for other organ systems, such as the cardiovascular and endocrine systems, remain rare.

In this chapter the available data on long-term neurological outcomes for survivors following amnioreduction and placental laser ablative therapies for TTTS are evaluated.

NEUROLOGICAL OUTCOMES IN MONOCHORIONIC TWIN GESTATIONS

Twin gestations constitute 2% of all deliveries and are increasing in frequency, primarily due to increasing maternal age and assisted reproductive technologies. Perinatal mortality is 3–7-fold increased in twins compared with singletons and constitutes 12% of all perinatal mortality, principally due to complications of preterm birth.[1,2] For monochorionic twins the perinatal loss rate is very high, with at least one loss after 24 weeks in 4.9% of cases compared with 2.8% of dichorionic twins.[3] Congenital anomalies occur with greater frequency in multiple pregnancies than singletons, with a relative risk of 1.25 (95% CI 1.21, 1.28).[4] The monochorionic twinning process is associated with an increased incidence of vascular abnormalities, such as acardiac twinning and TTTS.[5] In addition, single fetal demise in monochorionic twinning has been associated with ischemic intracerebral lesions such as hydrocephalus, periventricular leukomalacia, and microcephaly.[5]

Twin gestations also contribute significantly to adverse pregnancy outcomes, including neurological complications.[6] Cerebral palsy is increased 8-fold in twins compared with singletons.[7] The recognized antenatal risk factors for adverse neurological outcomes – prematurity, growth restriction and congenital anomalies – are all increased in twin gestations.

Monochorionic twins are at increased risk for adverse perinatal events compared with dichorionic twins, and accurate ascertainment of chorionicity in the first trimester is central to establishing appropriate obstetric surveillance strategies.[8] In a study of 52 preterm multiple gestations comprising 101 infants, antenatal necrosis of cerebral white matter was significantly more frequent in monochorionic compared with dichorionic twins (30% vs 3.3%).[9] Features associated with these cerebral changes in cases of monochorionic placentation were polyhydramnios, intrauterine co-twin demise, hydrops, and placental vascular anastomoses – all factors characteristic of TTTS. In a retrospective cohort study of 208 twin gestations, adverse neurological outcomes were reported in 6% of monochorionic twins compared with 1.9% of dichorionic twins alive at 12 months of age.[10] TTTS complicated the pregnancies in all adverse neurological cases for monochorionic twins. Adegbite and colleagues assessed 76 monochorionic and 78 dichorionic twin pregnancies delivered between 24 and 34 weeks, gestation to ascertain neuromorbidity rates.[11] There was a 7-fold greater neurological morbidity rate in the monochorionic survivors, related principally to TTTS, discordant growth restriction, and single intrauterine demise. The monochorionic infants had an 8% incidence of cerebral palsy compared with 1% for the dichorionic survivors. Additionally, a 15% incidence of neurological morbidity was present in the monochorionic compared with 3% in the dichorionic survivors. The intrauterine demise of one fetus complicates 2.5–5% of multiple gestations.[12] Intrauterine death of one monochorionic twin is associated with increased risk of neurological morbidity in the survivor.[5] In a retrospective study of 92 cases of single twin demise (42 dichorionic and 50 monochorionic), Bajoria et al reported the death of the co-twin in 26% of monochorionic and 2.4% of dichorionic pregnancies.[13] An abnormal neonatal cranial ultrasound was present in 46% of liveborn monochorionic single survivors. All dichorionic single surviving neonates had a normal cranial ultrasound. A major neurological handicap was present in 9.5% of monochorionic survivors compared with no cases in dichorionic single survivors. This group suggested that co-twin sequelae following the intrauterine demise of one fetus in a monochorionic twin pregnancy is dependent upon the placental vascular anastomotic anatomy. In those

cases complicated by TTTS, death of the recipient was associated with a poor outcome for the donor, but not the reverse. These data support the concept of placental anastomoses in cases of monochorionicity permitting transfer of blood from the surviving twin to the deceased twin, with secondary hypotension and cerebral hypoperfusion.

These data are supported by other studies demonstrating an increase in adverse neurological events following single intrauterine demise in like-sex twins compared with unlike-sex twins.[14,15] In a geographical cohort of 434 intrauterine single twin demise cases, Pharoah and Adi observed in same-sex pairs a cerebral palsy rate of 106/1000 survivors and other neurological sequelae in 114/1000. Of the different sex pairs a diagnosis of cerebral palsy was made in 29/1000 survivors and other neurological sequelae in 118/1000. The risk of serious cerebral morbidity in a surviving co-twin was calculated as 20% (95% CI 16, 25).[14] Further support for increased neurodevelopmental morbidity following intrauterine demise of a co-twin is provided by a population-based regional study of 111 children in a fetal co-twin demise compared with 142 from liveborn twin pairs with a single infant death. Fetal co-twin death cerebral palsy rates were 93/1000 infant survivors. Cerebral palsy rates were higher for like-sex pairs (114/1000) compared with unlike-sex pairs (45/1000).[15]

Thus, the available data indicate monozygous twins are at increased risk of intrauterine death (both or one co-twin). In cases of a monochorionic single twin death a secondary hypotensive episode may lead to brain or visceral injury in the survivor. The variation in response is most likely related to the type of placental vascular anatomosis.

NEONATAL CRANIAL IMAGING IN TWIN–TWIN TRANSFUSION SYNDROME

Neonatal cranial imaging with ultrasound is routinely performed to assess the neonate at risk of perinatal cerebral insults. Antenatal cerebral anomalies may be observed on imaging performed within 24 hours of birth, such as porencephalic and parenchymal cysts. High-grade intraventricular hemorrhage (Figures 17.1 and 17.2) and

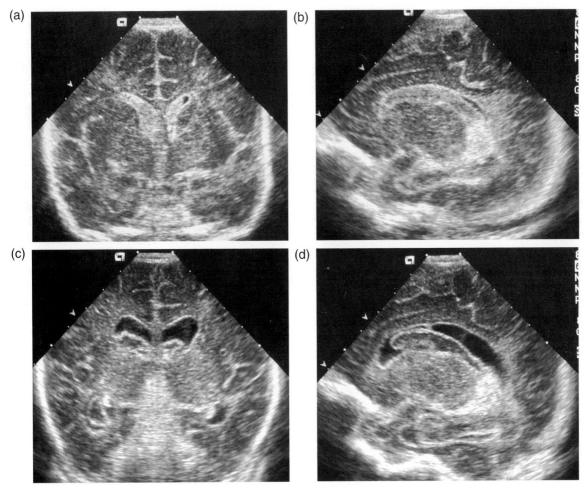

Figure 17.1 Neonatal cranial ultrasound demonstrating grade III intraventricular hemorrhage. Acute dilatation from hemorrhage, ependymal echogenicity, and secondary hydrocephalus are evident. (a) Coronal view, demonstrating ependymal echogenicity. (b) Sagittal view, hemorrhage in the lateral ventricle. (c) Coronal view, dilatation of the frontal horns secondary to intraventricular hemorrhage. (d) Sagittal view, hydrocephalus secondary to intraventricular hemorrhage.

periventicular leukomalacia (Figure 17.3) have been associated with increased rates of neurodevelopmental handicap, although the imaging appearances do not correlate directly with the clinical course. Unfortunately, most series of reporting perinatal outcomes of pregnancies complicated by TTTS have employed neonatal cranial ultrasound as a surrogate for adverse neurological outcome, which is not necessarily correct. Additionally, comparative gestation-matched imaging data of neonates from pregnancies not complicated by TTTS are lacking. Nonetheless, abnormal cranial ultrasound images have been

reported with a disturbingly high frequency in surviving neonates of pregnancies complicated by TTTS.

In a series of 17 pregnancies complicated by TTTS treated with amnioreduction therapy, 58% of neonates alive at 48 hours post-delivery had evidence of cranial ultrasound abnormalities.[16] The median gestation at delivery was 30 weeks. In 35% of these neonates the observed cranial sonographic anomaly was assessed to have been acquired antenatally. There was one case of cerebral infarction with tissue loss in a recipient twin. No neurodevelopmental outcome data

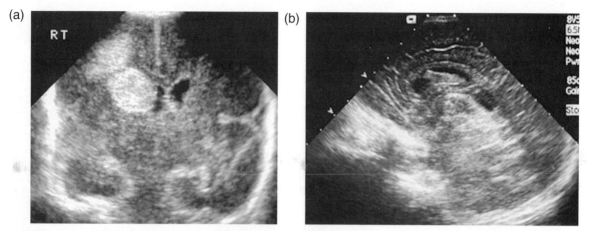

Figure 17.2 Neonatal cranial ultrasound demonstrating grade IV intraventricular hemorrhage with parenchymal hemorrhage. (a) Coronal view, intraparenchymal echogenicity secondary to hemorrhage in the right cerebral cortex. (b) Sagittal view, parenchymal hemorrhage.

were provided for these infants and therefore the clinical significance of these findings are uncertain, although the frequency is very much higher than that reported for preterm dichorionic twins.[9]

In the two large observational cohorts of TTTS,[17,18] neonatal cranial ultrasound abnormalities were common. An abnormal cranial ultrasound was present in 20.9% of survivors at 4 weeks of age in the series of Dickinson and Evans.[17] Periventricular leukomalacia, a strong marker for adverse neurodevelopmental outcome, was reported in 7.5% of neonatal survivors in this series. In 24.3% of perinatal survivors an abnormal neonatal cranial ultrasound was present in the International Amnioreduction Registry.[18] Abnormal cranial sonographic findings were observed in 24% of recipient twins and 25% of donors. Periventricular leukomalacia was reported in 5.1% of neonatal survivors, grades III and IV intraventricular hemorrhage in 6%, ventricular dilatation in 12.2%, and cerebral cysts in 5.1%.

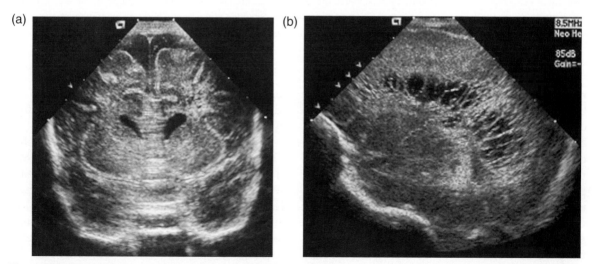

Figure 17.3 Periventricular leukomalacia. (a) Coronal view, cystic areas within the cerebral parenchyma. (b) Sagittal view, extensive cystic change within the brain parenchyma.

In 37 consecutive cases of TTTS, Reisner et al[19] reported a 19% incidence of intraventricular hemorrhage rate in survivors. Of those neonates treated antenatally by amnioreduction, 15.5% had grade III or IV intraventricular hemorrhage. It is important to note that only 56% of pregnancies treated with amnioreduction received antenatal corticosteroids, a therapy associated with a reduction in intraventricular hemorrhage in preterm infants. Cincotta et al[20] reported an incidence of 7% of intraventricular hemorrhage and 10% for periventricular leukomalacia in his series of 17 cases of TTTS treated principally with amnioreduction. Cerebral atrophy was present in 10% of cases. No lesions were present on the initial scans soon after birth, suggesting these lesions may have been acquired postnatally.

On the basis of the available data, it appears TTTS is associated with an increased incidence of antenatally acquired white matter damage and postnatal periventricular leukomalacia.

NEUROLOGICAL OUTCOMES IN CHILDREN TREATED WITH AMNIOREDUCTION THERAPIES

Given the available data on adverse neurological outcomes for preterm monochorionic twins and the high incidence of neonatal cranial imaging abnormalities described in the previous sections, it is clear the risk of long-term neurodevelopmental abnormality in survivors of TTTS is of concern. Whereas amnioreduction clearly offers the possibility of survival, it occurs at the cost of extreme prematurity in an environment where the pathophysiology of the disease process has exerted a profound hemodynamic stress to each fetus. Long-term neurodevelopmental data on survivors of TTTS treated with amnioreduction-based strategies consist of a few small cohort series with variable case ascertainment, potentially producing significant bias in the results. However, over the past 5 years, data have emerged to clarify the neurodevelopmental disability rates of this twinning complication. With placental laser ablation techniques gaining popularity, it may be that the available data on amnioreduction outcomes are virtually completed (Table 17.1).

Cincotta[20] compared the perinatal outcomes of 17 consecutive pregnancies complicated by TTTS with gestation-matched twin controls over a 3-year period. Unfortunately, the twin controls were not matched for chorionicity, limiting the comparability of the outcomes. The mean gestation at delivery was 29.1 weeks. Amnioreduction was the primary therapy and was employed in 12 cases (70.6%). Periventricular leukomalacia and cerebral atrophy were present in 17% of the TTTS cases and none of the controls. Twenty-three children survived to >24 months of age, with 13% diagnosed with cerebral palsy and 17.4% global developmental delay (see Table 17.1). Mari et al[21] reported on the non-controlled follow-up of 33 pregnancies with TTTS treated

Table 17.1 Neurodevelopmental outcomes for survivors with amnioreduction techniques

Author	Survival	IVH	PVL	CP	Developmental delay (non-CP)
Cincotta[20] (n = 34)	68%	0	3 (10%)	3/23 (13%)	4/23 (17.4%)
Mari[21] (n = 33)	60%	5 (9.8%)	3 (5.9%)	3/42 (7.1%)	12/42 (28.6%)
Haverkamp[22] (n = 94)	52%	3 (7.5%)	5 (12.5%)	9/40 (22.5%)	3/40 (7.5%)
Frusca[23] (n = 22)	70%	NS	NS	6/31 (19.4%)	8/31 (25.8%)
Lopriore[24] (n = 29)	50%	3 (10.3%)	3 (10.3%)	6/29 (21%)	5/23 (21.7%)
Dickinson[25] (n = 51)	62.5%	4 (7.7%)	2 (3.8%)	3/52 (5.8%)	5/49 (10.2%)

n, number of pregnancies potentially available for analysis; NS, not stated; IVH, intraventricular hemorrhage grades III and IV only considered; PVL, periventricular leukomalacia; CP, cerebral palsy.

with amnioreduction. The median delivery gestation was 30.5 weeks (range 18.5–37 weeks) and perinatal survival was 65.2% ($n = 43$). There were 8 cases of single intrauterine fetal death, of which only 1 surviving co-twin appeared normal. Forty-two children survived to >24 months of age with 65% neurologically normal, 24% demonstrated mild developmental delay and 5% attention deficit hyperactivity disorder. Cerebral palsy was proven or suspected in 7.1% (see Table 17.1).

Haverkamp et al[22] reported the long-term outcomes of 40/49 (82%) surviving cases of TTTS from a cohort of 94 pregnancies assessed at a mean of 24 months of age. The mean gestation at delivery was 31 weeks (range 24–36 weeks) with a 51% perinatal survival rate. The therapeutic interventions used were not stated. The neonatal cranial ultrasound was abnormal in 16/40 (40%) of those able to be assessed. On neurological examination, 70% (28/40) were assessed as neurologically normal. An integrated analysis of neurology and development classified 45% as having normal psychomotor development, 32% with minor neurological dysfunction, and 23% with severe psychomotor retardation. Frusca et al[23] conducted neurological assessments on 31 children at 24 months of age from 22 pregnancies complicated with TTTS treated with amnioreduction. No data were provided on cranial imaging results. Major neurological impairment was present in 8 cases and minor deficits in 5 (41.9%). In a neurological review of survivors who had reached school age, Lopriore et al[24] demonstrated a 21% incidence of cerebral palsy at a median age of 6.5 years. There was a high incidence (41%) of neonatal cranial ultrasound anomalies in this series, although IVH grades I and II were included. This work focused upon cerebral palsy as a major adverse neurological outcome, but did not mention behavioral disturbances, which can present a more difficult childhood management problem.

The most recent review of long-term neurological outcomes following prenatal detection of TTTS treated with amnioreduction therapies comes from Western Australia.[25] This study is notable for virtual complete ascertainment (94%) of all cases of TTTS within a geographically defined area, and thus avoids the bias of previous studies, which are derived from tertiary institutions with the more severe end of the disease spectrum over-represented. Additionally, a gestation-matched comparison between both twin and singleton pregnancies with TTTS children was made. From a total of 31 pregnancies with at least one liveborn infant aged more than 18 months, 52 children were identified and 49 assessed. A diagnosis of cerebral palsy was made in 3 children (5.8%). Gestation at delivery had a significant impact on IQ scores. Very preterm twins (≤32 weeks' gestation) demonstrated a 13-point reduction in IQ scores compared with non-TTTS gestation-matched controls. For those children born at later gestations (>33 weeks), this difference was not apparent. This is an important observation, given the increase in gestation at delivery noted with placental laser techniques compared with amnioreduction techniques. Assessment of childhood behavior showed no difference between children from TTTS pregnancies and gestation-matched controls.

It is recognized that without therapeutic intervention TTTS will result in perinatal mortality rates of 80–100%, depending upon the gestation at diagnosis. Utilizing amnioreduction strategies, it would appear the cerebral palsy rate varies from 6 to 22%. This wide variation is due to individual institution practices, gestation at delivery, and case ascertainment. Other, potentially more difficult, adverse neurological outcomes occur in a further 8–28% of cases. These latter anomalies have, in general, been poorly assessed. The major confounding variable in such studies has been a comparison group. Preterm birth is recognized as providing a significant impact on neurodevelopmental outcomes for children, and yet few studies have attempted to compare this confounding variable with outcomes from pregnancies complicated by TTTS. It would appear that a collaborative effort between obstetrician and pediatrician is required to provide accurate outcome data. In addition, less emphasis upon cerebral palsy as an adverse outcome and more upon other abnormal behavioral states is required.

The available data would suggest that with the use of amnioreduction strategies the more severe stage disease cases tend to result in perinatal death. In the cohort study of Quintero et al,[26] the outcomes for cases with stage IV disease demonstrated great differences in survival rates depending upon the therapy used. With amnio-reduction, a 25% survival resulted for stage IV disease, with a median gestation at delivery of 29 weeks. With placental laser ablation techniques, a 64% survival resulted with a median gestation at delivery of 31 weeks. Thus, any comparisons of long-term outcomes between these two therapeutic modalities will be confounded by gestation at delivery, in addition to inherent differences in the two techniques upon the pathophysiology of the disorder.

NEUROLOGICAL OUTCOMES IN CHILDREN TREATED WITH ENDOSCOPIC LASER SURGERY

The publication in 2004 of the randomized clinical trial of endoscopic laser surgery vs serial amnioreduction in the therapy of severe TTTS[27] demonstrated the superiority of the endoscopic surgical technique, leading to a rapid increase in the performance of placental laser ablation internationally. Although placental laser has not resulted in truly excellent outcomes, particularly in terms of dual-survivor rates, recurrence of TTTS, and feto–fetal transfusion, it offers a prolongation of gestation and resolution of hemodynamic changes not possible with amnioreduction. In keeping with contemporary research objectives, there are now a few series reporting longer-term neurological outcomes for surviving children following endoscopic placental laser.[28–30] As the median gestation at delivery is some 4 weeks greater with placental laser techniques compared with amnioreduction techniques, it would be predicted that neurological morbidity should be

lower, and indeed this appears to be the case (Table 17.2).

In a non-controlled study, Sutcliffe and coworkers reported the neurological outcomes of their cohort of surviving children following endoscopic placental laser in 2001.[28] Although the denominator is difficult to clearly ascertain in this study, 36 children from 54 pregnancies with at least 1 survivor were formally assessed by a pediatrician in addition to obtaining perinatal and sociodemographic data. The mean Griffiths mental development scores were within the normal range for all children assessed, although the dual survivors had a trend to lower scores than the single survivors (donor dual survivor 91.2, recipient dual survivor 97.7, and single survivors 101.6, $p > 0.05$). There was a significant difference in the locomotor subscale in the dual survivors compared with the single survivors (donor dual survivor 82.6, recipient dual survivor 85.3, and single survivors 99.1, $p < 0.05$), attributed to the increase in cerebral palsy in the dual survivors. A diagnosis of cerebral palsy was made in 13.9% (5/36) in the pediatric assessed group. There were a further 31 children surviving following laser who were assessed by their general practitioner; however, the data are unlikely to be as robust as those produced by formal assessment and therefore are not discussed in detail.

Two large prospective studies from the same research group in Germany assessing long-term neurodevelopmental outcomes following endoscopic laser surgery have been recently published.[29,30] Banek and co-workers reported on the first 73 consecutive pregnancies treated with

Table 17.2 Neurodevelopmental outcomes for survivors with endoscopic laser techniques				
Author	Survival	Normal development	Mild neurological handicap	Severe neurological handicap
Sutcliffe[28] (n = 67)	NS	NS	NS	6/66 (9%)
Banek[29] (n = 89)	61%	69 (78%)	10 (11%)	10 (11%)
Graef[30] (n = 167)	68%	145 (86.8%)	12 (7.2%)	10 (6%)

n, number of survivors; NS, not stated.

placental laser photocoagulation in Germany during the period 1995–1997.[29] All 89 survivors (31 dual survivors and 27 single survivors) were formally assessed with physical and neurological examinations, predominantly the Griffiths developmental scale. Normal development was present in 78%, minor neurological abnormality was present in 11%, and a major neurological abnormality in a further 11%. The donor/recipient status had no impact upon neurological outcome and, unlike the Sutcliffe et al study,[28] there was a trend to more favorable outcomes from the dual survivors. As expected, preterm birth was strongly associated with adverse neurological outcome. A recent study by the same German research team evaluating the subsequent cohort of survivors following placental laser (1997–1999) has been reported.[30] In this cohort were 167 surviving children from 127 consecutive pregnancies, the largest series of TTTS survivors reported to date, and the study is strengthened further by the almost complete ascertainment of cases. The survival rates of this cohort were improved compared with the previous publication, most likely reflecting increasing expertise with endoscopic laser techniques. Normal neurological findings were present in 86.8% of survivors when assessed at a median age of 3 years. Minor neurological abnormalities were present in 7.2% and major neurological abnormalities in 6% of cases.

The available neurodevelopmental outcome data following endoscopic placental laser from these three non-controlled series indicates an improvement compared with most studies of outcomes following amnioreduction techniques. These improved outcomes are most likely due to a combination of two important factors: first, the prolongation of gestation that is associated with successful placental laser ablative surgery; secondly, the alteration in the placental vascular architecture secondary to the occlusion of the majority of vascular anastomoses following endoscopic laser surgery. It is also important to recognize that cases of severe neurological abnormality will most likely persist with a 5–10% incidence rate due to the nature of monochorionic twinning and the stresses imposed on the fetuses prior to surgery. Until another therapeutic modality is introduced that can be implemented before the hemodynamic and endocrine

changes of TTTS occur, parents of monochorionic twins should be counseled about the potential adverse occurrences of this condition. The current challenge for the medical community is to ensure ongoing long-term follow-up of endoscopic surgical cases for TTTS, as it is unclear as to whether results from highly experienced centers such as the German unit can be replicated by smaller less-experienced units, which are now appearing with increasing frequency across the world.

REFERENCES

1. Gardner MO, Goldenberg RL, Cliver SP et al. The origin and outcome of preterm twin pregnancies. Obstet Gynecol 1995; 85:553–7.
2. Sherer DM. Adverse perinatal outcome of twin pregnancies according to chorionicity: a review of the literature. Am J Perinatol 2001; 18:23–37.
3. Sebire NJ, Snijders RJ, Hughes K, Sepulveda W, Nicolaides KH. The hidden mortality of monochorionic twin pregnancies. Br J Obstet Gynaecol 1997; 104: 1203–7.
4. Mastroiacovo P, Castilla EE, Arpino C et al. Congenital malformations in twins: an international study. Am J Med Genet 1999; 83:117–24.
5. Sperling L, Tabor A. Twin pregnancy: the role of ultrasound in management. Acta Obstet Gynecol Scand 2001; 80:287–99.
6. Nelson KB, Ellenberg JH. Childhood neurological disorders in twins. Paediatr Perinat Epidemiol 1995; 9:135–45.
7. Petterson B, Nelson KB, Watson L, Stanley F. Twins, triplets, and cerebral palsy in Western Australia in the 1980s. BMJ 1993; 307:1239–43.
8. Fisk NM, Bryan E. Routine prenatal determination of chorionicity in multiple gestation: a plea to the obstetrician. Br J Obstet Gynaecol 1993; 100:975–7.
9. Bejar R, Vigliocco G, Gramajo H et al. Antenatal origin of neurological damage in newborn infants II. Multiple gestations. Am J Obstet Gynecol 1990; 162:1230–6.
10. Minakami H, Honma Y, Matsubara S et al. Effects of placental chorionicity on outcome in twin pregnancies. A cohort study. J Reprod Med 1999; 44:595–600.
11. Adegbite AL, Castille S, Ward S, Bajoria R. Neuromorbidity in preterm twins in relation to chorionicity and discordant birthweight. Am J Obstet Gynecol 2004; 190:156–63.
12. Bajoria R, Kingdom J. The case for routine determination of chorionicity and zygosity in multiple pregnancy. Prenat Diagn 1997; 17:1207–25.
13. Bajoria R, Wee LY, Anwar S, Ward S. Outcome of twin pregnancies complicated by single intrauterine death in

relation to vascular anatomy of the monochorionic placenta. Hum Reprod 1999; 14:2124–30.

14. Pharaoh PO, Adi Y. Consequences of in-utero death in a twin pregnancy. Lancet 2000; 355:1597–602.

15. Glinianaia SV, Pharoah PO, Wright C, Rankin JM. Fetal or infant death in twin pregnancy: neurodevelopmental consequence for the survivor. Arch Dis Child Fetal Neonatal Ed 2002; 86:F9–15.

16. Denbow ML, Battin MR, Cowan F et al. Neonatal cranial ultrasonographic findings in preterm twins complicated by severe fetofetal transfusion syndrome. Am J Obstet Gynecol 1998; 178:479–83.

17. Dickinson JE, Evans SF. Obstetric and perinatal outcomes from the Australian and New Zealand Twin–Twin Transfusion Syndrome Registry. Am J Obstet Gynecol 2000; 182:706–12.

18. Mari G, Roberts A, Detti L et al. Perinatal morbidity and mortality rates in severe twin–twin transfusion syndrome: results of the International Amnioreduction Registry. Am J Obstet Gynecol 2001; 185:708–15.

19. Reisner DP, Mahony BS, Petty CN et al. Stuck twin syndrome: outcome in thirty-seven consecutive cases. Am J Obstet Gynecol 1993; 169:991–5.

20. Cincotta RB, Gray PH, Phythian G, Rogers YM, Chan FY. Long term outcome of twin–twin transfusion syndrome. Arch Dis Child Fetal Neonatal Ed 2000; 83:F171–6.

21. Mari G, Detti L, Oz U, Abuhamad AZ. Long-term outcome in twin–twin transfusion syndrome treated with serial aggressive amnioreduction. Am J Obstet Gynecol 2000; 183:211–17.

22. Haverkamp F, Lex C, Hanisch C, Fahnenstich H, Zerres K. Neurodevelopmental risks in twin-to-twin transfusion syndrome: preliminary findings. Eur J Paediatr Neurol 2001; 5:21–7.

23. Frusca T, Soregaroli M, Fichera A et al. Pregnancies complicated by twin–twin transfusion syndrome: outcome and long-term neurological follow-up. Euro J Obstet Gynecol Reprod Biol 2003; 107:145–50.

24. Lopriore E, Nagel HT, Vandenbussche FP, Walther FJ. Long-term neurodevelopmental outcome in twin-to-twin transfusion syndrome. Am J Obstet Gynecol 2003; 189:1314–19.

25. Dickinson JE, Duncombe GJ, Evans SF, French NP, Hagan R. The long-term neurological outcome of children from pregnancies complicated by twin-to-twin transfusion syndrome. BJOG 2005; 112:63–8.

26. Quintero RA, Dickinson JE, Morales WJ et al. Stage-based treatment of twin–twin transfusion syndrome. Am J Obstet Gynecol 2003; 188:1333–40.

27. Senat M-V, Deprest J, Boulvain M et al. Endoscopic laser surgery versus serial amnioreduction for severe twin–twin transfusion syndrome. N Engl J Med 2004; 351:136–44.

28. Sutcliffe AG, Sebire NJ, Pigott AJ et al. Outcome for children born after in utero laser ablation therapy for severe twin-to-twin transfusion syndrome. BJOG 2001; 108:1246–50.

29. Banek CS, Hecher K, Hackeloer BJ, Bartmann P. Long-term neurodevelopmental outcome after intrauterine laser treatment for severe twin–twin transfusion syndrome. Am J Obstet Gynecol 2003; 188:876–80.

30. Graef C, Ellenrieder B, Hecher K et al. Long-term neurodevelopmental outcome of 167 children after intrauterine laser treatment for severe twin–twin transfusion syndrome Am J Obstet Gynecol 2006; 194:303–8.

Anesthesia for surgical treatment of twin–twin transfusion syndrome

A Cristina Rossi and Marc A Kaufman

Introduction • Maternal safety • Avoidance of teratogenic agents • Avoidance of fetal asphyxia • Fetal anesthesia • Preterm labor • Anesthetic management

INTRODUCTION

Anesthesia for fetal surgery is unique in that it involves two patients, the mother and the fetus. Care of both of these patients must be considered during the perioperative period. For all fetal surgery some basic anesthetic objectives apply. They include maternal safety, avoidance of teratogenic agents, avoidance of fetal asphyxia, adequate fetal anesthesia, and monitoring for and prevention of preterm labor.

MATERNAL SAFETY

There is altered maternal physiology during pregnancy which results from increased concentrations of various hormones (human chorionic gonadotropin, progesterone, estrogen), mechanical effects of the gravid uterus, increased metabolic demand, and hemodynamic consequences of the low-pressure placental circulation.[1] Hormonal changes are probably responsible for most of the changes that occur in the first trimester. Mechanical effects become apparent when the uterus arises from the pelvis, which occurs during the second half of gestation.

All organ systems are affected. These changes have important perioperative implications.[2] The respiratory system, cardiovascular system, gastrointestinal system, changes in blood volume, and the altered response to anesthesia will be discussed.

Respiratory system

The respiratory system is altered in several important ways. Oxygen consumption increases because of the growth and metabolic needs of the fetus, placenta, and uterus. It rises approximately 20% during pregnancy. Alveolar ventilation increases 25% by the fourth month of gestation and 45–70% at term. Progesterone causes increased sensitivity to carbon dioxide. This results in a chronic respiratory alkalosis with a $PaCO_2$ of 28–32 mmHg.[3]

Functional residual capacity decreases approximately 20% as the uterus expands and results in decreased oxygen reserve and the potential for airway closure.

The decreased functional residual capacity and the increased oxygen consumption and diminished buffering capacity can account for the rapid development of hypoxemia and acidosis during periods of apnea or hypoventilation.

Capillary engorgement of the respiratory mucous membranes occurs, which may make mask ventilation, laryngeal visualization, and intubation more difficult.[4] Failed intubation is the leading cause of maternal death from anesthesia of the pregnant patient.

Cardiovascular system

The cardiac system undergoes changes to allow the mother to adapt to the needs of the fetus and to prepare her for delivery. Cardiac output increases by 30–50% during pregnancy as a result of increases in heart rate and stroke volume and decreases in systemic and pulmonary vascular resistance.[5]

During the second half of pregnancy, aortocaval compression occurs and can lead to hypotension in the supine position.[3] Compression of the vena cava may lower venous return to the heart, leading to a drop in cardiac output. Compression of the aorta decreases uterine blood flow as does a rise in uterine venous pressure.

Vena caval compression also results in the distention of the epidural venous plexus, which can increase the likelihood of an accidental epidural intravascular injection and increases the spread of spinal and epidural local anesthetics.

Gastrointestinal system

Pregnancy is associated with a decrease in lower esophageal sphincter tone and gastric motility.[6] This decrease results from mechanical factors with the gravid uterus that distort the pyloric and gastric anatomy and from hormonal changes retarding gastric emptying. Thus, all pregnant patients are at risk for regurgitation of gastric contents and the development of aspiration pneumonia.

Changes in blood volume and blood constituents

Blood volume expands up to 30–45% at term. A smaller increase in red blood cell volume than plasma volume results in a dilutional anemia.[7]

Pregnancy induces a hypercoagulable state, with an increase in fibrinogen, factors VII, VIII, X, and XII, and fibrin degradation products. It is also associated with an enhanced turnover of platelets, clotting, and fibrinolysis. During the postoperative period, there is a high risk for thromboembolic complications.

Altered response to anesthesia

Pregnancy decreases the minimal alveolar concentration in all inhalation agents and increases the sensitivity of nerves to blockade from local anesthetics because of hormonal factors.[8]

There is a decrease in thiopental requirements and more extensive spread of epidural and spinal anesthesia.

There is decreased protein binding associated with low albumin concentration during pregnancy which may result in a greater fraction of unbound drug with the potential for greater drug toxicity during pregnancy.

AVOIDANCE OF TERATOGENIC AGENTS

A valid concern for a pregnant woman about to receive an anesthetic for fetal surgery is whether any of the drugs to be used will have teratogenic effects on her fetus. In humans, it is generally believed that the most vulnerable period for the teratogenic effect of drugs is the first trimester.

Teratogenic effects of anesthetic drugs have never been conclusively demonstrated. The anesthetic drugs of most concern are nitrous oxide and the benzodiazepams.

Nitrous oxide

In animal studies, nitrous oxide may vasoconstrict the uterine vasculature and decrease uterine blood flow if not combined with another inhalation agent. Nitrous oxide can also inhibit methionine synthetase, which could result in reduced DNA synthesis and decrease in methylation reactions.[9] However, no adverse effects of nitrous oxide administration have been demonstrated in human pregnancy.

Benzodiazepines

Benzodiazepines have been anecdotally associated with cleft lip anomalies, but usually in association with abuse of substances such as alcohol and never in a controlled study. The present consensus among teratologists is that diazepam is not a proven human teratogen and there are few data to suggest that a single dose of a benzodiazepine during the course of an anesthetic would prove harmful to the fetus.[10]

The inhaled agents, narcotics, intravenous agents, muscle relaxants, and local anesthetics have a long history of safety during pregnancy.

AVOIDANCE OF FETAL ASPHYXIA

Maternal oxygenation

Fetal oxygenation is a function of maternal oxygen content and placental blood flow. Maintaining normal partial pressure of oxygen, partial pressure of carbon dioxide, and uterine blood flow are the best protection against fetal asphyxia.

Transient mild to moderate maternal hypoxemia is well tolerated in the fetus, secondary to fetal hemoglobin being present in high concentration and it having a higher affinity for oxygen. Severe maternal hypoxemia results in fetal hypoxia and, if persistent, may cause fetal death. Complications that cause profound maternal hypoxia include difficult intubation, esophageal intubation, pulmonary aspiration, high level of regional anesthesia, and toxic reactions to local anesthetics.

Hyperventilation should be avoided. It can cause respiratory or metabolic acidosis, which can cause umbilical artery vasoconstriction. Hypocarbia can also produce a shift in the oxygen–hemoglobin dissociation curve to the left, and decrease movement of oxygen across the placenta to the fetus.[11]

Uteroplacental perfusion

The uterine vasculature is almost fully dilated during pregnancy, receiving about 10% of the cardiac output at term, with 70–90% of that going to the placenta. This means that uterine perfusion cannot be increased by vasodilation and depends on perfusion pressure, i.e. the maternal blood pressure. Maternal hypotension from any cause can jeopardize uteroplacental perfusion and cause fetal asphyxia. The most common causes of hypotension during surgery of the pregnant patient include deep levels of general anesthesia, sympathectomy with high levels of spinal or epidural block, aortocaval compression, hemorrhage, or hypovolemia.

Recent evidence has challenged the view that the mixed adrenergic ephedrine is better than the α agonist phenylephrine for the treatment of hypotension during administration of regional anesthesia in pregnant patients. A meta-analysis of a randomized controlled trial of ephedrine vs phenylephrine during spinal anesthesia for cesarean sections resulted in the following conclusions:

1. No difference for prevention and treatment of maternal hypotension.
2. Maternal bradycardia was more likely to occur with phenylephrine.
3. Women given phenylephrine had higher neonatal arterial pH.
4. No difference in the incidence of true fetal acidosis of fetal pH of <7.2.[12]

Preoperative anxiety and light anesthesia can increase circulating catecholamines, which may impair uterine blood flow.[13] Clinical evidence does not support avoiding inhalation agents, provided maternal hypotension is avoided. Opioids and induction agents may decrease fetal heart rate variability, which may signal the presence of an anesthetized fetus. There are no reported effects of muscle relaxants on uteroplacental perfusion.

FETAL ANESTHESIA

Studies about fetal pain are controversial. The rationale of providing anesthesia derives from studies in preterm infants or in fetuses undergoing invasive procedures without prior anesthesia.[14] A suppression of insulin secretion and an increased release of catecholamines, cortisol, β-endorphins, and other hormones had been reported. The endocrine response, stimulation of the autonomic nervous system, alterations of the fetal heart rate, and increased fetal movements are abolished by administration of anesthetic agents.[2] In addition, a redistribution of blood flow to the heart, kidneys, and brain occurs as a response to noxious stimuli as early as 18 weeks.[15,16]

Studies about the fetal perception of pain present two limitations. First, stress responses, which are used as an indicator of fetal pain, do not necessarily imply pain and do not involve the cerebral cortex, which is an important step of the neuroanatomic pathway of pain perception.[17] Secondly, the period of gestation at which the human fetus is able to respond to noxious stimuli is still unknown. The development of the sensory system and of neural structures and functions, and the integration of the thalamic connections to the cerebral cortex begin at about 22 weeks' gestation. Therefore, it is unlikely that the fetus is able to perceive pain at earlier gestational ages.[18]

PRETERM LABOR

The prevention of preterm labor is the most difficult problem to surmount perioperatively. Preterm delivery is the greatest cause of fetal loss and is probably not related to anesthetic management, but to the underlying disease and surgery itself. Prevention and management of preterm labor are discussed elsewhere in this text.

ANESTHETIC MANAGEMENT

General guidelines

Preoperative assessment

Preoperative medication to allay anxiety or pain are appropriate, since elevated catecholamines may decrease uterine blood flow. Midazolam is commonly used in small incremental dosing for anxiety.

Aspiration prophylaxis is indicated for gestational age >14 weeks. A combination of a non-particulate antacid, metoclopramide (speeds gastric emptying and increases lower esophageal sphincter tone) and an H_2 receptor antagonist is indicated.

NPO guidelines are followed for non-emergent surgery. A minimum of 4 hours for clear liquids and 6 hours for solids is recommended.

Discussion of perioperative tocolytics with the obstetrician is important. Magnesium sulfate use can potentiate the effects of muscle relaxants and make hypotension more difficult to treat during blood loss or volume shifts. Terbutaline can cause hypotension, tachycardia, myocardial ischemia, hyperglycemia, pulmonary edema, and hypokalemia.

Intraoperative management

Twin–twin transfusion syndrome (TTTS) occurs in 10–15% of monochorionic multiple pregnancies and is associated with a high level of perinatal morbidity and mortality if left untreated.[19] The etiology of TTTS is commonly believed to be related to the net imbalance of blood flow between the twins through placental vascular anastomosis. The treatment of choice is the selective laser photocoagulation of communicating vessels (SLPCV), which is a minimally invasive technique. These procedures have been performed under general, regional, and intravenous sedation techniques.[20]

Because SLPCV is a minimally invasive technique, it can be speculated that the adverse effects of general anesthesia on the mother and the fetuses can be avoided. There are no studies investigating if local anesthesia/conscious sedation is as efficacious and safe as general anesthesia. A study in Tampa, Florida was conducted to compare maternal and fetal outcomes of local anesthesia/conscious sedation vs general anesthesia administered to patients undergoing fetal endoscopy for TTTS.

Materials and methods

Patients undergoing SLPCV for TTTS were enrolled. Preoperative assessment consisted of both obstetric and anesthetic examinations. The obstetric examination consisted of a physical examination and ultrasound for biometry, anatomy, amniotic fluid volume, and placental location. The ultrasound was completed by Doppler studies of the umbilical vessels, the middle cerebral artery, the ductus venosus, and the tricuspid valve. TTTS was diagnosed if the maximum vertical pocket (MVP) was >8 cm in the recipient's sac and <2 cm in the donor's sac and was classified according to Quintero's staging system.[21] The anesthetic examination consisted of a complete history and physical examination, complete blood count, blood chemistry analysis, electrocardiogram, and basic blood pressure (BP) assessment. Blood pressure was measured on the day of admission and 1 hour prior to surgery. All the patients were classified according to the American Society of Anesthesiology physical status guidelines.

According to protocols, approved by the local Institutional Review Board (IRB) patients underwent general anesthesia (GenA) or total intravenous anesthesia (TIVA) in the period between 1998 and 2002 and local anesthesia/ conscious sedation (LocA) anesthesia from 2002 to August 2004.

GenA consisted of the administration of induction agents (thiopental sodium 4 mg/kg or propofol 2 mg/kg) with fentanyl (100 µg) followed by muscle relaxant (succinylcholine 1.5 mg/kg) and intubation. Maintenance of anesthesia comprised muscle relaxation (vecuronium 1 mg/kg or atracurium 0.4 mg/kg), inhalation agents (isoflurane 1–2% or Ethrane (enflurane) 2–4%, combined with nitrous oxide–oxygen (50:50) and intermittent doses of Demerol (meperidine; 25 mg) or morphine (2–4 mg).

TIVA consisted of the same induction drugs, and maintenance was achieved with a propofol infusion (100–200 µg/kg/min) and intermittent doses of fentanyl (50 µg), midazolam (1 mg) and Demerol (25 mg) or morphine (2–4 mg).

LocA was performed with intermittent doses of fentanyl (50 µg) and midazolam (1 mg) before Foley catheter insertion and the use of morphine (2–4 mg) before trocar insertion.

Pre-admission testing (PAT) BP was measured on the day before surgery; preoperative (preop) BP was assessed 1 hour prior to surgery. Intra- and postoperative BP measurements were recorded. Intraoperative hypotension was promptly corrected with ephedrine administration. Hypotension was defined as a systolic BP <100 mmHg or a decrease of >20% of basal values. During surgery, the lowest systolic (SYS) and diastolic (DIA) BP measurements and their corresponding heart rates (HR) were obtained. Operating time and maternal complications such as bleeding and amniodetachment were recorded. Maternal blood loss was estimated by comparing preoperative hemoglobin (HB) and hematocrit (HCT) values to the postoperative ones. After surgery, the first measurement of SYS and DIA pressure and HR were recorded.

Fluctuations of BP in the perioperative period were calculated as follow:

- (PAT BP – LI)/PAT BP%
- (preop BP – LI)/preop%
- (LI – post)/LI%.

where LI is the lowest intraoperative blood pressure.

After surgery the first measurement of SYS and DIA BP (postop BP) and HR were recorded when the patient arrived in the post-anesthesia care unit.

SLPCV was performed as previously described.[22] If surgery could not be completed for any reason, umbilical cord ligation of the apparent sick twin was offered to the patient.

Fetal monitoring during surgery consisted of continuing ultrasound visualization of fetal heart beat, and fetal heart rate (FHR) measurements were collected both before and during surgery. For each patient, gestational age (GA) at surgery, any postoperative maternal complications, blood transfusion, premature rupture of membranes, and survival rates were also collected.

Data are expressed as number (%) for categorical variables and mean (± standard deviation) for continuous variables. Statistical analysis was performed with GraphPad InStat Version 3.05. Categorical variables were compared with χ^2 for independence test with Yates' continuity correction; whenever the frequency was ≤5, GenA and TIVA were considered as a single group and compared with LocA by the Fisher exact test. Quantitative variables were tested for normality with the Kolmogorov–Smirnov test. In case of normality, variables were analyzed with unpaired or paired Student's t-test, one-way analysis of variance (ANOVA), and repeated measures ANOVA. Data not normally distributed was assessed with the corresponding nonparametric test. If a significant difference was noted, the post test (Tukey–Kramer multiple comparisons test after ANOVA and repeated measures ANOVA and Dunn's multiple comparisons test after Kruskal–Wallis and Friedman test) was performed in order to detect an intergroup or intragroup (LocA vs GenA vs TIVA) differences. A $p <0.05$ was considered statistically significant.

Results

A total of 368 patients underwent SLPCV for TTTS from February 1998 to February 2004. One patient was excluded for termination of pregnancy due to cardiac malformation, 1 for a monoamniotic gestation, and 2 for premature

Table 18.1 Maternal complications

	LocA	GenA	TIVA	p value
Number of patients	139 (40%)	103 (30%)	103 (30%)	
Stop surgery for bleeding	0	0	1 (1%)	1
Amnioinfusion for bleeding	2 (1.4%)	16 (15.5%)	13 (12.6%)	<0.0001
Blood transfusion	1 (0.7%)	3 (3%)	1 (1%)	0.0002
Pulmonary edema	3 (2.1%)	2 (2%)	0	1
Chorioamnionitis	0	1 (1%)	1 (1%)	0.5175

GenA, general anesthesia; LocA, local anesthesia; TIVA, total intravenous anesthesia.

rupture of membranes before surgery, leaving 345 patients eligible for analysis. 19 had a triplet pregnancy. In pregnancies with twins, LocA was performed in 139 patients (40%), GenA in 103 (30%), and TIVA in 103 (30%). Patients did not differ in age, and stage of disease, were classified as ASA I or II with the same frequency and underwent surgery at the same gestational age. The operating time was shorter ($p = 0.0002$) in the LocA and TIVA (46.63 ± 23.24 minutes, 47.82 ± 18.88 minutes) than in the GenA group (63.70 ± 40.35 minutes). Bleeding caused termination of surgery in only 1 case of TIVA (1%), while in 31 (9%) it required an amnioinfusion. Among these 31 patients, 2 (1.4%), 16 (15.5%), and 13 (12.6%) underwent LocA, GenA, and TIVA, respectively ($p < 0.0001$). Blood transfusion was necessary in 5 (1.4%) of patients: LocA 1 (0.75%), GenA 3 (3%), and TIVA 1 (1%); $p = 0.6519$. Five (1.4%) patients had pulmonary edema, 3 (2.1%) in LocA and 2 (2%) in GenA ($p = 0.0849$). Two chorioamnionitis, 1 in GenA and 1 in TIVA, were reported. The complications are summarized in Table 18.1.

During surgery both the SYS and DIA blood pressures decreased significantly relative to the preoperative values in all three groups (Tables 18.2 and 18.3), but the fluctuations before, during, and after surgery were more evident in the GenA and TIVA groups than in the LocA group.

Table 18.2 Systolic blood pressure (mmHg) by anesthetic method

	LocA	GenA	TIVA	p	post test
PAT	118.24 ± 11.26	115.43 ± 12.67	116.00 ± 11.41	0.2366	
preop	114.98 ± 12.85	114.30 ± 15.84	115.87 ± 13.78	0.7591	
LI	105.17 ± 13.18	89.24 ± 10.69	91.78 ± 10.13	<0.0001	LocA vs GenA and TIVA
postop	115.94 ± 14.20	121.19 ± 16.60	116.29 ± 19.41	0.0039	GenA vs LocA
p	<0.0001	<0.0001	<0.0001		
post test	PAT vs preop and LI preop vs LI LI vs postop	PAT vs LI and postop preop vs LI and postop LI vs postop	PAT vs LI preop vs LI and postop LI vs postop		

LocA, local anesthetic; GenA, general anesthetic; TIVA, total intravenous anesthesia; PAT, pre-admission testing; LI, lowest intraoperative blood pressure.

Table 18.3 Diastolic blood pressure (mmHg) by anesthetic method

	LocA	GenA	TIVA	p	post test
PAT	60.87 ± 10.51	65.52 ± 11.58	59.76 ± 9.08	0.0001	LocA vs GenA and TIVA
preop	60.44 ± 9.62	68.63 ± 13.65	65.10 ± 11.43	<0.0001	LocA vs GenA and TIVA
LI	50.76 ± 9.55	47.71 ± 9.96	44.93 ± 9.17	<0.0001	LocA vs GenA and TIVA
postop	57.75 ± 15.56	61.84 ± 14.32	60.81 ± 14.27	0.0843	
p	<0.0001	<0.0001	<0.0001		
post test	PAT vs LI preop vs LI and postop LI vs postop	PAT vs LI and postop preop vs LI LI vs postop	PAT vs LI and postop preop vs LI and postop LI vs postop		

LocA, local anesthetic; GenA, general anesthetic; TIVA, total intravenous anesthesia; PAT, pre-admission testing; LI, lowest intraoperative blood pressure.

In particular, in LocA, GenA, and TIVA, during surgery SYS decreased, respectively:

- 10.81%, 22.64%, and 20.29% from the basal values (p <0.0001; post-test: LocA vs GenA and TIVA)
- 8.2%, 20.83%, and 19.86% from the preoperative values (p <0.0001; post-test: LocA vs GenA and TIVA).

After surgery, SYS increased 11.58%, 37.83%, and 27.93%, respectively (p <0.0001; post-test: LocA vs GenA and TIVA).

Similarly, during surgery DIA reduction was:

- 15.02%, 26.10%, and 22.93% from the basal values (p <0.0001; post-test: LocA vs GenA and TIVA).
- 14.98%, 28.46%, and 29.55% from the preoperative values (p <0.0001; post-test: LocA vs GenA and TIVA).

After surgery, DIA increased 16.55%, 33.71%, and 40.96%, respectively (p <0.0001; post-test: LocA vs GenA and TIVA).

Furthermore, during surgery, SYS decreased more than 20% of basal values in 23 (16%), 53 (51%), and 53 (51%) cases of LocA, GenA, and TIVA, respectively (p <0.0001) and more than 20% of preoperative values in 16 (11%), 53 (51%), and 48 (34%) cases of LocA, GenA, and TIVA, respectively (p <0.0001). In addition, intraoperative SYS was <100 mmHg in 43 (31%), 80 (77%), and 76 (73%) patients treated with LocA, GenA, and TIVA, respectively (p <0.0001).

The maternal HR changed significantly in GenA and TIVA, but was constant in LocA (Figures 18.1–18.5).

Although maternal hemoglobin and hematocrit were significantly decreased after surgery, the maternal blood loss did not differ among the three groups.

Four patients had miscarriages at 20.41 ± 2.19 weeks without any difference in the three groups. Premature rupture of membranes was diagnosed in 122 (35%) patients, of which 44 (31.6%) were in LocA, 28 (27.1%) in GenA, and 50 (48.5%) in TIVA (p = 0.0029). Amniodetachment occurred in 17 (5%) patients and equally in the three groups both during and after surgery. Leakage was reported in 25 (7.2%) of patients, more in the GenA 11 (10.6%) and TIVA 9 (8.7%) than in LocA 5 (3.6.%) (p = 0.0347). However, gestational age at delivery was independent of the type of anesthetic administered. Pregnancy outcomes are reported in Table 18.4.

Fetal heart rate of both donor and recipient was decreased after surgery in all groups, but the intergroup analysis revealed that the postoperative recipient FHR was higher in the LocA than in the TIVA and GenA. However, fetuses of patients undergoing GenA had a FHR lower than the other groups before surgery. Survival of at least one twin was independent of the anesthetic technique.

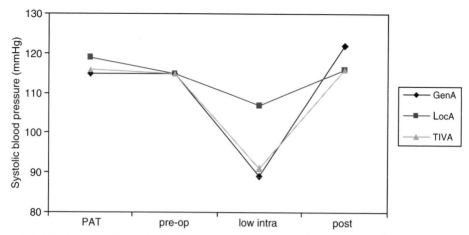

Figure 18.1 Systolic blood pressure fluctuation in the perioperative period. GenA, general anesthesia; LocA, local anesthesia; TIVA, total intravenous anesthesia; PAT, preoperative blood pressure; pre-op, blood pressure 1 hour before surgery; low intra, lowest intraoperative blood pressure; post, blood pressure 1 hour after surgery.

Gestational age at delivery was independent of the type of anesthetic administered. Delivery before 34 weeks was different between the groups and occurred with less frequency in the LocA group ($p = 0.02$). Survival of at least one twin was independent of the anesthetic technique.

Conclusion

Although endoscopic laser photocoagulation of placental vessels has been performed under general, epidural, and local anesthesia,[19,23,24] the preferential use of any technique has still not been established.

Maternal adaptation to pregnancy is characterized by an increased sensitivity to carbon dioxide, increased oxygen consumption, and hypotension in the supine position. General anesthesia can exacerbate these adaptations. Prior to induction, patients should be well oxygenated to avoid hypoxia secondary to decreased functional residual capacity, increased oxygen consumption, and increased maternal metabolism.[25]

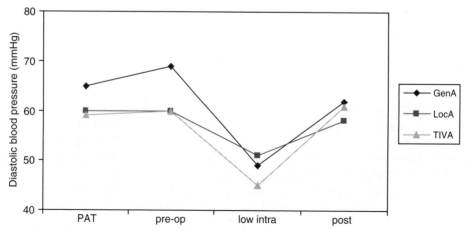

Figure 18.2 Diastolic blood pressure fluctuation in the perioperative period. GenA, general anesthesia; LocA, local anesthesia; TIVA, total intravenous anesthesia; PAT, preoperative blood pressure; pre-op, blood pressure 1 hour before surgery; low intra, lowest intraoperative blood pressure; post, blood pressure 1 hour after surgery.

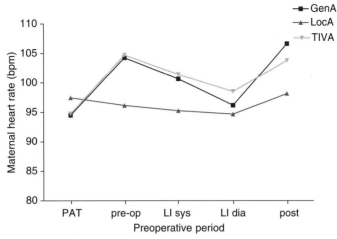

Figure 18.3 Heart rate fluctuation in the perioperative period. GenA, general anesthesia; LocA, local anesthesia; TIVA, total intravenous anesthesia; PAT, preoperative heart rate; pre-op, heart rate 1 hour before surgery; LI sys, maternal heart rate corresponding to the lowest systolic intraoperative BP; LI dia, maternal heart rate corresponding to the lowest diastolic intraoperative BP; post, heart rate 1 hour after surgery.

Our study showed that in patients undergoing general anesthesia, either with a balanced anesthetic or with total intravenous anesthesia, the blood pressure fluctuated more before, during, and after surgery than with local anesthesia. The intraoperative blood pressure remained in the normal ranges in the local/conscious sedation group, but not in the general anesthesia groups.

Similarly, the maternal heart rate varied widely in the general anesthesia groups but was constant in the local/conscious sedation group. These findings suggest that local anesthesia/conscious sedation allows a constant and optimal blood perfusion to the mother and fetus that cannot be achieved with the administration of general anesthesia. Furthermore, although not

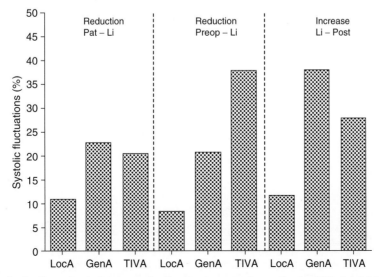

Figure 18.4 Systolic fluctuations. LocA, local anesthesia; GenA, general anesthesia; TIVA, total intravenous anesthesia; PAT, pre-admission testing; LI, lowest intraoperative blood pressure; preop, preoperative; post, postoperative.

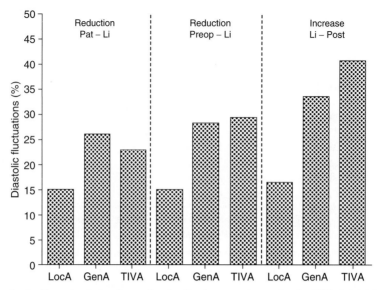

Figure 18.5 Diastolic fluctuations. LocA, local anesthesia; GenA, general anesthesia; TIVA, total intravenous anesthesia; PAT, pre-admission testing; LI, lowest intraoperative blood pressure; preop, preoperative; post, postoperative.

statistically significant, a trend towards maternal complications when general anesthesia was performed was noted.

The pregnant patient is susceptible to fluid retention and pulmonary edema as a result of decreased oncotic pressure secondary to the reduction of total serum proteins.[26] Moreover, tocolytic medications that are often required to prevent preterm labor can interact with anesthetic drugs.

Beta-adrenergic agents, nitroglycerin, and magnesium sulfate can all make the patient more susceptible to pulmonary edema. In our study, pulmonary edema complicated the postoperative status, regardless of anesthetic administered. The incidence of pulmonary edema has dropped to zero after the recognition of these factors and diligent fluid management with the proper use of colloids to maintain colloid osmotic pressure.

Table 18.4 Pregnancy outcomes

Outcome	LocA	GenA	TIVA	p value
Miscarriage	7 (5%)	5 (4.8%)	2 (2%)	0.4287
PROM	44 (31.6%)	28 (27%)	50 (48%)	0.0029
Amniodetachment	8 (5.7%)	5 (4.8%)	4 (3.8%)	0.6163
Leakage	5 (3.6%)	11 (10.6%)	9 (8.7%)	0.0347
Gestational age at delivery	32.47 ± 4.15	31.74 ± 5.21	31.70 ± 5.22	0.7346
Delivery before 34 weeks	63 (45%)	59 (57.2%)	64 (62%)	0.0247
Postoperative FHR donor	135.71 ± 14.11	132.58 ± 20.36	130.68 ± 22.27	0.114
Postoperative FHR recipient	135.54 ± 16.57	129.66 ± 14.02	131.22 ± 14.97	0.011
At least 1 survival	112 (80%)	80 (77%)	91 (88%)	0.1154

GenA, general anesthesia; LocA, local anesthesia; TIVA, total intravenous anesthesia, PROM, premature rupture of membrane, FHR, fetal heart rate.

Since SLPCV improves the hemodynamic status of both fetuses after surgery,[27] the postoperative reduction of FHR associated with LocA and TIVA, but not with GenA, may be related to the pathophysiology of the disease rather than the anesthetic technique. The alteration of the FHR can be attributed to the adaptation of the twins to the new circulation established after surgery.[27] The fetal survival rate did not differ according to the type of anesthesia.

The advantage of general anesthesia vs local anesthesia is that the former provides analgesic effects not only to the mother but also to the fetus through the placental transfer of halogenated agents. However, there is some concern that before thalamic connections form at 22 weeks, fetal response to noxious stimuli does not involve consciousness, but is just a reflex.[2] The neuro-anatomical connections necessary to feel pain develop after 26 weeks.[17] While it has been shown that premature infants undergoing minimal anesthesia for surgery develop responses with the elevation of stress hormones[28–30] and that such responses are abolished with administration of adequate anesthesia,[31] there are no data to demonstrate that fetal anesthesia is necessary or beneficial. When local anesthesia is administered, analgesia and amelioration of autonomic and stress responses secondary to potential painful procedures on the fetus can be achieved by infusion of parenteral opioids.[2] Moreover, laser endoscopic photocoagulation of vascular anastomosis of TTTS and cord ligation have to be considered as placental or cord procedures, rather than fetal procedures, and therefore only maternal anesthesia is required.[2]

In conclusion, our study shows that endoscopic laser therapy for TTTS can best be performed under local anesthesia with conscious sedation. Local anesthesia/conscious sedation is associated with the same pregnancy outcomes as general anesthesia, but with less incidence of maternal complications. This anesthetic also provides a constant hemodynamic status in the perioperative period that guarantees adequate oxygenation and perfusion to both the mother and fetuses. Patient acceptance of local anesthesia/conscious sedation is also appealing, since it allows the mother to watch her unborn babies during surgery.

REFERENCES

1. Barron WM. The pregnant surgical patient: medical evaluation and management. Ann Int Med 1984; 101: 683–91.
2. Rosen M. Anesthesia for fetal procedures and surgery. Yonsei Med J 2001; 42:669–80.
3. Cauldwell CB. Anesthesia for fetal surgery. Anesthesiol Clin North America 2002; 20:211–26.
4. Leontic EA. Respiratory disease in pregnancy. Med Clin North America 1977; 61:111–28.
5. Capeless EL, Clapp JF. Cardiovascular changes in early phase of pregnancy. Am J Obstet Gynecol 1989; 161: 1449–53.
6. O'Sullivan CM, Sutton AJ, Thompson SA et al. Noninvasive measurements of gastric emptying in obstetric patients. Anesth Analg 1987; 66:505–11.
7. Pritchard JA. Changes in the blood volume during pregnancy and delivery. Anesthesiology 1965; 26:393–9.
8. Palahniuk AJ, Shnider SM, Eger EL 2nd. Pregnancy decreases the requirement for inhaled anesthetic agents. Anesthesiology 1974; 4:872–83.
9. Baden JM, Serra M, Mazze RI. Inhibition of fetal methionine synthase by nitrous oxide. Br J Anaesth 1984; 56:523–6.
10. Koren G, Patuazak A, Ito S. Drugs in pregnancy. N Engl J Med 1998; 338:1128–36.
11. Motoyama EK, Rivarg G, Acheson F, Cook CD. The effect of changes in maternal pH and pCO_2 on the pO_2 of fetal lambs. Anesthesiology 1967; 28:891–903.
12. LaPorta RF, Arthur GR, Datta S. Phenylephrine in treating maternal hypotension due to spinal anaesthesia for caesarean delivery: effects on neonatal catecholamine concentrations, acid base status, and Apgar scores. Acta Anaesthesiol Scand 1995; 39:901–5.
13. Shnider SM, Wright RG, Levinson G et al. Uterine blood flow and plasma norepinephrine changes during maternal stress in the pregnant ewe. Anesthesiology 1979; 50: 524–7.
14. Anand KJS, Hickey PR. Pain and its effects in the human neonate and fetus. N Engl J Med 1987; 317:1321–9.
15. Giannakoulopoulos X, Sepulveda W, Kourtis P, Glover V, Fisk NM. Fetal plasma cortisol and beta-endorphin response to intrauterine needling. Lancet 1994; 344:77–81.
16. Lloyd-Thomas AR, Fitzgerald M. Do fetuses feel pain? Reflex responses do not necessarily signify pain. BMJ 1996; 313:797–8.
17. Smith RP, Gitau R, Glover V et al. Pain and stress in the human fetus. Eur J Obstet Gynecol Reprod Biol 2000; 92:161–5.
18. Kallen B, Mazze RI. Neural tube defects and first trimester operations. Teratology 1990; 41:717–20.
19. Ville Y, Hecher H, Gagnon A et al. Endoscopic laser coagulation in the management of severe twin–twin

transfusion syndrome. Br J Obstet Gynaecol 1998; 105:446–53.

20. Quintero RA, Dickinson JE, Morales WJ et al. Stage-based treatment of twin–twin transfusion syndrome. Am J Obstet Gynecol 2003; 188:1333–40.

21. Quintero RA, Morales WJ, Allen MH et al. Staging of twin–twin transfusion syndrome. J Perinatol 1999; 19:550–5.

22. Quintero RA, Comas C, Bornick PW, Allen MH, Kruger M. Selective versus non-selective laser photocoagulation of placental vessels in twin-to-twin transfusion syndrome. Ultrasound Obstet Gynecol 2000; 16:230–6.

23. Zikulnig L, Vetter M, Hackeloer BJ. Endoscopic laser coagulation of placental anastomosis in 200 pregnancies with mid-trimester twin–twin transfusion syndrome. Eur J Obstet Gynecol Reprod Biol 2000; 92:135–9.

24. Galinkin JL, Gaiser RR, Cohen DE et al. Anesthesia for fetoscopic surgery: twin-reverse arterial perfusion sequence and twin–twin transfusions syndrome. Anesth Analg 2000; 91:1394–7.

25. Gaiser RR, Kurth CD. Anesthetic consideration for fetal surgery. Semin Perinatol 1999; 23:507–14.

26. Myers LB, Cohen D, Galinkin J et al. Anesthesia for fetal surgery. Pediatr Anesth 2002; 12:569–78.

27. Ishii K, Chmait RH, Martinez JM, Nakata M, Quintero R. Ultrasound assessment of venous blood flow before and after laser therapy: approach to understanding the pathophysiology of twin–twin transfusion syndrome. Ultrasound Obstet Gynecol 2004; 24:164–8.

28. Anand KJ. Hormonal and metabolic function of neonates and infants undergoing surgery. Curr Opin Cardiol 1986; 1:681.

29. Anand KJ, Brown MJ, Bloom SR, Aynsley-Green A. Studies on the hormonal regulation of fuel metabolism in the human newborn infant undergoing anesthesia and surgery. Horm Res 1985; 22:115–28.

30. Anand KJ, Brown MJ, Causon RC et al. Can the human neonate mount an endocrine and metabolic response to surgery? J Pediatr Surg 1985; 20:41–8.

31. Anand KJ, Sippel WG, Aynsley-Green A. Randomised trial of fentanyl anaesthesia in preterm babies undergoing surgery: effects on the stress response. Lancet 1987; 1:62–6.

Index